▼▼▼

PATIENT SATISFACTION PAYS

▼▼▼

QUALITY SERVICE
FOR PRACTICE SUCCESS

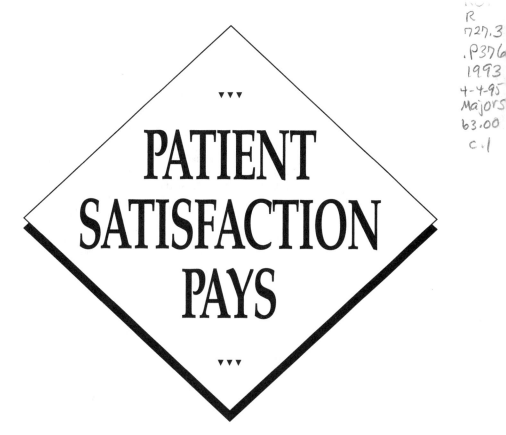

PATIENT SATISFACTION PAYS

QUALITY SERVICE FOR PRACTICE SUCCESS

Stephen W. Brown, PhD
Director
First Interstate Center
for Services Marketing
Arizona State University
Tempe, Arizona

Sheryl J. Bronkesh, MBA
President
The HSM Group, Ltd.
Scottsdale, Arizona

Anne-Marie Nelson
Vice-President
The HSM Group, Ltd.
Scottsdale, Arizona

Steven D. Wood, PhD
Professor, College of Business
Arizona State University
Vice Chairman
The HSM Group, Ltd.
Scottsdale, Arizona

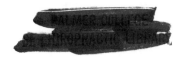

AN ASPEN PUBLICATION®
Aspen Publishers, Inc.
Gaithersburg, Maryland
1993

Library of Congress Cataloging-in-Publication Data

Patient satisfaction pays: quality service for practice success /
Stephen W. Brown . . . [et al.].
p.   cm.
Includes bibliographical references and index.
ISBN: 0-8342-0394-4
1. Patient satisfaction.   2. Medical personnel and patient.
3. Medical care—Quality control.   I. Brown, Stephen Walter, 1943-
[DNLM: 1. Patient Satisfaction.   2. Quality Assurance, Health
Care.   W 85 P29883   1993]
R727.3.P376   1993
362.1'068'8—dc 20
DNLM/DLC
for Library of Congress
93-20094
CIP

Editorial Resources: Ruth Bloom

Library of Congress Catalog Card Number: 93-20094
ISBN: 0-8342-0394-4

Printed in the United States of America

2 3 4 5

Table of Contents

---a---

Foreword

We all intuitively agree that patients are the foundation of our medical practices and that our efforts should be focused on satisfying the needs of those who seek our care. Yet, evidence that we don't always succeed abounds. *Patient Satisfaction Pays: Quality Service for Practice Success* is **the** book that will make us more sensitive to our patients and more successful in our practices by helping us understand and meet the wants and needs of our patients. Those who read this book will find dozens of ideas for nurturing loyalty in current and new patients as well as for developing and motivating staff members who are as committed as we are to patient satisfaction.

This is the first time I've read a book intended for physicians and other health care professionals that uses the term *customer* to refer to patients. This may initially shock some of us because we may consider it unprofessional to think of our patients as customers. In reality, patients are consumers of our services, and, like customers everywhere, they measure us according to the quality of our service. It is incumbent upon us to ensure that the nonmedical component of the service we provide (which is the component that patients use to evaluate our medical care) meets and even exceeds the expectations of our patients.

Patient Satisfaction Pays is much, much more than just another tome about smiling, having a pleasant receptionist to answer the phone, and being nice to patients. It's a practical handbook for motivating the medical practice to become a patient-sensitive, harmonious team. This book emphasizes the important role each individual plays in the provision of quality service. The authors clearly demonstrate that, if you aren't directly taking care of the patient, then you better be serving someone who is. As a result, the insurance clerk, the office manager, and the transcriptionist will learn the importance of teamwork, cross-training, and going the extra mile for the patient, referral sources, another employee, and even the payer. *Patient Satisfaction Pays* should be required reading not only for physicians seeking to create successful practices but for all staff members as well.

Many practices have the attitude that, if it ain't broke, don't fix it. The truth is, in this rapidly changing health care environment, if we wait until it breaks, it will be too late. This book makes the point that we should be continually evaluating our services, activities, and actions, looking for ways to make them better. Although I have been an active manager and marketer in my practice for several years, I found numerous practical suggestions in the following pages to incorporate in the day-to-day operation of my practice.

Don't just read this book, enjoy it. Use it. You will find ideas that you can readily implement in your practice, ideas to share with your staff, and ideas to discuss with colleagues. Just as constantly improving your clinical expertise requires ongoing effort, enhancing your patient satisfaction skills takes study and practice. *Patient Satisfaction Pays* is the perfect handbook for any medical practice, including yours. ❧

Neil Baum, MD

Acknowledgments

Among other bits of maternal wisdom, Mom taught us never to forget to say "thank you." Mom usually is right; this is no exception. Completing this book was a project for which we owe a great deal of appreciation to a great many people. We want to thank all of the physicians who took the time to talk with us and share their ideas and thoughts in order to give you, the reader, the benefit of their success at creating satisfied patients and profitable practices. We also thank the office managers, practice administrators, and staff members who shared their knowledge and tips. And we couldn't have written about patient satisfaction without consulting the countless patients who told us their perceptions of what's satisfying and what's not when it comes to service in the medical practice.

We collected an assortment of medical encounter anecdotes from friends, acquaintances, and colleagues. These personal experiences bring to life the points made throughout the book. Thanks to all of you who contributed your stories and views.

No matter how compelling a topic may be, how vital the content, a book reaches no one without a publisher. We couldn't have asked for a stronger proponent at Aspen than Elizabeth Thompson, acquisitions editor, who believed in the merits of our topic and our approach. Thanks, Liz! Also, thanks to Ruth Bloom and the copyeditor, whose red pens honed our words.

Another Liz—Liz Krauch, research assistant—also deserves special thanks and a meritorious badge of honor for organization, teamwork, and devotion above and beyond the call of duty. She manned the FAX machine and computer with efficiency, pulled the pieces together, tied up the loose ends, and helped us deliver a professionally prepared manuscript.

Our colleagues at The HSM Group, Ltd. provided insight and assistance throughout the process of research, writing, and manuscript preparation. A big thank you to Leslie Scott, Stan Kleiner, Patricia Pritchard, Sharon Flanagan-Hyde, Sue Matteson, and Diana Ryan. And special mention goes to our medical consultant, Marc Lato, MD.

We also wish to recognize the influence of colleagues at Arizona State University and specifically individuals associated with the First Interstate Center for Services Marketing.

And finally, our thanks to our families for their love and encouragement. An extra special recognition to Steve Nelson and Ed Buchbinder, who read passages and chapters, gave us opinions and support, and seldom uttered a discouraging word as deadlines approached and one of us grew cranky. ❧

Stephen W. Brown
Anne-Marie Nelson
Sheryl J. Bronkesh
Steven D. Wood

Part 1

If the Patient Isn't Your Customer, Who Is?

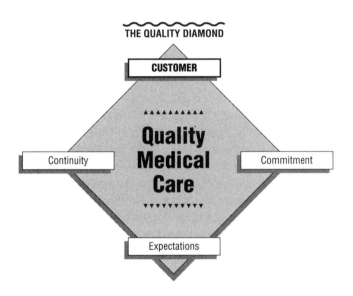

THE QUALITY DIAMOND

CUSTOMER

Continuity

Quality
Medical
Care

Commitment

Expectations

We're somewhat brazen, starting out this book on patient satisfaction by calling your patients your customers. But as the title of this section indicates, if the patient isn't your customer, who is? Your patients use your services. The service you provide happens to be medical care, which makes it somewhat more personal than, say, getting a haircut or buying a car. The personal, even intimate aspect of medical care makes satisfying your patients—knowing what your customers' wants and needs are—even more critical for the health of your practice as well as for your patients.

As you'll learn in the chapters in this section, patient opinions are getting closer scrutiny. Payers are asking how patients feel not only about the care they receive but about how their physicians communicate with them, how the practice staff treat them, and the kind of information they are given. Savvy physicians are asking their patients the same questions and are using what they learn to improve the quality of their service, to anticipate and exceed patient expectations. They are reaping the rewards of putting the patient at the top of their organization, just as the Quality Diamond, our framework for patient satisfaction, puts the customer first.

The rewards of putting the patient first? Patient loyalty. Staff loyalty and motivation. Improved productivity. Better compliance. Fewer malpractice suits. Whether you call it patient satisfaction or customer service, as you'll discover in the following chapters, it does pay. ❧

1

Patient Satisfaction Does Pay

We have a good friend who is a physician. He's an excellent doctor who went into medicine because he cares about people and believes he can make a difference with his medical education, training, and expertise. He tries to stay current with all the changes in medical technology, pharmacology, diagnosis, and treatment. Using his medical skills and knowledge to help people and nurturing a relationship with his patients is rewarding, he says. "As a doctor, you go home at the end of the day and look in the mirror and you can feel good about what you've done."

He strives to achieve the best possible outcome for every patient. He is a concerned, competent clinician. But like many of you today, he sometimes feels overwhelmed with the financial, legal, and contractual obstacles that seem to get in the way of quality care. He feels frustrated with the encroaching demands from third party payers, health plan reviewers, government regulations, and employers.

Like you, our physician friend knows what **he** believes quality service to be. He has a simple philosophy: "I try to treat every one of my patients as I would my mother or father." He believes this approach helps personalize the care he and his staff provide. But sometimes, he says, medicine seems to have traded the physician-patient relationship for paperwork, forms, regulations, more forms, more paperwork—and oh, by the way, the CPT-4 codes have changed for that procedure, and Medicare says you owe $4,562 in overcharges. Also, you have a family practice committee

3

meeting on Thursday, and Mrs. Ames wants you to call her about her husband's angina, and six of your patients have changed insurance because their deductible is lower; do you want to sign up with their new health plan? It pays about 70% of billed charges. And the GenTex sales rep is here; he has a new drug he wants to show you, says it'll only take 5 minutes, can you squeeze him in? And don't forget you've got a board meeting tonight to discuss the loan for the new surgery center. And your wife called. She wants to know if you're going to Amy's soccer game this evening. It's the playoffs. Also, John and Emily are having a disagreement about who's running the staff meeting tomorrow; do you want to mediate? But don't handle any of that until you talk to the book-keeper. She says you and Dr. Jones have got to meet with her about the accounts receivable; she wants to know if she can hire a collection agency. And by the way, the head of the hospital qual-ity assurance committee wants to know if you'll join the commit-tee. She says she's heard you're very quality oriented and you'd be a great addition.

PATIENT SATISFACTION IS A CRITERIA FOR EVALUATION

Everyone wants a chunk of our friend's time, he says, which leaves less and less time for his patients. No matter what, he'll never sacrifice quality medical care. But he knows that there's a growing demand for physicians to **prove** that they understand and strive to meet patient needs. Patient satisfaction is becoming one of the criteria by which physicians are chosen and retained and practices are rated—by business and industry, the govern-ment, managed care, and patients, too.

"What patients want is the feeling that their doctor is there for them. They want me to listen to them and not make them feel rushed. And I do—most of the time! I try to create rapport with my patients. But sometimes I feel like I'm standing at one end of a paperwork maze, and my patient is at the other, and I'm trying to make that personal connection and meanwhile I'm wondering how I'm going to jump through all the hoops his health plan requires to get him referred to the specialist I think he needs. You know, the nonmedical stuff is what wears you down!"

CLINICAL QUALITY + SERVICE QUALITY = PATIENT SATISFACTION

We wrote this book for all of you who, like our friend, know that patient satisfaction is not an option. You understand and practice clinical quality, but you could use help and ideas for improving service quality and patient satisfaction. You read endless medical journals, attend CME conferences, review product literature on new technology, consult with colleagues, and most of all make time for your patients because you know that quality is more than the technical component of medicine. It's listening, and touching, and making contact in a hundred different ways.

We wrote this book for everyone who wants to provide the best care and the best service possible. We believe, and numerous physicians have confirmed, that patient satisfaction pays, economically and clinically. It solidifies loyalty and compliance, attracts new patients, and can improve practice productivity and efficiency. (Trust us on this. We'll prove our point.) We believe, as you do, that quality service is not a fad but a long-term reality that directly affects medical care, patient outcome, and the success of your practice.

This book is designed to guide you and your staff in improving service quality so that you will achieve patient satisfaction in your practice. Within these pages, we offer direction, ideas, and strategies that have worked for other physicians in private practice. This is not a book about how to implement total quality management (TQM), which is a systematic, comprehensive **process** for improving the quality of every activity and interaction in an organization (however, you may recognize some of the principles of TQM sprinkled through the chapters). This is a book about **patient satisfaction**—what it is, who is responsible for it, who defines it, and how to provide, measure, and ensure it. It's about **quality service** in medical practice, what it means, where it counts, how to provide it and how to improve it. And how it contributes to the bottom line.

WHAT IS QUALITY SERVICE?

Like our friend the physician, you know that quality is the underpinning of good medical care and patient satisfaction. But it's a nebulous term when you take it out of the medical arena. You're confident about your diagnostic, medical and surgical skills. But what is quality *service*? Where and when do your patients expect it? How could you do a better job of providing it? And how can you and your staff possibly fit any more activities into a schedule that's already overflowing with too many people, too much paperwork, and too little time?

Over the years, we've worked with enough physicians and practices to see that some stay in control, maintain professional satisfaction, and keep growing numbers of patients happy even while wave after wave of change and upheaval washes over health care. We felt there was something to be learned from practices with a powerful commitment to patient satisfaction, what their attitudes and methods are, and what the results are. We believe, as you do, in improving service quality. We wanted to get the message out that *patient satisfaction pays*. But, if we were going to talk to doctors through this book, telling you how to provide quality service and patient satisfaction, we felt we ought first to **talk to physicians.**

WE LISTENED TO YOU AND YOUR IDEAS

So we did. We interviewed physicians like you across the country: physicians in multispecialty group practices with 175 or more physicians; solo physicians in rural, urban, and suburban practices; specialists in practice with one, two, or twenty others; physicians with one office and one staff member; and others with satellite offices networked like lace throughout their service area. We spoke to cardiologists, neurologists, family physicians, internists, ophthalmologists, gastroenterologists, surgeons, orthopedic surgeons, pediatricians, plastic surgeons, urologists. . . . We spent time in their offices, observing them with patients, questioning them about their attitudes and beliefs as well as their activities and interactions. We spoke to their staff members—office managers, nurses, receptionists, medical assistants, technicians, physicians' assistants, bookkeepers, billing clerks. . . . We sat in their waiting rooms, listening and observing. In addition to the extensive health care research we've done over the years with consumers via focus groups as well as by developing, implementing, and analyzing thousands of patient surveys, we asked numerous patients what they expect from their doctors.

Some of the physicians we interviewed are heavily contracted with managed care networks. Some are in areas with less than 2% managed care penetration. We interviewed physicians employed by staff model health maintenance organizations (HMOs) and physicians who are independent practice association (IPA) or preferred provider organization (PPO) providers. Like many of you, most of those we spoke with have a mix of fee-for-service and managed care clients and must balance the specific requirements of managed care contracts with the sometimes unrealistic demands of patients. We queried everyone about communication, patient expectations, and the role of their staff, and we probed about reimbursement, managed care, and Medicare. All fretted about the cumbersome restrictions, regulations, limitations, and documentation requirements that cobweb their participation with these third party payers, complicating their ability to provide the highest quality of care.

DESPITE CHALLENGES, QUALITY QUEST CONTINUES

But like you, none of these physicians has burned out or given up. They vow to continue to improve their service and their care and to find ways to meet and even surpass patient expectations despite the complexities of medicine today. One physician cited a litany of concerns, including overhead costs, Medicare reimbursement, and other factors that have limited her practice growth and financial success. Expressing disappointment that she hadn't reached her projected goals by age 40, she nevertheless rated her satisfaction with medicine "a 10."

The physicians we interviewed and visited for this book were chosen because they deal with the same issues and concerns you deal with. We don't hold them out to you as the best clinicians or practices. They're not necessarily superior to other physicians. We include them because they demonstrate quality service in all or some important part of their practices. And they were willing to spend some time with us, offering their opinions, insights, and ideas for improving quality service.

You may recognize some of their names, but most of them are unknown except in their own communities. They are like you. They read the *Journal of the American Medical Association*, *American Medical News*, *Medical Economics*, the *Medical Tribune*, and their specialty journals. They talk (and occasionally complain) to colleagues. They encourage their practice staff to learn and grow. They listen to their patients and sometimes worry about them.

WE TALKED TO ALL KINDS OF PHYSICIANS

As we visited with these physicians, we noticed—as you will—that although there are similarities among them, every practice has a unique style and a different approach to patient care and satisfaction. For example, we visited a pediatrician with a staff of eight, all part-timers, who takes and returns **every** telephone call himself. He sees up to 50 patients a day.

We met with an internist who spends an hour with every new patient. We visited a busy cardiology group whose physicians' homes are linked via computer to patient records so that evening and weekend calls are handled as efficiently and thoroughly as they are in the office. In this same practice, the medical director was recently offered (and accepted) a metal lathe in barter from a patient who wanted to pay on his account but didn't have the money. We talked to a family physician who takes his patient's medical history on a laptop computer in the examination room. His patients love it, and him.

We spoke with physicians in Bremerton, Washington; in Manchester, New Hampshire; in San Francisco, California; and in New Orleans, Louisiana. We asked them to define quality service and patient satisfaction, and we got answers that ran the gamut. No surprise. You know that each of your patients defines patient satisfaction according to his or her own needs, experiences, and expectations (we'll talk about that in Chapter 13). In fact, this shifting view of what satisfies is part of the perplexity in health care.

Because health care takes place in a world in which patients have countless service encounters every day, we reviewed what's happening and what works best in other service organizations, including Marriott, Federal Express, and Xerox, as well as in the neighborhood restaurant and car repair shop. And we leaned heavily on our own experiences in working with numerous physicians and specialty societies over the past 20 years.

PATIENTS HAVE THE LAST WORD

Opinions and definitions of quality service and patient satisfaction are as numerous as CPT-4 codes. But first, our opinion: Patient satisfaction is what each patient says it is. What your patient ultimately says, however, is in your hands, in the words you speak, and in the belief you have in yourself, your profession, your staff, and your patient. Patient satisfaction is determined by each individual according to his or her needs and experiences and according to your actions and interactions and those of the people and processes that surround your practice. You can't always meet a patient's every need or expectation, but if you show personal concern, creating the relationship with your patients mentioned at the beginning of this chapter by our friend, your patients will usually be satisfied nevertheless.

Patient Satisfaction Pays. Here's How:

These are just a few of the payoffs gained from investing in quality service:

- Greater profitability
- Improved patient retention
- Increased patient referrals
- Improved compliance
- Improved productivity
- Better staff morale
- Reduced staff turnover
- Improved collections
- Greater efficiency
- Reduced risk of malpractice suit
- Personal and professional fulfillment

And the effort is worth it. Patient satisfaction is the interest earned on an investment of quality service. Patient satisfaction is a dollars and **sense** issue. It's an economic success factor. Give service and quality careful, continuous attention and connect with each patient, and your practice will reap the benefits listed below.

You're reading this book because you're interested in improving the health of your practice through better service. Our prescription: Take the advice of the colleagues whose ideas you'll read in the chapters to come. There's no quick treatment, no single, instant remedy. But when you focus on service quality and inoculate your practice against a "who cares?" attitude, "adequate" standards, or "good enough" efforts, you'll see proof day by day, week by week, that patient satisfaction pays.

---

*"Quality service? I don't ask for much from my doctor." The woman, a business professional in her late 30s, seemed pleased to be asked. "I don't want to wait endlessly, but I understand if something comes up in the schedule to cause a delay—just **tell** me about it! I'm much more forgiving if someone keeps me informed." She paused, leaning forward in her chair.*

*"I like to feel that I have my doctor's attention during the visit. I don't expect a half hour of his time, just a sense of concern. My gyn is wonderful. I only see him about once a year, but he always seems to remember something personal about me. It's probably written in the chart—but at least he's read the chart! When he talks to me, he **looks** right at me—not at his paperwork, or forms. . . .*

"His staff is friendly. They seem to enjoy each other and the work they do. They make me feel welcome. That's so important—I can't tell you the doctors' offices I've been to where they make you feel like an interruption in their day." A frown creased her forehead. She continued, "I've noticed my doctor always shakes my hand when he comes in the exam room. Like we're partners, you know? He asks me my opinion. He explains things so they make sense, and he gives me information that I can take home and read. I'm not just a 'case' to him.

"When I first started going to this doctor years ago, his office was very convenient—right across the street from where I worked. Now I have to drive 30 minutes across town because I changed jobs—but I don't mind. Over the years, I've recommended him to all of my friends." ❧

—— ào ——

2

The Bottom-Line Benefits of Top-Line Performance

I saw a new patient last week who must have gone right back and talked to her co-workers. Thirty minutes after she left my office, I got a phone call for an appointment from a friend of hers. She's already referred six new patients to me.
—Carol Gilmore, MD, Denver, Colorado

Dissatisfied members have feet—they'll walk away from you.
—Leonard Abramson, President, U.S. Healthcare[1]

It's a Darwinian jungle out there. The practices that don't improve quality and meet their patients' needs will be absorbed by those that do.
—Harley Negin, MD, San Jose Medical Group, California

When you get to the bottom line, the benefit of improving patient satisfaction **is** the bottom line. And the top line. Practices that pay special attention to when, where, and especially how service is provided see results on the bottom line in lower costs and greater profitability and at the top in increased revenues. There's proof in practice. We accumulated an assortment of testimonials from physicians about the value and benefits of paying personal attention to patients.

Further evidence that quality service pays off:

- One dissatisfied patient who leaves a practice can result in the loss of $238,018 in income over the lifetime of the practice, according to an analysis of the revenue potential from a lifetime of patient visits, referrals, and hospitalizations.[2]
- Companies that successfully satisfied all their client groups—customers, employees, and stockholders—increased sales over an 11-year period by an average of 682% compared to 166% for those that only satisfied one or two of these groups.[3]
- Failure of patients to keep appointments (a ramification of dissatisfaction) ranges from 19% to 52%.[4] Missed appointments directly affect practice efficiency and the bottom line.
- A comprehensive quality improvement process implemented at the San Jose Medical Group in California yielded happier patients and dramatically improved staff morale as well as $50,000 in annual savings in medical records retrieval and another $157,000 in denied claims.[5]
- More than 200 Texas physicians who have never been sued for malpractice credit their flawless records to positive patient relations.[6]
- A large group practice in Houston that has made total quality management a way of life has seen staff morale soar as processes were streamlined. Today, even with Medicare cuts under the Resource-Based Relative Value System (RBRVS), "we're more profitable than we were two years ago," the administrator reported with delight.

Marvin Korengold, MD, founder of the 20-physician Neurology Clinic in Chevy Chase, Maryland, is one of the many physicians we interviewed who are convinced that putting the customer first reaps economic rewards. Like others, Dr. Korengold attributes thriving referrals, high patient volume, low staff turnover, and a positive bottom line to the practice's never flagging commitment to the patient. The physicians and staff demonstrate their commitment in a variety of ways, from responsive scheduling to a general "can-do" attitude.

Physicians and medical groups across North America have heard the call for better service. They have concluded, "Good enough isn't. Quality assurance doesn't necessarily mean quality care to our customers." These physicians and practices are listening to their patients' demands for personal concern and information. They see managed care firms measuring not only cost but patient satisfaction. They are paying attention as employers tell providers, "We want proof of value."

At Arthritis and Rheumatism Associates in Silver Spring, Maryland, Herbert Baraf, MD, believes that the practice's top-down, bottom-up attitude that *patient satisfaction counts* has had a measurable impact in improved patient loyalty. "We see it in the form of return business and increased patient referrals," Dr. Baraf says. Other physicians we interviewed and worked with point to improved cash flow, prompter payments, reduced staff turnover, and a better bottom line as tangible results of focusing on quality improvement and attention to the customer.

> *Q.* What is patient satisfaction?
> *A.* Whatever the patient says it is.

THE BOTTOM LINE STARTS AT THE TOP

A better bottom line starts at the top with the customer: your patients. You'd better believe they notice the difference in a practice that puts them first. Consider the contrasting experiences of a woman who consulted two surgeons recommended to her:

> *I had to have my spleen removed due to a very rare splenic cyst. Needless to say I was very anxious about the prospect of surgery, particularly because splenectomies not resulting from trauma are uncommon. Prior to the examination, I was left in a cold exam room for 35 minutes with nothing but year-old medical journals to read. Surely a consumer magazine would have been more appropriate! When the surgeon finally arrived, he introduced himself but there was no eye contact. He merely slapped my CT scans on the view box and said, "Gotta come out. . . interesting case." And still no eye contact. So much for building rapport with the patient.*

After that experience, she visited another surgeon:

He gave me a warm greeting upon my arrival, and devoted considerable time to carefully explaining the technical aspects of the surgery as well as the postoperative recovery. He also demonstrated, without my asking, great sensitivity when describing the cosmetic impact of an abdominal incision, which was not going to be pretty. His style, coupled with his reputation in the medical community, convinced me he was a surgeon I could have confidence in.

There's a welcoming warmth in customer-first organizations. We knew we were on to a first-class practice while writing this book when we made plans to visit the Heart Center in Manchester, New Hampshire. We were impressed even before we arrived with the attention to detail as letters and phone calls were traded between Manchester and Scottsdale, during which the Heart Center staff provided information, recommendations for accommodations, flights, and directions to the practice. We arrived at our hotel late in the evening, hungry and weary after a long and busy day, and found in the room a basket of fruit, cheese, and juice as well as an arrangement of flowers. When we visited the practice the next day, we discovered that this welcoming attitude is standard for every customer. Although we may have received extra-special attention as out-of-town guests, the gift basket and flowers symbolized the friendliness, warmth, and "we go out of our way" feeling that staff members and physicians in the practice demonstrate to patients and each other.

SERVICE IS A BUSINESS STRATEGY

Providing service that is outstanding, memorable, and customer focused has long been a competitive business strategy for non–health care organizations. Several examples that come instantly to mind: Disney, Nordstrom, Federal Express, the Ritz-Carlton and Marriott hotel companies, and Wal-Mart. These companies have built success on service that stands out. In recent years, the health care industry has discovered that quality service not only is expected by patients but makes sound business sense. U.S. Healthcare, CIGNA, Prudential, the Cleveland Clinic, Carle Clinic, Hospital Corporation of America, and the two-doctor practice down the street . . . there are few major providers today who are not closely scrutinizing their attitudes, activities, and processes and taking steps to improve them.

Just as hotels and packaged goods marketers have for years, health care organizations now understand how important the customer's perception is in measuring and determining quality. Moreover, they're using patient satisfaction as an economic incentive. The idea is discomfiting to some physicians. Upon learning that CIGNA Corporation planned to poll his patients, an Illinois internist characterized his reaction as "abject fear. . . I was accustomed to evaluation by appropriateness of therapy and by outcome, not by *patient perception* of treatment and outcome."[7]

In 1987, U.S. Healthcare, an IPA-style health plan, began linking physician bonuses to patient evaluation of their doctor's personal interaction with them. Individual pay for U.S. Healthcare providers is adjusted according to the results of patient satisfaction surveys, medical record audits, and compliance with the company's managed care philosophy. U.S. Healthcare's ranking system places its 3,500 primary care physicians in one of five categories, with those in the top ranking categories earning 25% more per patient than those who score in the middle. Physicians whose satisfaction, audit and other scores put them at the bottom earn 25% less than the base capitation rate.

How do U.S. Healthcare providers come out in the rankings? In 1991, six of ten were rated average (category three). One-third (32%) were category two physicians, proving themselves upwardly mobile in achieving patient satisfaction and overall quality. The high-earning 4% at the top are patient-pleasing physicians. Another 4% evidently could benefit from quality improvement and patient communication training; their scores put them in the below-average category. Fortunately, none of the U.S. Healthcare providers was at the bottom.

Emphasizing its commitment to quality, U.S. Healthcare has increased the weight given to quality indicators in its incentive formula. Previously the ratio of quality to cost-saving was 50% to 50%. In 1992, it was 80% to 20% in favor of quality indicators.

OTHERS FOLLOW SUIT

Other national health plans are using similar approaches to penalize or reward physicians for poor or excellent performance and patient relationship-building skills. About 9% of managed care patients were asked to evaluate their doctors in 1990.[8] That number is rising as health plans, seeking to keep their members from walking away, measure their providers' rapport-building skills as well as their medical expertise. Prudential and CIGNA evaluate consulting physicians according to board certification, peer rating, and by making visits to their practices to evaluate office ambience, staff skills, documentation and clinical practice patterns, **and** patient satisfaction criteria.[9] Intergroup, a large Arizona health plan with 224,000 members and 1,675 physician providers, regularly queries patients about their reaction to physician communication, waiting time, staff courtesy, and other nonclinical issues. Intergroup then reports its findings to physicians and group medical directors and, if needed, requests a plan for improvement—and the results.

Employers such as Xerox Corporation are demanding that their medical providers measure patient satisfaction with their physicians. "We don't want to lose sight of how the patient feels," said the benefits director of Xerox.[10(p.1)]

Regulatory, economic, and social factors are causing this heightened awareness of and interest in quality service, particularly in health care. Among the most influential change agents are patients. Within the past 15 years, the patient persona has changed. Our physician friend has noticed it. You've probably noticed that many of your patients are no longer passive, unquestioning recipients of medical benevolence. This is especially true of the baby boomers, who tend to be less familiar with and less tolerant of the patriarchal, autocratic-style physician. More educated and more demanding, these patients have a liberated, interactive view of their role. They see themselves as participants with a voice in the health care encounter. Reinforcing this self-perception (or perhaps because of it), patients today are often characterized by the media as health care *consumers.* This description affirms their new assertive role and has further colored their attitude toward the medical service they receive. Compare the definition of *patient* with the definition of *consumer:*

> **Patient** *From the Latin* patiens, *from the present participle of* pati, *to suffer. Capable of bearing affliction with calmness; capable of bearing delay and waiting for the right moment.*
> **Consumer** *From the Latin* consumere, *to take completely, to take up. One who acquires goods or services; a buyer.*

YOUR PATIENTS ARE YOUR CUSTOMERS

The concept may be initially tough to accept, but believe it: Health care consumers—your patients—are your **customers.** Increasingly, they see themselves as **buyers** of health care services. This attitude, along with more education, marketplace competition, employer requirements, the fitness and self-help health movements, and the media, have all helped make your patients more quality conscious and sophisticated in their selection of physicians.

Don't be intimidated or put off by our use of customer in referring to your patients. It's only to emphasize and encourage a frame of reference—an attitude that may be somewhat different from what you may have learned in medical school or in practice. Patients traditionally were deferential; customers can be demanding. By viewing patients as customers, providers acknowledge patient equality and rights in the health care relationship. Viewing patients as customers encourages an effort to understand and meet their needs. As *customers* or *consumers* rather than merely *patients,* individuals seeking medical care want to participate actively in decisions, including the selection of providers and even to some extent the treatment that may be required. As consumers, they believe that they have rights and that providers and their agents have responsibilities. They seek value for their medical dollar, even though many do not pay directly for the cost of their care. As customers and consumers, they want to be informed before, during, and after the medical service takes place.

As *customers,* patients are more sensitive to quality and value in health care. A 1988 survey found that 50% of consumers were

Exhibit 2-1

Whose Needs Come First in Your Practice?

If Practice Needs Come First		*If Patient Needs Come First*

A practice that puts patients after the needs of the physician(s) and staff may respond in the following way:

A practice that views patients as customers takes this approach:

Often the patient is made to feel like an intrusion on a busy practice. Patient calls are seen as interruptions and patient visits as disruptions which must be tolerated.

♦ ♦ ♦
Service Orientation

"How can we serve you?" is the guiding principle for how physicians and staff deal with each other, referral sources, and patients—all of whom are considered customers.

Telephone calls are answered and returned as it meets the needs of practice and staff. Patient calls are placed on hold or transferred indiscriminately until the staff has the time to handle them.

♦ ♦ ♦
Telephone

Every telephone call is viewed as a person with a need to be met, not just a voice. The caller's permission is requested before moving him or her along in the communication process (e.g., transferring, placing call on hold, or calling back.)

Schedule is set up according to the convenience of the physician, staff or a rigid appointment book. There is no flexibility or consideration of patient needs.

♦ ♦ ♦
Scheduling

Office hours are determined with the needs of the practice's patients in mind. If early morning, evening, or weekend hours are preferred, the practice will attempt to accommodate within reason. Surveys may be periodically taken to ensure that current hours of operation are convenient.

(continued)

A patient requiring several lab tests, X-rays, and other diagnostic tests may be scheduled at widely spaced intervals, with large time gaps between tests, or at inconvenient locations. Testing site policies, practices, and attitudes are not considered to reflect on the practice.

Convenience

Diagnostic tests are scheduled according to patient condition, age, health, and preference whenever possible. Testing sites are viewed as extensions of the practice; patient opinions are sought of these sites, their policies, and their staff.

Patients are moved from reception area to exam room to holding room to lab just to keep them moving and to free up rooms, not due to real progress in their visit interactions.

Comfort

Patients are moved from one area to another only as necessary, and then as conveniently as possible.

Office decor, furnishings, layout, lighting, and temperature are designed to meet the needs of physician(s) and staff, because they are the ones who spend the most time in the practice.

Environment

Office decor, furnishings, layout, lighting, and temperatures, etc., are designed with patient comfort as the primary consideration along with the functional needs of the physician(s) and staff.

Paper gowns instead of cloth are considered appropriate because they are cheaper. Patient dignity or preference is not a factor.

Dignity

Personal dignity and comfort is a major consideration in selecting gowns, exam room furnishings, and equipment.

Physicians park in a clearly marked "Physicians only" covered parking area closest to the practice entrance. Patient parking is in an open lot.

Parking

Patient parking is located as close to the entrance as possible. If no parking is available nearby, valet parking or validation of parking vouchers is offered.

(continued)

The physician focuses primarily on obtaining information quickly during the medical history taking. Little consideration or time is allotted to patient concerns or questions. If a patient requests additional information, the physician may offer a pamphlet without discussing it; this is viewed as "patient education."

♦ ♦ ♦
Interaction

Physicians and staff seek to understand and meet (or exceed) patient needs during the medical history and interview. Patients are asked open-ended questions that encourage them to express concerns or questions. Printed or video information is important but secondary to face-to-face education.

Quality care is viewed as consisting only of accurate diagnosis, appropriate treatment, and the best possible outcome for the circumstances and patient condition. The appearance of the office, waiting time, staff attitude, and physician interaction are considered noncritical to "quality medicine."

♦ ♦ ♦
Quality

Quality care is understood by physicians and staff to encompass surrogate indicators and relationship issues as well as technical skills.

Patient follow-up is considered unnecessary except for serious conditions. Physicians and staff expect patients to call the office answering service after office hours only if a "real" emergency occurs.

♦ ♦ ♦
Follow-up

Follow-up is critical, providing feedback and opportunity for patients to bring up forgotten or unaddressed issues or symptoms.

Physicians to whom patients are referred are viewed as separate and distinct from the practice, not an extension and reflection of the practice.

♦ ♦ ♦
Referral Physicians

Physicians to whom patients are referred are viewed as reflecting on the quality of the practice. Patient opinion of consultants is solicited.

Physician is considered to be "the highest authority." Patient opinion counts only peripherally.

♦ ♦ ♦
Patient Perception

The patient is considered to be "the ultimate authority" in evaluating the medical experience.

aware of high-quality physicians, compared with 42% only a year earlier. Moreover, these discriminating, quality-conscious consumers say that better quality care has greater value. More than seven of ten said they were willing to pay an extra $15 per visit out of their own pockets to be seen by better quality physicians.[11]

How does it affect your medical practice when you view patients as customers? Exhibit 2-1 may help you understand the actions and attitudes of a practice that treats its patients as customers compared with a practice that takes a more traditional view of patients.

CHANGE IN ATTITUDE BENEFITS EVERYONE

Both physicians and patients benefit from a change in attitude in which the patient is viewed as a customer. We know this is a paradigm shift for many in medical practice, and it requires stepping out of your traditional health care box to make this shift. It's not easy. Even our physician friend believes that "consumerism has jaded many people in their view of physicians." Consumerism, however, is not to be blamed for the tenuous nature of some doctor-patient relationships. Rather, there is a failure to acknowledge the critical role of this relationship in the medical encounter.

The personal relationship **is** the heart of quality health care, and creating a customer-first focus enhances rather than diminishes the human aspect. The actions and attitudes of the physicians and staff at the Manchester Heart Center reflect this. Many physicians and practices we encountered in researching this book understand this. They have lifted customer service ideas out of car dealerships, hotels, and airlines and are using them in meeting, greeting, and treating their patients. Many of these physicians quoted Sir William Osler, who said "patients don't care how much you know until they know how much you care" to illustrate the importance of an empathic relationship.

Although our friend the doctor has difficulty accepting the concept of the patient as customer, like you he recognizes that personalized care—which is nothing more than paying careful, caring attention to the customer's needs—ensures better medicine, better outcomes, and a better bottom line. **You** understand the value of improving practice processes, activities, and interactions with patients. Some of you are doing it because you intuitively recognize that efficiency, consistent service, and patient satisfaction are related to practice success. Some of you have always brought business principles into the management side of your medical practices, and service improvement is viewed as simply another logical strategy for practice growth, especially as external pressures increase and reimbursement declines.

DOCTOR, YOU HAVE A CHOICE

Just as patients have a choice of health care providers, you have a choice. You can create a practice environment that encourages and rewards improvement, innovation, and personal attention to your customers. You can lead your satisfied patients to better health and in the process improve the health of your practice and your satisfaction with medicine. Or you can adopt the John Paul Sartre school of thought, the "quality is existential" perspective (we don't recommend this, however). The "quality is existential" philosophy reflects the belief of a few physicians we interviewed who said, "I **am** quality!", who believe that quality resides in the medical degree. Although they are providing technical quality of care, many of these physicians and their practices are foundering in a health care environment that is constantly changing and demands change to achieve progress, satisfaction, and success.

Change is constant in medicine, as it is in every industry. Choices are everywhere. Your customers, patients as well as health plans and employers, are making choices every day that affect **your** bottom line. You, too, have a choice. You can choose to put your customer at the top of your organization, making patient satisfaction the guiding principle of your practice and motivating your staff to give your customers superior medical care and service. Or, by refusing to change, you can allow external forces to direct your future and determine your success.

What's your choice? ❧

References

1. M. Freudenheim, Patients' grades help to set pay for health-plan doctors, *New York Times* (May 26, 1990): 1.
2. R.W. Luecke, V.R. Rosselli, and J.M. Moss, The economic ramifications of "client" dissatisfaction, *Group Practice Journal* (May/June 1991): 8–18.
3. B. Dumaine, The corporate culture connection, *Fortune* (May 4, 1992): 119.
4. W.M. Macharia, G. Leon, B.H. Rowe, B.J. Stephenson, and R.B. Haynes. An overview of interventions to improve compliance with appointment keeping for medical services, *JAMA* 267 (1992): 1813–1817.
5. J.G. Shaw, Making quality improvement work, *Group Practice Journal* (January/February 1992): 6–23.
6. L. Mangels, Tips from doctors who've never been sued, *Medical Economics* (February 18, 1991): 56–64.
7. C. Morain, HMOs try to measure (and reward) "doctor quality," *Medical Economics* (April 6, 1992): 206–215.
8. Freudenheim, *New York Times* (May 26, 1990): 1.
9. H. Larkin, Networks boost office oversight, *American Medical News* (October 14, 1991): 11–12.
10. Freudenheim, *New York Times* (May 26, 1990): 1.
11. Voluntary Hospitals of America, Special report: Quality care. *Market Monitor* (1988): 11.

3

The Inside Story: What You Say about Patient Satisfaction

There was a time when patient satisfaction was fairly uncomplicated. The physician diagnosed the problem and prescribed medication or surgery or some other treatment, and the patient either got better or didn't. If the physician did his or her best, the patient was satisfied. The relationship was the satisfier. A good outcome wasn't always expected; it certainly wasn't demanded.

Today, the proliferation of technology and technodrugs has changed expectations as well as techniques. Perfect health (or, at minimum, significantly improved well-being) is too often viewed as the patient's right and the physician's responsibility, no matter what the patient's fitness or condition. Anything less is viewed as substandard medicine.

"People expect absolute cure without any risk, complications, pain, or pressure to leave the hospital before **they** are ready to leave. There's a belief that the more technology is applied, the better the outcome," said Donald Parsons, MD, a Denver, Colorado surgeon. Not only that, while you're diagnosing, testing, probing, medicating, and operating—all with no-risk, no-pain, 100% guaranteed results—you're expected to keep the customer satisfied with super service.

Satisfaction: *The fulfillment or gratification of a desire, need, or appetite.*
Satisfy: *1. To gratify the need, desire or expectation of. 2. To fulfill (a need or desire). 3. To relieve of doubt or question;*

25

assure (from Latin satisfacere: satis, *sufficient, enough +* facere, *to do, make).*

Quality service depends first and foremost on the quality of your medical care. But as we've pointed out earlier, patients can't judge your diagnostic acumen, your medical knowledge, or your surgical precision. They don't have the expertise to make a trained evaluation. Instead, they use surrogate indicators and the individual "moments of truth" to decide how good you are.

In the chapters ahead, you'll discover how and why satisfaction occurs during the health care encounter. You've already learned in the previous chapter that patient satisfaction is whatever the patient says it is. However, even though your patient is the only one who can decide if he or she is satisfied, your opinion does count. In fact, your opinion—your evaluation of the encounter—is critical to patient satisfaction. As you will see, if there is a gap between your perception and your patient's perception of your mutual encounter, there's a problem that can affect satisfaction (more on this later in this chapter).

WHAT DO YOUR COLLEAGUES SAY ABOUT PATIENT SATISFACTION?

Because your opinion does count, we asked physicians—your colleagues—how they determine if their patients are satisfied and how they define quality service. Ophthalmologist Joseph Noreika, MD, of Medina, Ohio, understands that perception is reality. He says that satisfaction depends on perspective. "Patient satisfaction is different depending on whether you're the provider, the patient, or the payer. Like the three blind men describing the elephant, it depends on what part of the elephant each is 'seeing' at the time." Dr. Noreika believes that patients use *surrogates of quality* to evaluate the total health care experience. These surrogates—a friendly greeting, a comfortable office, a reasonable wait, and a caring attitude—stand in for the clinical characteristics such as diagnostic skill or surgical technique that patients are unable to judge.

James Nuckolls, MD, internal medicine specialist in Galax, Virginia, believes that patient satisfaction is determined by whether patients show up for appointments and pay their bills. These actions, he says, are symptoms of an "ongoing, established relationship." According to Jerry Meltzer, MD, a Denver ophthalmologist, patient satisfaction is "meeting the patient's perceived needs." How do you know what the patient's needs are? "You **listen**!" Dr. Meltzer relies on his staff to gather insights that patients don't always share with their physicians. "My staff communicates with me about patient concerns. And I listen visually and verbally to the patient. When I engage in what may seem like superfluous conversation, I'm probing for things the patient may not want to tell me, things they may be embarrassed or afraid to tell me."

Dr. Herbert Baraf, the Maryland rheumatologist, believes "the quality of the physician-patient relationship lies in hearing and addressing the patient's complaint," even if the condition can't be cured or the medical problem solved. Like many of you, Dr. Baraf understands that patients are satisfied if they feel that someone has paid attention to their concerns.

For family practitioner Robert Bright, MD, of Bremerton, Washington, patient satisfaction occurs through "a series of small friendly gestures; the result is that patients feel comfortable in the practice." And for David Silverman, MD, a gerontologist in West Hartford, Connecticut, "going the extra step" in providing quality service is the path to patient satisfaction. According to Harley Negin, MD, of San Jose, California, satisfaction results when patients experience "ready access to the right person at the right time, no long wait, no equivocal answers when they're anxious, and a sense that things are operating smoothly."

Charles Inlander, president of the People's Medical Society, an Allentown, Pennsylvania advocacy group for health care consumers, believes "patient satisfaction is a 50-50 relationship in which the physician gives 70%." The first burden Inlander places on the physician in the relationship is "competence. Patient satisfaction is secondary to medical outcome. You can die liking your doctor."

SINCERE DISCUSSION, COMPLETE EXAMINATION SATISFIES PATIENTS

One of the most thorough explanations of what creates a satisfied patient was offered by Thomas Zink, MD, former medical director of Sanus Health Plan in St. Louis, Missouri:

*It comes from being a sincere listener to the patient's com-
plaint, followed by earnest discussion about symptoms and
issues surrounding the complaint. After the discussion,
there should be a gentle, complete exam given in an
unhurried fashion. Then, nailing the diagnosis with good,
complete history taking and cost-effective tests—enough to
give the physician a confidence factor without testing just
for the sake of it.*

*Then you make sure that the patient understands the risks
and benefits of therapy and treatment and has an opportunity for follow-up with the doctor. And finally, you show
sincere interest through your actions and words that you
really care about the patient, that you're on their team.*

Reading Dr. Zink's description, with its emphasis on *slow, complete, sincere* discussion and examination, you may be thinking,
"That's the ideal. What about the real world, where the schedule
falls apart if you spend too much time with one patient, where
patients don't disclose everything you need to know, and where
managed care and lack of insurance limit your diagnostic testing
and treatment?" We acknowledge that patient personality and
limitations in access, reimbursement, and hours in the day may
sometimes prevent satisfaction—your patient's **or** yours—from
reaching the level you'd like. But we hope you'll gain ideas and
strategies in this book to maximize satisfaction and, ultimately,
practice success despite the limitations and restrictions of health
care today.

MANAGED CARE: A SIGNIFICANT FACTOR

It's probably not news to you that one of the trends most
significantly affecting the way you practice medicine is the growth
of managed care. As increasing numbers of employers switch
from indemnity to managed care coverage for their employees,
physician-patient relationships are often disrupted and sometimes severed. As the number and strength of these health plans
continues to grow, the influence they exert grows as well, affect-

ing physician and patient choices in everything including the primary provider, referral physician, diagnostic tests, medication, and even the treatment ordered.

Two significant issues arise out of the growth of managed care:

- The critical role that physicians have in educating health care consumers about the importance of a healthy relationship between physician and patient. A long-standing knowledge, respect, and communication between provider and patient can do much for the quality of care. On the other hand, tenuous relationships without depth or mutual trust can lead to excessive tests, patient dissatisfaction, and poor compliance. Physicians can do much to help their own patients and the public understand that good medical care requires a solid relationship that is nurtured with time and trust.
- The need for physician understanding that ensuring satisfaction for capitated or contract patients is vital to practice success. As you've seen, payers are asking your patients what they think of you, your staff, and your communication style. Their opinions can carry significant weight at contract negotiation time.

Certainly, within managed care there are situations over which you have no control. Restrictions may limit the type or extent of care or service or the referrals you believe are appropriate. Some patients will change physicians because you do not participate in their employer's new health plan. But within a particular plan, whether a patient chooses Dr. Goodhealth as his or her primary care physician over Dr. Getwell is strongly influenced by what he or she hears from other plan members. If you participate in a certain health plan because you wish to attract new patients, you must provide a level of service to patients (and to plan consultants) that generates satisfaction and favorable comments if you wish to retain those members and bring new ones to your practice.

We consulted a foremost expert in the health care industry to learn what this entails. Our expert's response is fairly typical of how patients describe what satisfies them:

Ninety-year-old May, a veteran of multiple surgeries and physician encounters, is a currently pleased but not uncritical judge of medical providers. She says of her own surgeon, "He's the best doctor ever. He really cares. He takes the time to explain things. I have all the confidence in the world in him." She adds a telling comment: "Liking your doctor has a lot to do with getting better."

Confidence. Trust. Caring concern. Over and over we hear (and research proves) that these are the minimum daily requirements for patient satisfaction, and for all of the other benefits that patient satisfaction brings to your practice. They are the surrogates by which patients judge your technical quality. They are the qualities that count with the ultimate evaluators: your patients.

INTERPRETING SIGN LANGUAGE

How do you cultivate these qualities? How do you really know if your patients are satisfied? They don't always tell you. You and your staff must *interpret* outward signs from each patient that indicate whether the encounter was gratifying and met his or her expectations. To interpret those signs, it helps to know what influences your patient's assessment of his or her interaction with you and your staff. According to Zeithaml, Parasuraman, and Berry, a complex set of factors colors any experience. They describe them as *past experience, word of mouth, external communications,* and *personal needs.*[1] In a medical practice, these influencing factors for patients are the following:

- the patient's prior experience with other physicians and other health care settings as well as with you and your practice
- portrayals of and evidence about physicians and health care from newspapers, magazines, television news and network programs, movies, books, and educational materials
- what he or she has heard about you, as well as about other physicians, from friends, family, co-workers, and other patients
- the patient's current medical condition and health care needs

These factors combine to create a preconceived notion about what **may** or **should** happen during the visit; these constitute the patient's *expectations.* This mental picture contains images of people and their actions and attitudes as well as outcomes that the patient anticipates occurring. The patient's *experience* is what he or she sees, hears, and senses in your office in the reception area, in interactions with you and your staff, experiences in the exam room and upon leaving. But this experience doesn't stand on its own. The patient's *perceptions* of the experience determine how he or she rates the visit and you. You and your staff may comment when a patient leaves your office, "That went well." Your favorable view, however, doesn't alter your patient's reality if his or her perception of the experience is negative. In this case, perception is reality. Your goal is to equalize the perceptions, so that both you and your patient have the same favorable picture.

The following example depicts how perceptions may differ:

> *Mr. Philips called to schedule an appointment with an ophthalmologist. A precise and organized person, he asked a number of questions, including details about the visual field test for which he had been referred. The receptionist carefully explained that a complete eye examination also would be necessary, and the caller agreed to the two procedures. When he arrived for his appointment, Mr. Philips asked at the reception desk how long the examination and visual field test would take. "Oh, you're only having the eye exam today," he was told. "We don't schedule the visual field test until after the eye exam. You'll need to come back another day for that. In fact, we don't do those tests in this office— they're done at our other location."*
>
> *Irritated, Mr. Philips said, "Why didn't you tell me I'd need to schedule a separate appointment?" Convinced she was right, the receptionist insisted that she **had** told him. Mr. Philips **knew** he had specifically asked her about scheduling both tests when he called.*

Earlier, we said that physicians must accept and understand the reality that patients are customers. It's equally important to patient satisfaction that you strive to make **your** perception match your patient's. A study by Brown and Swartz that compared patient and physician perceptions showed that the wider the gap (*Doctor:* "I gave quality care;" *Patient:* "He doesn't care about **me**"), the more unhappy the patient is likely to be.[2]

Patients compare their expectations (what they anticipate will occur) with *how they perceive the encounter.* This can be expressed in a simple equation. If perception (the patient's personalized view) exceeds expectations (the preconceived picture), satisfaction occurs. If expectations are greater than perception, the outcome is dissatisfaction, no matter what the clinical outcome may be. The following is a formula depicting patient satisfaction:

> **Experience + Needs + Communication = Expectations**
>
> **If Perception Exceeds Expectations: Satisfaction**
>
> **If Expectations Are Less Than Perception: Dissatisfaction**

As you can see, satisfaction is a unique and personal state that is complicated by factors over which you and your staff may have limited control: external communication, previous experience, and the patient's needs. This makes management of those factors over which you have some control critical to patient satisfaction.

Whew! Tall order. How do you close this gap? Let's go back to our earlier assertion. While your patient determines whether he or she is satisfied, you and your staff interpret these "satisfaction signals." They may include immediate feedback such as verbal response, facial expression, or body language. Whether the patient complies with your treatment regimen, returns for scheduled follow-up visits, seems comfortable asking questions, refers others to the practice, completes a survey with favorable responses, or gives positive feedback to a referring physician can also be interpreted as signs of satisfaction.

SATISFIED PATIENTS RATE MEDICAL CARE MORE FAVORABLY

Physicians today must acknowledge **and understand** the factors that determine patient satisfaction and the role that satisfaction plays in the success of their practice. You must step into your patient's shoes and look at your practice from his or her perspective, because it's the one that counts. Then, with your staff, you must determine how best to create an optimal experience for your patients. What are the steps and standards needed to ensure a favorable encounter? This is not an insignificant matter. Research has documented a connection between a patient's satisfaction with the physician, staff, and practice and his or her willingness to follow the treatment plan; satisfaction may even affect the clinical outcome. (Remember 90-year-old May's comment: "Liking your doctor has a lot to do with getting better.") Patients who are satisfied perceive the medical care they receive as higher quality. Satisfied patients are loyal to a practice; they also refer others more readily and more frequently.

It's not always simple knowing what your patients want or expect or knowing what satisfies them. Needs vary from one individual to another, and the same patient may have different needs from one visit to the next. Yet understanding patient expectations is so critical to quality service and to meeting or exceeding needs that we've devoted several chapters to the subject. Some of the techniques you'll read about in more detail include patient focus groups, Mystery Shopper Surveys, a postvisit question card, and a simple one-question technique for eliciting patient concerns. You need to know patient expectations because people aren't always logical when it comes to their health and your ability to make them better. Some patients may have unrealistic expectations. Some patients don't know themselves what they want, or they may bury their deep-seated concerns in cryptic questions and comments while expecting you to decipher their needs. If you and your staff don't probe for the "hidden agenda," your patient may hold you responsible for not realizing the *real* reason for the visit.

Despite the complexities of patient personalities, surrogate indicators, and external influences, over and over again physicians we interviewed said and demonstrated that it is possible to provide a level of service that results in satisfied patients. They understand the importance of clinical expertise, and of meeting patient needs. Says Flagstaff, Arizona family physician Lana Holstein, MD, "A patient's evaluation of the quality of care comes

down to what the doctor does and says in the exam room—
whether the doctor understands the patient's fear, discomfort,
and need for reassurance. Whether the doctor validates their
wish to better their lives."

Ophthalmologist Dr. Noreika agrees: "High tech **needs** high
touch. You must convince patients that nothing else matters but
them. It's a yardstick for success—if you do it well, your practice
continues to grow, and your growth is generated by your exist-
ing, satisfied patients." ❧

References

1. V.A. Zeithaml, A. Parasuraman, and L.L. Berry, *Delivering Quality Service: Balancing Customer Perceptions and Expectations* (New York, N.Y.: The Free Press, 1990): 19–23.
2. S.W. Brown and T.A. Swartz, A gap analysis of professional service quality, *Journal of Marketing* 53 (April 1989): 92–98.

4

Mining Diamonds: Investing in Patient Satisfaction

Quality service means a whole lot of things to a whole lot of people. You may interpret it differently from your partner or the physician next door. And as long as quality **medical care** is at the heart of it, there are a variety of acceptable ways to provide good service. Just keep four words in mind:

Customer

Commitment

Expectations

Continuity

These are the four key elements of quality service. These are the elements necessary for the clinical and economic outcome you seek. The *customer* is the reason for all your efforts. Without *commitment*, you will achieve nothing that is meaningful. You must know your patient's *expectations* to satisfy, manage, or exceed them. And like a diabetic dependent on insulin, service demands *continuity* through daily attention and continual improvement.

We call these four facets of quality service the Quality Diamond because a focus on quality is like mining diamonds (see Figure 4-1). The gems you bring forth are patient satisfaction, staff motivation, professional fulfillment, and practice success.

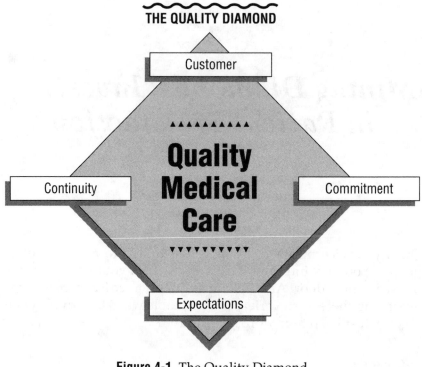

Figure 4-1 The Quality Diamond

We know that most physicians and practices understand quality in general and quality medical care in particular but that
you're not always clear on the finer points of quality *service*: how,
where, when, who, and even sometimes what and why?

We developed the Quality Diamond as a framework for explaining the who, how, where, when, what, and why of service quality.
The Quality Diamond is based on the belief that quality must be
inherent in every thought, attitude, action, and process, with the
needs of the patient foremost. Quality isn't always innate; it most
assuredly takes planning, thought, and intent. To make quality second nature and to provide quality service, you must *plan* to do so. It's
a lack of planning as well as the "quality is a slogan" or "Wednesday
is Quality Day" mentality that defeats efforts to provide quality
service. Quality consultant Tom Vanderpool was quoted in the *Wall
Street Journal* as saying that many companies don't see results and

may tire of trying because they isolate quality programs from daily operations. "They tend to put it off as something special, as an objective with 10,000 activities unto itself," he says. "It is not. It's a way to meet business objectives."[1(p.B-1)] If you or your staff think of quality as a program or a slogan rather than a habit and an attitude, it'll doom you to defeat every time.

YOUR TIME IS PRECIOUS—AND FILLED WITH ACTIVITY

We know you haven't got time for nonessential activities. We listened to our physician friend describe a typical frenetic day in his practice as he brandished stacks of mail and phone messages and pointed to piles of charts to be reviewed and signed. We know your schedule is chock-full of meetings, patients, hospital and nursing home visits, phone calls, forms, regulations, conferences, and consultations. Only by squeezing something or someone out of your appointment book do you make time for family, self, and leisure.

You and your staff simply want to take care of patients and to be paid a reasonable amount for your time, expertise, and emotional investment. You believe it's important to meet your patient's needs (you wouldn't be reading this book if you didn't). When your patients leave your office, you want them to be satisfied with your diagnosis and treatment but also impressed enough with the overall service attitude and actions to recommend you to others. You're distressed when someone departs your practice because they were unhappy with you or your staff. (Our friend says that in his early days of practice he used to tear his hair out over every patient who requested a medical records transfer. Today, with third party payers causing frequent patient shifts, he doesn't agonize. He takes action, sending a letter to patients who request a release of medical records to ask if there is a problem so that it can be corrected. This communication and correction have brought disgruntled patients back, he says.)

The Quality Diamond describes what we believe are the four critical elements of quality service. But first, the caveats:

- Don't ignore or minimize the importance of any of the elements of the Quality Diamond. Each is critical.

- Accept that *how* care is delivered is as important as the clinical care itself in creating patient satisfaction.
- Include all the practice staff. Your staff is so important that we've devoted several chapters just to their role.
- Be willing to give new ideas and new methods time to work.

OVERCOMING BARRIERS TO QUALITY SERVICE

The Quality Diamond is designed to help you overcome the biggest barriers to service quality:

- Misplaced practice priorities
- Lack of commitment
- Not knowing where to start
- Treating quality as an add-on
- Trying to do too much too quickly

Says Steven Walleck of McKinsey & Co., a national consulting firm, "Most [quality programs] require so much groundwork before results can be expected that you're almost systematically doomed."[2(p.B-9)] We believe one of the surest routes to failure is trying to turn quality service into a program. (One staff member in a large practice described it this way: "Oh yeah, they gather us all together for a rah-rah session, and they pass out the buttons and give us the slogans and tell us, 'This time we really mean it! We're gonna be a quality practice!' And meanwhile we're thinking, This too shall pass and then we can get back to our jobs!")

A belief in quality must be an internal attitude, not a slogan on a poster. If you're not burning with the belief that patient satisfaction is the reason your practice exists, you're not truly committed to quality service. Go back to Chapter 1 and start over. Come back when you believe.

If you're convinced and committed, let's take a closer look at the elements of the Quality Diamond.

THE CUSTOMER

The patient as customer: The idea puts things in a whole new light, doesn't it? When you view your patient as a customer, suddenly he or she has rights that might have been waived or considered unnecessary for the *patient*. Customers can be demanding, annoying, unrealistic, loud, and objectionable. They can be pleasant, easygoing, intelligent, accommodating, and knowledgeable. They also can be timid, questioning, unprepared, lacking knowledge, and uncertain about what they want or need. (Hm-m-m. Sounds very much like your patients, doesn't it?) But because business depends on them to stay in business, *customers* are given the benefit of the doubt. They get good service no matter who they are or how they act (within reasonable limits).

Notice that in our discussion of the customer we use the singular reference: the *customer*. There's a reason for this: We want to reinforce the idea that each patient should be viewed as an individual, not an anonymous member of a demographic, psychographic, or other group with aggregate needs, concerns, and experiences. Each patient is unique, with specific personalized needs and expectations. When you begin to categorize, compartmentalize, or pigeonhole your patients, you depersonalize them. When this happens, your patient becomes "the gallbladder on the phone" or "the anterior cruciate in exam room 2." In turn, you may begin to tune out individual needs and concerns in the mistaken belief that you know what all patients with that condition or ailment want or need. You may have treated thousands of lupus patients, but each is singular and unique.

In businesses and practices with a service orientation, the customer is at the top of the organization chart, just as we've placed the customer at the top of the Quality Diamond. It's where your primary customer, the patient, belongs in the organization chart for your practice.

COMMITMENT

Commitment begins with the physician. This holds true whether you're a solo practitioner (and thus the titular as well as acting head of the practice) or the newest physician in a group of forty. Commitment means making an emotional and intellectual pledge to a *course of action*. Commitment signifies belief that has depth and substance. If you truly believe in quality service, if you believe that patients have rights that extend beyond accurate diagnosis and treatment, you can't help but be committed, because it's the only way to demonstrate your belief. If you are committed to your patients and to quality in practice, you will embrace quality improvement as a necessary ongoing behavior and attitude in your practice, and you will convey this attitude to your staff.

> If you're **interested** in something, you do it when you have time.
>
> If you're **committed** to something, you make time to do it.

Whether you are the head of the practice or one of many physicians in a group, your commitment to quality service must be 100%—as much a part of the care you provide as your clinical quality, your skilled surgical technique, a well-researched diagnosis, and treatment that's clinically effective and appropriate for your patients. If you are half-hearted or hesitant about the importance of service excellence, you are not truly committed. Employees and practice colleagues will know that you don't mean what you say and they are likely to reflect your attitude in their behavior toward each other and with patients.

By the way, when we speak of you or your practice, we're referring to every kind of practice: solo or group, 2 physicians or 200, single specialty, primary care, multispecialty, or subspecialty. And when we speak to *you*, we mean **every physician** in the practice. (We mention this because a physician in a group practice, in response to a question about his role as leader, replied, "I'm not the leader—that's Dr. Jones, the medical director." He may not view himself as the leader, but his patients and staff do.) The examples you set and the decisions you make as well as those of your partners or associates are carefully observed. And like it or not, your example and decisions are what employees will heed, believe, and emulate. We mention this as both disclaimer and encouragement. Understand your influence and power. Use it ethically and effectively to achieve results.

In most practices, the administrator or office manager is the second tier of influence. The individual in this position is viewed by employees as the physician's surrogate when it comes to management issues. A receptionist in a four-physician pediatric practice commented, "The message about the practice philosophy and mission comes through our supervisor, but we know it's from the physicians." The physicians accomplish this by being visible with staff—eating lunch with them, stopping to chat about their weekend, offering comments and compliments when they observe positive interactions, and participating in staff meetings and practice activities.

EXPECTATIONS

In a study at Boston City Hospital, physicians and patients in the primary care center were asked to name the most important medical problem addressed during their visit. In less than half the cases did physicians and patients agree that the problem even involved the same organ system.

What we have here is a failure to communicate, an inability by patients to voice their needs and a lack of understanding of patient expectations by physicians. Perhaps these physicians assumed they were familiar with their patients' problems because they had textbook knowledge and experience with similar cases. Perhaps the patients interpreted their physicians' confidence to mean that their questions or comments would be viewed as an interruption or unnecessary. Whatever the circumstance, it's evident that neither patient nor physician listened to the other. Miscommunication like this demonstrates the need for understanding patient expectations about the medical process and all of the related activities and evidence that surround it. If you **don't** take the time and effort to discern what your patients anticipate from their health care encounter and what their needs and concerns are, you may make the mistake of assuming that you know what they want or what they hope to gain. This is inefficient from a productivity standpoint and can result in less effective clinical outcome.

On the other hand, with accurate knowledge of patient expectations, physician and staff time and effort are invested in doing things superbly rather than constantly fixing things that went wrong. This is certainly more productive and satisfying for everyone. Certainly, your experience can help speed the diagnostic process: It lets you know immediately what a set of symptoms may point to, allowing you to eliminate certain possibilities, but it also acts as a filter. You see only what your experience tells you to expect. Experience, especially after countless patients and years of practice, can block change and new beliefs or attitudes.

Over the years, many physicians have told us, "I **know** what my patients want and what they need." When we survey their patients to learn how satisfied they are and what they expect, the responses always surprise these physicians. As Albrecht and Zemke point out in *Service America*,[3] the longer you've been in business, the more likely it is that you really don't know what your customer wants. Setting aside assumptions and putting a ruler to reality allows you to develop measurable service parameters, that is, standards that yield more predictable and consistent service outcomes. There are a number of ways to measure and evaluate patient expectations; you'll learn about them in the chapters in this section.

CONTINUITY

Continuity is the loop-closer. It is the method for making certain that attention to service quality is continuous, consistent, ever improving, and never ending. Continuity encompasses all the ways and means for measuring, evaluating, and monitoring your progress. Continuity makes quality a built-in attribute of every activity. It becomes a habit. And habits, as we all know, are hard to break.

Think of continuity as the superhighway for quality. Habit, or tradition, is the cul-de-sac, a dead-end street where nothing moves or improves. Continuity is service that gets better day after day. It's continuous improvement in practice. Continuity formalizes the act of examining every practice activity and asking, "Is there a better way? Can we do this with more care, faster, slower, or more thoroughly? Are we doing everything possible to keep our patients comfortable, educated, and informed? Should we speed up? Slow down? Eliminate steps? Add steps? Can someone else do this better?"

Continuity means understanding that what you do today may not be appropriate or effective tomorrow. Things change. People change. Health plans change. Continuity requires continuous measurement: asking questions, seeking answers, updating your beliefs, and changing behaviors. It means doing every little thing a little bit better every day and looking for little things as well as big things to improve. It means making *status quo* a couple of dirty words and praising mistakes if they result from trying new ideas. It also means making amends when mistakes occur and seeking ways to avoid them in the future.

Continuity means looking beyond health care at what other industries are doing to ensure excellent service and customer satisfaction. This concept, called benchmarking, brings innovation into the practice. It leads to paradigm shifts, that is, stepping out of the health care box that contains all the activities and beliefs surrounding what is typical or expected in a medical practice. Benchmarking helps you open the windows of your mind, letting in the breeze of new ideas.

Continuity begins by setting standards for service. We call them minimum requirements for maximum performance. Like practice parameters for clinical care, standards are service parameters, specific requirements that ensure consistency.

Continuous improvement requires commitment and participation from everyone in the practice. In this section, you'll learn how other practices encourage enthusiastic participation and knowledgeable decisions from their staff. You can't do it by yourself. Effective change calls for effective, motivated people.

THE QUALITY DIAMOND: A FRAMEWORK FOR PRACTICE SUCCESS

The Quality Diamond is a framework for understanding service quality and the important components of it. It gives structure to a concept—quality—that sometimes can seem as difficult to touch, feel, or describe as clouds in the sky. The Quality Diamond brings quality down to earth and makes it tangible. It starts with the customer. It needs your commitment, an understanding of expectations, and continuity: continuous improvement day by day, year in, year out. It isn't simple, but it's manageable. And it has rewards: On the bottom line, in professional fulfillment, in staff satisfaction, and especially, in satisfied patients. ◆

References

1. G. Fuchsberg, Quality programs show shoddy results, *Wall Street Journal* (May 14, 1992): B-1.
2. Fuchsberg, *Wall Street Journal* (May 14, 1992): B-9.
3. K. Albrecht and R. Zemke, *Service America* (Homewood, Ill.: Dow Jones-Irwin, 1985).

—— ❧ ——

Part 2

If You Don't Show Commitment, Will Your Staff?

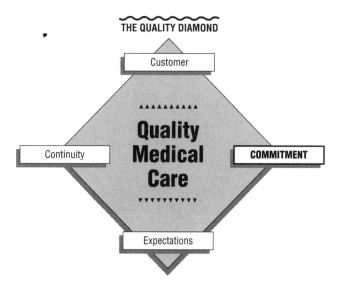

THE QUALITY DIAMOND

Customer

Continuity

Quality Medical Care

COMMITMENT

Expectations

Commitment—whether it's to quality medical care, a motivated staff, or satisfied patients—starts and ends with the leader of the practice: the physician. We discovered the power of commitment in visiting practices and talking with physicians. Physicians who *believe* in patient satisfaction and quality service don't just talk it. They do it. That's commitment.

The staff members in their practices follow the lead of these committed physicians. Not because they have to, not because they're paid to, but because they, too, believe in patient satisfaction. They believe fervently that they have an important role in ensuring that patients receive quality care. As a result, the pa-

45

tients in these practices get attentive personal service from people who have been taught, trained, and continually encouraged to care.

The physicians and employees in these practices aren't perfect. Like everyone, they make mistakes, work longer hours than they might like, and deal with the entanglements of regulations and reimbursement limitations. But they have a vision, a goal that keeps them going and keeps them committed. ⁊

5

Lighting and Leading the Way

What you are speaks so loudly I cannot hear what you say.
Ralph Waldo Emerson

Leader: *1. A person who leads others along a way; a guide.*
2. One in charge or in command of others.

Joel Barker, author of *Future Edge,* says that a leader is "a person you will follow to a place you wouldn't go by yourself."[1(p.163)] That's a pithy definition, but we would modify it: A leader is someone you'll follow. Period.

This explains why there are plenty of CEOs, presidents, managers, and titular heads of kingdoms, countries, states, businesses, and practices, but not many leaders. Leadership is an attribute *and a skill,* not a title. Leaders are born, but they're also made. Often, they are former followers who have been taught, encouraged, and inspired to lead by other leaders.

Every organization needs a manager—someone to ensure structure, continuity, and consistency. Someone to maintain the framework. Every organization also needs a leader, someone its constituents confidently follow and in whom they believe. In some organizations, the manager and leader are the same person. In extremely fortunate organizations, there is more than one manager/leader. Leadership is vital to an organization's viability; a

47

group cannot function without a leader. When the person who occupies the leader's position (the president, CEO, or other "authority" figure) does not demonstrate leadership traits and actions, the group will informally elevate or appoint someone to leadership status, or someone from within the group will assume the role by demonstrating the required leadership skills.

In a medical practice, the leader(s) ought to be the physician(s). We say ought to be because, as a rule, your staff looks to you for leadership, guidance, and vision. They expect it of you because you occupy the designated leadership position. You are the ultimate authority, and your words and actions carry weight. Your staff will listen intently to what you say, but they'll observe even more critically what you do. If your words and actions don't match, your staff will be confused; they may begin looking elsewhere for someone to follow. Or they will take their cue from your behaviors—the way you interact with patients, your colleagues, and other employees—rather than heed your words.

SOMEONE MUST LEAD THE WAY TO QUALITY SERVICE

Leadership is critical in medical practice not only because a line-up of patients and staff expect it but because quality improvement **demands** leadership. As we've pointed out, quality, particularly quality service, doesn't just happen. It must be planned and guided. That's your role: to inspire and guide.

The physician in the practice (whether you're **it** or one of many) inherits the position as well as the title of head of the practice. Whether you are also the **leader** of the practice depends on several things:

- What you say (What are the words?)
- How you say it (What is your tone?)
- Whether you mean it (Do you burn with belief?)
- How you act it out (Do your actions match your words?)

Washington, D.C. radiologist Lawrence Cohen, MD, spoke for many of the physicians we interviewed in describing the physician's leadership role: "The physician has the ultimate responsibility for [his or her] office, and therefore ensuring patient satisfaction. The doctor must be the model for the office, setting an example for the staff *and showing leadership.*" He defined this in part as "making sure the people in the office observe how you handle different patient personalities. For example, cancer patients may be very angry and take it out on staff. I will explain to my staff that this person is not angry with us; he or she is dealing with a frightening diagnosis and their words or actions have nothing to do with us personally, and we therefore shouldn't respond in anger or hostility, but with compassion." To reinforce his leadership by example, every 2 or 3 weeks Dr. Cohen brings his staff together to discuss topics related to patient satisfaction and quality improvement. One time the discussion might be appropriate ways to respond to or deal with an offensive patient, who commonly spews vulgarities in the office; another time the discussion might be ways to identify and solve office inefficiencies as they arise rather than letting them magnify and grow.

"I think it's important that the physician show by example how [he or she] expects patients to be treated. You lead from respect, not authority. You have to be involved in what's going on. I will solicit the opinions of my staff on certain issues, and I expect them to consult with me when they're not sure what's the best decision." Dr. Cohen believes it's important for all employees, from the receptionist to the radiology technician, to understand the significant impact they have on patient satisfaction. "It's their interaction with the patient that sets the entire foundation for the relationship between the office—especially the doctor—and the patient."

As Dr. Cohen pointed out, the cohesion of the physician's words and actions determines leadership, that is, whether you instill in your employees trust, confidence, and willingness to follow you **and** whether patients comply with your instructions.

LEADERS BEGET NEW LEADERS

A leader instills action, continued innovation, and results by encouraging the growth of new leaders. This happens when staff members are given firm guidance, a voice in the action, and the information necessary to make knowledgeable decisions. As Denver ophthalmologist Jerry Meltzer, MD, says, "I'm the leader, but our practice is a participatory democracy. I'm the captain of the ship, but the staff makes it go." Like Dr. Cohen, he understands that leaders involve and educate others, seek and implement the opinions and ideas of others, encourage **them** to lead, and allow them the possibility of making a mistake. (The leader also encourages responsibility, accountability, and recovery, so that if someone does screw up he or she accepts the error and immediately makes amends.)

It's said that General Dwight Eisenhower used to demonstrate the meaning of leadership with a piece of string lying on a table. He would say, "Pull it and it will follow wherever you wish. Push it and it goes nowhere." Eisenhower understood that leaders motivate others by making them **want** to reach organizational goals and by inspiring people, not by threatening or coercing them (inspiring and motivating others is the subject of Chapter 11).

For service quality to be the accepted standard and attitude throughout the practice, it must be demonstrated at the top. Through your leadership, you show your staff what service looks, sounds, and feels like. By participating actively through leadership, you demonstrate your belief in the process, the act and the **fact** of quality. Participation makes your commitment visible. Participation doesn't mean that you must attend every meeting or that you must put your *imprimatur* on every document. Nevertheless, leaders make their presence felt even when they are not around. They do this by becoming familiar faces, by their familiarity with people, policies, and events, and by making their beliefs strongly known to those who turn to them for guidance: managers and line staff.

Leaders practice "management by walking around." Get out in the field with your staff. Talk to them; find out what they're working on, what they're concerned about, what excites and energizes them (as well as what bores and enervates them). While you're wandering around, listening and learning, you can also provide information and education, verbally and by your example reinforcing the mission, values, and beliefs that ensure quality service. Become involved, but don't take over. You can, and should, delegate decisions and management tasks when appropriate.

Unfortunately, in delegating management tasks to their office managers or practice administrators, physicians often delegate leadership. Or, more correctly, they abdicate leadership. Writing in the *New England Journal of Medicine* about quality in health care, Donald M. Berwick, MD, MPP, observes, ". . . Physicians, for example, seem to have difficulty seeing themselves as participants in processes, rather than as lone agents of success or failure."[2(p.55)] He points out that quality pioneers Juran and Deming, in determining the source of problems in quality, found that "the problem was not one of motivation or effort, but rather of poor job design, failure of leadership, or unclear purpose."[3(p.54)] Physicians, Berwick says, must be more than observers of problems; they must lead toward solutions if they wish to achieve "gratitude and loyalty of more satisfied patients."[4(p.56)]

Fortune magazine writer Walter Kiechel III, in reviewing a book on leadership, outlined what he believes are the qualities of leaders. He said a leader is a *servant* to those he leads. He also cited the following qualities of leaders:[5]

- They take people and their work seriously. They value those who follow them.
- They listen, taking their lead from the troops. They understand that those who do the work know it best.
- They heal. They share in mistakes and pain; they are vulnerable, and thus they are trusted.
- They are self-effacing. They don't glorify themselves; they recognize others.
- They see themselves as stewards. They share their vision but also listen to the needs and vision of others. From this, says Kiechel, emerges "a shared vision, and a better one."

There are many ways to demonstrate leadership, and leaders have an assortment of traits unique to their individual personalities and styles. Yet we observed some common leadership characteristics among physicians in practices that have strong, effective teams with a commitment to patient satisfaction. Measure yourself against the traits we observed in the physician leaders in these patient-centered practices, as shown in Exhibit 5-1.

Kansas City, Missouri ophthalmologist Timothy Cavanaugh, MD, believes that being a leader means "modeling quality. It's important that the staff and patients understand that the physi-

Exhibit 5-1

Is There a Leader in Your Practice?

A leader demonstrates the following traits:

1. Passionate about his or her vision and shares it with others
2. Appeals to the best in each person
3. Encourages and rewards people for achieving goals
4. Manages by walking around
5. Solves problems by encouraging others to seek solutions
6. Is a good listener
7. Gives honest, frequent feedback
8. Confronts nasty problems
9. Is fair and decisive
10. Is tolerant of open disagreement that fosters innovation
11. Has strong convictions and commitment
12. Gets down in the trenches when necessary
13. Trusts the skills and decisions of staff
14. Delegates complete, complex and/or significant jobs
15. Admits mistakes and takes blame when appropriate, gives credit to others
16. Sees patient satisfaction as a **means** and an **end**
17. Respects everyone at every level
18. Is straightforward
19. Is consistent and credible
20. Keeps promises
21. Has integrity and expects it of others
22. Sees mistakes as learning opportunities
23. Is empathic
24. Sees self as "with" others rather than "above" them, yet recognizes the need to be in command

How do you rate as a leader? Are you nurturing other leaders among your staff?

cians see themselves as part of the [quality] process. I believe in showing the staff that I'm interested in their input about how we provide our services." Smart doctor. He knows that staff see and hear patients more and are involved more with them and thus can offer ideas and improvements that directly affect how patients view the practice. He also knows that modeling quality, service, and the personal and professional values that are important to the physician and the practice is how new leaders are developed from within the troops.

In the practices we visited, employees demonstrated a sense of purpose, participation, and *ownership*. We attribute this to the abundance of formal and informal communication, instigated or encouraged by the physician(s) and office managers, that occurs in these patient-focused practices. This communication from the top down, bottom up, and across all boundaries fosters understanding, commitment, and self-worth by staff. The leaders in these practices are both seen and heard; they keep people informed in staff meetings, social settings with staff, informal deskside conversations, and memos and letters.

This view of the leader as empathic and involved is a far cry from the traditional image of the Napoleonic commander-in-chief exhorting his or her troops to battle from the safety of the command post. If you are to inspire your team, you must demonstrate an internalized belief in quality and communicate it actively and often.

The administrator of a large Midwestern group practice with a quality improvement campaign acknowledges that "getting physicians tied into the corporate attitude about quality is difficult." The practice, he says, needs a formal training program to inoculate the physicians. Yet he is skeptical about the possibilities of creating such a program. Others acknowledged the difficulty of getting physicians to accept directives, or even advice, even from those they pay to give them advice. The associate medical director of a California group practice currently engaged in a quality improvement process said, "The toughest thing is to garner widespread physician participation."

LEADERS LISTEN AND CREATE NEW LEADERS

This medical director speculated that quality improvement is a "nondictatorial, nonhierarchical" process that may diminish physician status. "Some doctors don't like that." Leadership conveys status, but a lack of leadership traits will diminish status, even (or especially) in someone occupying the designated leadership spot. You must listen to be a leader. Recognize that the best ideas come from those directly engaged in a process. Listen to the reception-ist with an idea about changing the schedule, to the medical assistant who sees a better way to ensure patient compliance, and to the patient who feels that he or she doesn't have enough information about the arthritis medication you've prescribed.

"I'm not anything special because I have an MD degree," insists Lorin Swagel, a physician with Swagel Wootton Eye Care in Mesa, Arizona. He and his partner have a staff of 42. "I want to be approachable," Dr. Swagel says. "I want my staff to feel they can let me know if I make a mistake." His leadership goal: to hire good people and help them become better. "In return, I get good employees who help me to be successful."

That's what leadership is all about: creating new leaders. ✎

Ten Leadership Action Steps

1. Acknowledge and accept your role and responsibility as leader.
2. Read about leaders and leadership in all fields and endeavors.
3. Ask others for their opinions and ideas.
4. Listen to the opinions and ideas of others, both solicited and unsolicited. Implement them when you can.
5. Don't be afraid to delegate.
6. Participate in processes when possible. Demonstrate interest and enthusiasm for staff events and activities.
7. Recognize the participation and contributions of others.
8. Be enthusiastic. Enthusiasm can be quiet and subtle as well as rah-rah and boisterous. Pick the approach that best suits you and the occasion.
9. Make decisions. Then explain them—before, during, or afterward, depending on the timing and circumstances.
10. Let others make decisions. Give them authority and accountability.

References

1. J.A. Barker, *Future Edge* (New York, N.Y.: Wm. Morrow & Co., 1992), 163.
2. D.M. Berwick, Sounding board: Continuous improvement as an ideal in health care. *New England Journal of Medicine* 20, 1 (1989): 53–56.
3. Ibid., 54.
4. Ibid., 56.
5. W. Kiechel III, Office hours: The leader as servant, *Fortune* (May 4, 1992): 121–122.

ᴥ

6

Commitment: Doing It with Conviction

"Just do it."

This was Nike's slogan for the 1990s, urging people to quit contemplating fitness and take action. This get-it-done approach may work fine for running, weight lifting, and aerobic exercise—and for selling shoes. But when it comes to a long-term quality service strategy, "just doing it" without a little planning first may not be the most desirable way to achieve patient satisfaction. Not if you want lasting results and employees who provide a high level of service along with you.

You're already committed to quality medical care. Quality service calls for equally strong commitment and action. But before action comes planning and awareness. Commitment without these elements is a disciple without a prophet. It's the eggshell without the egg. It's empty. If you are truly committed, and if others are to believe in you and follow you, then it's necessary to understand what a commitment to quality service requires and to plan for it. Thus we offer the Commitment Commandments:

1. **Thou shalt have vision.**
   What are you committed to? What's your purpose, your goal, the treasure at the end of the treasure map? This is a step in planning for quality service improvement. Chapter 7 will help you define and refine your vision.
2. **Thou shalt have conviction.**
   You must believe in your heart that your patients deserve

full satisfaction. You must believe firmly and devotedly that attitude and action can make a difference in service and medical care. If you do not have this conviction, you won't convince anyone, and you won't achieve a superior level of patient satisfaction.

3. **Thou shalt be passionate.**

   True commitment is not passive or remote. If you're committed to quality, you get emotional about it. You must be passionate in describing your vision of quality service to staff members, because they can't share a feeling if it isn't there. Your passion will show when you see lackadaisical or sloppy service (although you'll channel your anger in constructive, positive ways). It will show when you observe especially caring or attentive service, and you will comment on it to reinforce it.

4. **Thou shalt make thyself visible.**

   Commitment makes itself known. To express your commitment, demonstrate it (this is where "just do it" makes sense). Make yourself seen and heard in exemplifying the kind of service you expect of others. Marvin Korengold, MD, of the Neurology Center in Chevy Chase, Maryland, walks and talks service throughout the 20-physician, 300+ staff practice. He's not the only one: Each of the organization's 10 offices has a managing physician who "owns" the responsibility for ultimately ensuring service quality. Dr. Korengold is visible and vocal about quality service. When he had a medical problem requiring numerous physician visits and hospitalization in 1992, he spoke during a staff meeting to Neurology Center employees about his experience and what he had learned (and what they could learn) from his physician-as-patient role reversal.

5. **Thou shalt learn and grow.**

   If *all* members of the practice are not continually learning new things, exploring new opportunities and new ways of expressing commitment, the passion for quality will slowly burn out. Continual education—both clinical and service related, personal and professional, through seminars, conferences, journals, and networking—stokes the fire.

6. **Thou shalt celebrate!**

   Commitment requires an occasional pep rally, a visual, verbal, active renewal and reminder of what you and your staff are committed to. Those who show their belief in quality service through sincere concern for patients and extraordinary efforts need and deserve recognition and rewards to confirm and renew their commitment. Celebrations affirm the "rightness" of the belief. A celebration doesn't have to be long, loud, or noisy. Bremerton, Washington physician Robert Bright and his staff go to lunch once or twice a month to talk about how things are going and to share pats on the back. The four-physician internal medicine group practice of which Dr. Richard Abrams is a member has quarterly luncheons and twice-yearly parties that give physicians and staff a chance to interact in a social setting. For a recent spring celebration, the office closed at noon, and everyone boarded a charter bus for Central City, a Rocky Mountain gambling town, for frivolous fun.

7. **Thou shalt regularly review and re-up thy commitment.**
   Making a commitment to quality service is not a one-time event. Physicians and staff must continually re-up commitment, confirming beliefs and methods for achieving the level of service that will exceed customer expectations.

8. **Thou shalt review thy progress at least once a year.**
   How are we doing? Do we really believe what we say? Does it show? What are our "signs of success?" An annual review keeps you on track and helps everyone evaluate progress and results. It's also a good time to re-up. A number of practices we encountered hold retreats away from the office in a comfortable environment that stimulates intelligent and innovative thinking and nonjudgmental comment. A retreat can involve only physicians, but the most effective ones bring physicians and staff together for 6 or 8 hours of dialogue and renewal.

ARE YOU COMMITTED? TAKE THIS TEST AND SEE

Now that you know the Commitment Commandments, your next questions may be: How do we express commitment? Is now the time to jump into it and "just do it?"

No. First, test your commitment. Is it solid and heartfelt? Ask yourself these questions:

1. Are you willing to practice what you preach, to become a role model for quality service? Dr. Abrams views his responsibility in role modeling as encompassing "everything. How the patient is greeted, the schedule, the appearance of the office, it all comes back to me. I have to set the tenor for everything in order to direct it. If I call in on my day off and I'm put on hold, I clock how long I'm on hold. If it's too long, I make sure I call attention to it."
2. Can you see yourself in the role of cheerleader, or leader, in encouraging quality service? (You may recall from the previous chapter that every physician has a role as leader from the staff's perspective, no matter where he or she is in the professional hierarchy of the practice.)
3. Are you willing to take time via staff meetings, one-on-one discussions, memos, verbal praise, and your own example to scatter the seeds of quality and then to water, feed, and help them flourish in the practice?

We don't want to minimize or oversimplify commitment. We know that, especially in larger group practices (and sometimes even in smaller ones), there are quality cheerleaders with strong conviction, there are those whose belief is strong but not as overt, and there are always one or two or a few physicians (those who believe that quality is packaged with the medical degree) who are skeptical or even unbelievers regarding the impact that quality improvement can have. "It's tough to convince some doctors to change their ways," says Harley Negin, MD. He is associate medical director of the San Jose Medical Group, a 90-physician multispecialty group practice that implemented a formal quality improvement program in late 1990 led by Cupertino, California consultant James Shaw.

Results in the practice have been consistent and in some cases dramatic, yielding savings of more than $200,000 in streamlined processes and more productive employees. Despite the economic proof of the pudding, Dr. Negin says, getting widespread physician commitment is difficult. "Ultimately, we need to make doctors see that a quality process is a part of medicine. It's a duty, like treating a sore throat or doing an appendectomy. First we have to establish the culture. Then new doctors [in the practice] would become entrenched in it."

For physicians who are sometimes set in old habits, Dr. Negin says, "It's a matter of unlearning old ways. We're asking people to jump through hoops they never thought they'd be doing."

GAINING COMMITMENT ISN'T ALWAYS EASY, BUT IT'S WORTH IT

Gaining commitment is not always easy, but it's worth the effort. Dr. Negin offered a testimonial to its value: "Our group is much better off than 2 years ago, economically and otherwise. There's a sense of moving forward rather than floundering. We have a structure and a process in place; we have a quiet confidence where before we were out of control. We believe we will survive and even prosper."

> **Commitment:** 1. A pledge to do something. 2. The state of being bound emotionally or intellectually to some course of action.

If you could honestly answer "yes" to the previous test questions, you are ready to go public with your staff, gaining their commitment, participation, and involvement. This is where action by example is important. No matter how heartfelt and intense your commitment to service may be, it is meaningless until you demonstrate it. Your commitment must be evident and credible if you expect others to become committed as well.

WHAT YOU ARE SPEAKS LOUDLY

"I think we send a message to our staff about what we believe by what we do and what we say," says Dr. Baraf, the rheumatologist. For example, Dr. Baraf tells staff not to "guard" him from patients. "I don't want my patients to think I'm not accessible. If a patient calls when I'm unavailable, my staff will take a message and let me know what the patient is concerned about. I want to respond personally, not through my staff." This communicates to staff **and** patients his philosophy of personal attention and interest in the patient, Dr. Baraf believes. (By the way, patients appreciate this. One man commented to us about his annoyance at being asked to describe his symptoms and problems to the nurse before being seen by the physician. "I feel like some of the things I say are filtered out as nonessential and never reach the doctor," he said. To get around this problem without losing the efficiency of staff prescreening, physicians should summarize to the patient the information noted by the staff member on the chart and then ask, "Is there anything the nurse missed that's important for me to know?")

Commitment without action is cocktail party chatter—talk without substance. Worse, if you recycle the same words later on, people remember their previous emptiness. So follow your verbal commitment with ongoing and consistent demonstration of the meaning behind it. In many organizations, it takes a catastrophe such as declining profitability to shock leaders into action. But why wait for catastrophe? Why wait for staff to quit, health plans to withdraw or patients to leave to recognize the value that good service adds to quality medical care?

For Childress Buick in Phoenix, Arizona, it took a new computer system that bombed to wake up general manager Rusty Childress, but he awoke in a hurry. "The system was a disaster, and customer satisfaction reached rock bottom. So did sales. From that point forward, we got on the bandwagon of preventing problems before they occur, and giving our employees and customers the best possible service," Childress said. The dealership put its commitment in writing with a detailed employee handbook, *Creating Service Excellence*. The manual describes the company's service philosophy and the expectations and responsibilities of employees (or partners, as they are called). It also outlines customer needs, expectations, and rights. It offers techniques for improving telephone courtesy, attitude, interpersonal communication, stress and time management, and goal setting. A lengthy policy handbook is one way to verbalize commitment, but it's not the only way. Nordstrom's customer service policy for employees consists of one statement: "Use your good judgment in acting in the best interests of your customer."

To activate the words in the handbook, Childress Buick involves all staff and customers in a comprehensive effort to ensure customer satisfaction from the first moment of contact. *Project First Impressions* includes a quarterly focus group of 8 to 12 customers, a VIP Motor Club for new customers with special benefits and discounts, and a Buyer's Appreciation Night at which new car owner questions are answered. Childress has quality teams of front-line employees who meet monthly to identify and solve problems in specific areas. Other surrogate indicators of the Childress quality commitment include its in-house newsletter (titled *Squeaks and Rattles*), a quarterly publication sent to 20,000 customers and potential customers; customer amenities such as free coffee in the service lounge; a service hostess who greets service customers on arrival; a full tank of gas upon delivery of a new car; a toll-free phone line; and a full-time customer relations department.

DO YOU KNOW THE VALUE OF *YOUR* CUSTOMERS?

Childress Buick demonstrates its commitment with activities and attention to processes that focus equally on employee and customer needs and satisfaction. The dealership understands that poor quality costs. They've calculated the lifelong value of each customer ($142,000) so that they know the revenues lost when someone leaves dissatisfied. (Do you know the value of a patient in your practice? As you saw in Chapter 2, when you factor in the average number of visits in a year calculated over a lifetime plus the patient's potential referrals and **their** average potential visits, the total is significant.) At Childress, service do-overs required because of errors or process foul-ups show up on the financial statement as a "policy adjustment." Thus the bottom-line impact of not doing it right the first time—or less than superior service—becomes very clear.

Dr. Baraf was jolted to action a number of years ago when the office manager in his practice quit abruptly. The minor cataclysm forced Dr. Baraf to deal with everything from insurance billings to scheduling. It was eye-opening, he said. "I took a call from a patient who was requesting for the eighth time that an insurance form be submitted. She told me, 'I used to think you were a quality doctor, but if this is the way you run your practice, I'm not so sure.' It made me see that there are a number of ways that patients evaluate us as doctors." The event focused him on the need to improve service in his practice. Today, he not only preaches quality service, he lives it. "Our staff knows how to act just by watching Dr. Baraf," said practice administrator Margaret Dieckhoner.

Stephen Hales, MD, a pediatrician in New Orleans, Louisiana, believes that commitment has helped him achieve the kind of practice he wants. A solo practitioner, Dr. Hales has a unique practice style that he readily admits would not work for everyone. It includes a fanaticism about waiting time (patients shouldn't have to wait, Dr. Hales believes), about patient phone calls being returned (he calls everyone himself), and about personal attention to children and their parents. Many of his patients drive past more conveniently located pediatricians to see him. His style works, Dr. Hales says, because "everybody in the practice is committed to making things work. You can't have the doctor think it's a great idea and the folks up front not committed to it."

Timothy Cavanaugh, MD, of the Hunkeler Eye Clinic in Kansas City, Missouri, is another believer. "The whole idea [of quality] has to be embraced at the upper level, and also from the bottom up. It will fall apart at any level if there's not total commitment."

Commitment at the Hunkeler Clinic was made visible when the practice became the first medical group to join the quality committee of the local Chamber of Commerce. The goal of the committee is to promote quality in business throughout Kansas City to attract new businesses to the city. The goal of the Hunkeler Clinic in joining was to gain ideas and information about service improvement from other members, a diverse group that included a long-distance telephone service company, AT&T, a railroad, and other local businesses.

Intending that quality seep into every crevice and pore of the practice, the Hunkeler Clinic is going about the process slowly, understanding that it **is** a process and not a program. Task groups made up of employees and physicians are assigned responsibility for specific quality problems. For example, when Dr. Cavanaugh felt that his patients were waiting "entirely too long," his first instinct was to fix the problem. "I wanted to tell my staff what to do," he said. Instead, he suggested to his tech that she and others come up with a solution. Directed only to solve the problem rather than being told how, staff members tackled the waiting time situation. "They now see each patient as 'theirs', and take a personal interest in giving their patients a good experience."

SHOW WHAT YOU MEAN; WALK THE TALK

Make your commitment meaningful by talking to your staff about what quality service means to you and encouraging them to look for ways to demonstrate it themselves. Encourage employees to listen to patients and to look for processes that can be improved. Then reward them for their ideas and implementation. Most of all, walk the quality talk if you want others in step with you. If you don't act out your words, you may find yourself falling into a chasm of your own creation. A study by the American Society for Quality Control reported that employees perceive a gap between what CEOs say about quality as a company priority and what they actually do. Employees said that what CEOs say and what they do doesn't necessarily match up.[1] When words and deeds don't match, the deed is believed every time.

Close the gap. Exemplify your words with your behavior, but also deputize your office manager and staff to seek out and destroy actions that impair effectiveness and words that convey convenience rather than concern. Deputize staff to carry out quality. In deputizing others, you are not turning over responsibility but sharing it. This conveys to **everyone** that patient satisfaction is everybody's business.

A commitment to quality service means trusting others to carry it out. This is a big step, and a tough one for many physicians. It means giving your staff the latitude to make meaningful decisions. Help them to have **impact** in your practice. Show that you have trust and confidence in them. Yes, occasionally they'll make a mistake, but who doesn't? (We are referring to service mistakes that do not affect clinical care; we are not encouraging empowerment that impairs diagnosis or treatment!) Your staff needs to know that you, too, make mistakes; in fact, initiating change in the practice is bound to produce missteps and errors at first.

Service recovery, discussed in Chapter 28, helps you learn from the mistakes. Through training and ongoing education, you can help staff avoid serious mistakes (you'll read more about empowering staff effectively in Chapter 10).

SHOW PATIENTS YOU CARE: THAT'S QUALITY SERVICE

Commitment is not convoluted or complex. It's incredibly simple. New Orleans plastic surgeon Gustavo Colon has done a lot of things in his solo practice: bringing in a consultant, surveying patients, hiring a patient coordinator to spend time with new patients, and creating a video to explain cosmetic procedures . . . lots of stuff. It works. His overall commitment is simple: "What we're trying to do is show our patients that we care and that we're interested."

Commitment means finding, or making, a path around obstacles. If you're committed to quality, you won't let barriers and pitfalls deter you. Your superb office manager, an ally and leader in your quality process, quits after 10 years with your practice? Find out why, then use the information to improve. Your patient survey results say that patients don't feel you spend enough time with them? Good. You've got a project that calls for innovation and change and for which you can measure results. Bring a team together to investigate and come up with solutions.

Commitment takes planning, but it doesn't necessarily take big deeds. Scandinavian Airlines president Jan Carlzon once said to his team, "We don't seek to be 1,000% better at any one thing. We seek to be 1% better at 1,000 things."[2(p.59)] Believe strongly in providing patient satisfaction, plan for it, and **do** what you believe every day. ❧

Action Steps To Inspire Commitment

1. Define your personal and professional values, that is, what you believe in.
2. Know what you want to accomplish personally and professionally and why.
3. Define your personal style of achievement, whether in work or in play.
4. Help your staff understand where you and the practice have been so that they can help you determine where you wish to go.
5. Through discussion, develop a unified understanding of the business you're in, who your customers are, what their expectations are, and what your current and desired image is.
6. Use the responses to the questions and discussions to frame a mission statement that is realistic, optimistic, and achievable but requires continual stretching.

References

1. F. Rose, Now quality means service too, *Fortune* (April 22, 1992): 99–108.
2. T. Peters and N. Austin, *A Passion For Excellence* (New York, N.Y.: Random House, 1985): 59.

---
§

7

Share the Vision

"If you don't know where you're going, you might end up there."
—*Yogi Berra*

You may have read about the Ivy League college class whose members were surveyed 20 years after they had graduated. The 5% of students who had a well-defined long-term goal when they graduated had achieved a significantly higher level of professional and financial success than the rest of their classmates.

The successful students had a vision. A vision gives you a sense of direction, a purpose, and a place to go. Defining and communicating a vision for your practice is like turning on the light after stumbling around a room in the dark. With the light out, you may eventually figure out how to get from one end of the room to the other, but only after stubbing your toe on the sofa, knocking over a lamp, and stepping on the cat's tail. Your vision lights the way and makes the path clear. And since you're usually not the only one trying to make your way through the room (you've got all those staff and patients trying to get through the door and to the other side without stubbing **their** toes or irritating the cat), turning the light on makes sense.

Nevertheless, many physicians, banded together in a group practice or making their way on their own, grope along in the dark. Perhaps it's because defining a direction for the practice is made to seem a mysterious, lengthy, and difficult task that calls for A CONSULTANT (or a whole pack of them) to whisk you away to some expensive resort for 3 days of solemn talk about the ghosts of health care past and future. At the end of the 3 days, by which time your ears resonate with phrases such as *paradigmatic axioms* and *process-directed organizational futility,* you will have come up with a VISION (bells ringing, angels singing) designed to send you soaring exultantly into the future.

TO CREATE A VISION, KNOW YOUR VALUES

Guess what? You don't necessarily need a consultant (although a consultant or objective outside expert can be helpful in guiding and melding diverse points of view). And it shouldn't take 3 days to come up with a vision and goals for achieving the vision. What you need are:

- Some idea of your values—what's important to you in your practice and in serving your patients
- A sense of purpose (i.e., why you want to accomplish what you want to accomplish)
- Belief and confidence in those you've chosen to help you achieve your goals
- Innate and realistic understanding of your personal and professional style, that is, the way you work and play
- Understanding the threats, opportunities, and trends in your specialty and in health care that may affect how you practice medicine in the future.

You can do this portion of your mission description (which is what this introspective process is designed ultimately to come up with) on your own if you are a solo practitioner or with your partners if you are in a group practice. Examine your beliefs, attitudes, and core values for each of the points above, and come up with written statements that clarify each point. If you've been in practice for some time, you may wish to do a little historical research first. What have your style, activities, and results been in the past? How have you behaved? Behavior is a reflection of belief. What changes or improvements do you plan, or wish, to make? Dr. Negin, associate medical director of the San Jose Medical Group in California, said that not long ago his group decided to develop a mission statement for the practice. Upon searching in the files, they found not one but **two** previous mission statements.

Remember Dr. Baraf, the Maryland neurologist whose office manager's departure jolted him into the reality of how patients judge quality? That's when he defined his vision for medical practice: "What I wanted for my practice was a loyal staff of competent personnel, a good business foundation with good management, and to be able to see patients and provide the sort of ancillary services rheumatology patients need: a lab, X-ray, physical therapy. I wanted to be able to provide good care in a pleasant environment."

Dr. Baraf's mission statement was specific and extensive. It clearly defines and determines decisions and behavior. Your mission statement can be broader and less specific. Nevertheless, his shows that he thought seriously about his goals, particularly in terms of service to his patients.

GATHER THE TROOPS AND GET THEIR IDEAS

Bring the practice staff together for the next phase of the process. If you are a group practice with an extremely large staff, you may wish to select representative members to gather ideas and offer input on behalf of the whole group. Or hold departmental meetings to gather input, then select the best ideas from these. Remember, your staff members are your deputies, carrying out the quality mission along with you. You need to know what **they** are thinking and what their beliefs are as much as they need to know what you think and believe.

At the meeting with your staff, take some uninterrupted time to discuss and come up with answers for the questions in the next few pages. Try to get away from the office. A meeting room at a local hotel or a community room of the library will work well. Close the office at noon or all day, or devote a weekend morning to this discussion. But if you ask your staff to give up a Saturday morning, pay them for it at normal overtime rates. Put the discussion in a positive context (e.g., "I need your help in moving into the future with the practice. We're going to take a look at where we've been and figure out where to go and how best to get there. You know my patients and my style and the problems and opportunities as well as I do—maybe better. Will you help me plan where we're going?").

The day arrives. The room is equipped with chairs comfortably grouped around a table. Refreshments are available in a corner of the room. You have a flip chart and marker pens, and you've designated a recorder (someone to take good notes from the discussion). Now your staff—2 sets of eyes, or perhaps 10 or even 20—are focused eagerly on you.

To put things in perspective, start by recounting to your staff a history of the practice. It doesn't have to be long and detailed. Make it upbeat and include anecdotes and humorous mistakes to make your history come alive and to help everyone understand your beliefs and values. This oral history will help those charged with moving you into the future understand how you and they have arrived at this point. If you have one or more long-time staff members, encourage them to help tell the history, particularly some of the significant highlights or amusing moments that involved them.

EXPLAIN WHAT YOU BELIEVE AND WHY 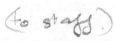 (to staff.)

In your review of the practice, explain why you became a physician (for a group practice, have a few physicians do this):

- Why you chose your medical specialty.
- What you like about medicine and your specialty.
- What you don't like about both.
- What, if anything, you would change about your decision regarding your specialty, practice location, office environment, and type of patients you treat.
- What you hope to change or improve in the future.

In other words, give your staff a sense of who you are and what you believe in. This may be hard for you; it's a little like your first kiss. You may wonder, "What if I say too much? Too little? What if they think I'm self-indulgent or sentimental? What if they don't understand why I'm telling this to them?"

Don't worry. If you explain your intentions ("We're going to create a quality road map for the practice"), your staff will appreciate and enjoy your review. Explain that it helps to know where you've been when you're planning a trip so that you don't take the same detours and forks in the road and stop at the same bad roadside restaurants as the last time you made the trip.

When you've finished your history, you will need to answer a few questions to develop a vision. For this you will need your staff's input, for a vision must be shared if it is to be believed and acted out. (It's that commitment thing again!) You can start by distributing sheets of paper on which the following questions are printed. Ask each person to answer the questions from his or her perspective, according to their own beliefs about the correct answer, not as they believe you want them to or as the practice now exists (unless the question specifically asks that).

Here are the questions to answer:

- *What business are we in?*
- *Why are we in this business?*
- *Who are our customers? (Remind people that more than one answer is possible.)*
- *Who should our customers be?*
- *What are the expectations of our customers?*
- *What image do we want, (i.e., what do we want our customers to think of when they think of us)?*
- *What should we be doing and saying to meet our customers' expectations and to reinforce our desired image?*

Both physicians and employees are likely to find this exercise extremely interesting and enlightening. Depending on the type of employees you have, how well you've educated them about your practice and values, how well and how often you reinforce this message, and the length of time they've been with you, you may discover that their answers are similar to yours. On the other hand, you may discover a broad chasm separating your views and theirs.

If staff members are hesitant to respond, it may be helpful to use the brainstorming technique to get people thinking creatively. Sometimes a group situation can inhibit individual expression of new ideas or opinions; brainstorming can overcome this. The following is a description of how to brainstorm effectively.

How To Brainstorm Effectively

Brainstorming is a method of encouraging the free flow of creative ideas in a group setting. Because the group may inhibit creativity and imagination, these guidelines should be followed:

1. No criticism or negativity is permitted. There are no bad or dumb ideas.
2. Ideas should be recorded exactly as stated by the individual.
3. Ideas should focus on processes, not people.
4. Give the group several minutes for each question or topic to think about and/or jot down their ideas.
5. The discussion leader should prime the pump by offering a few ideas if needed.
6. For each issue or question, first solicit thoughts and ideas randomly. When spontaneous suggestions trickle off, encourage ideas from any group member(s) who has not offered one. Some people are naturally shy or inhibited in this setting.

It's important not to use this exercise as a punitive measure. No person's views should be held against him or her. The purpose of this discussion is to first brainstorm, then come to agreement: "We are in the business of making people feel good about their health," or "We are in the business of good vision," or whatever you decide your business is.

GAIN A CONSENSUS OPINION OF ATTITUDES AND VALUES

Once you discuss and agree on what business you're in and who your customers are—patients, physicians, family members, each other, employers, insurance companies, and/or members of the community—go through each of the remaining questions and come up with a set of reasonable responses that reflect consensus attitudes and beliefs.

> **Consensus:** *An opinion or statement that reflects the majority of the group and that can be supported by all. Consensus is a majority opinion but does not entail a show of hands or other vote counting.*

You may have an outlier, a staff member whose views are divergent from those of the rest of the group. Avoid letting this individual's opinions color or overpower the rest of the group's thinking. If his or her views are negative (for example, if he or she holds a dim view of patients and their expectations), you or a senior staff member must work closely with him or her in the future to encourage participation. If after extensive discussion this individual cannot, or chooses not to, share the consensus perspective, it will probably be wise to suggest that he or she look elsewhere for an employer with a more similar outlook and set of beliefs.

When you've completed this exercise, you will have the basis for developing a mission statement. Exhibit 7-1 shows the mission statement developed by Arthritis and Rheumatism Associates in Silver Spring, Maryland, where Dr. Baraf practices. Compare it to the mission statement in Exhibit 7-2 of the Hunkeler Clinic in Kansas City, Missouri, and use the two statements to stimulate discussion and ideas for developing a mission statement for your practice.

A SAMPLE APPROACH TO DEVELOPING A MISSION

Let's look at developing a mission statement from the perspective of an orthopedic practice with a subspecialty in knee surgery. The answers to these questions reflect the consensus values and opinions of the practice staff:

- *What business are we in?*
  Helping patients achieve physical mobility or helping them ensure maximum flexibility.

Exhibit 7-1

Mission Statement
Arthritis and Rheumatism Associates
Silver Spring, Maryland

The goals of our practice are:

1. To provide the best possible medical care for our patients.
2. To treat each patient with dignity, respect, kindness, and courtesy.
3. To serve our community through preventive medicine and education.
4. To have a smoothly functioning practice where staff and physicians work together in a spirit of harmony and cooperation.
5. To have highly qualified, motivated personnel who are interested in their work and our patients and find our practice professionally pleasing and rewarding.
6. To have a practice that recognizes its responsibilities to its employees and understands that the work of the office is most productively and efficiently done in an environment of mutually understood guidelines.

Source: Courtesy of Arthritis and Rheumatism Associates, Silver Spring, Maryland.

- *Why are we in this business?*

  To satisfy a personal need to help others, and to make a reasonable profit for the practice.

- *Who are our customers?*

  People with bone, joint, and muscle problems; other physicians; health plans; employers; insurance companies and third party payers; and each other.

- *Who should our customers be?*

  All the above, and in particular people with knee problems.

- *What are the expectations of our customers?*

  To have their needs, **as they define or perceive them,** met.

- *What image do we want (i.e., what do we want our customers to think of when they think of us)?*

  A practice made up of compassionate, skilled professionals who have the most current technical knowledge and who go out of their way to satisfy patients. We want not only to

Exhibit 7-2

Mission Statement
Hunkeler Clinic
Kansas City, Missouri

The primary mission of the Hunkeler Eye Clinic is to provide quality eye care with care, concern, and compassion for each of our patients.

We remain committed to continuing improvement in quality through adaptation of technological advances and continuing education.

The Hunkeler Eye Clinic will be involved in clinical evaluation of state-of-the-art technology. However, the focus will remain on quality treatment for each patient.

The Hunkeler Eye Clinic is also committed to continuing education of our physicians and staff to assure improvements in patient care. Furthermore, it is important to adequately inform our patients about their eye condition and the appropriate alternatives to preserve a lifetime of good vision.

Source: Courtesy of the Hunkeler Eye Clinic, Kansas City, Missouri.

provide the highest quality of clinical care but also to give our customers **more** than they want, need, and/or expect whenever we can.

- *What should we be doing and saying to meet our customers' expectations and to reinforce our desired image?*

    We must unify our words and actions toward our patients, referral sources, and each other. We must always try to look at our practice, our actions, and our words through the eyes and ears of our customers.

On the basis of this discussion, the physicians and staff created the following statement:

Our mission is to help our patients become as physically independent and fit as possible by providing superior orthopedic care and personal attention. We will listen to our patients and communicate with them about their condition and treatment, and we will treat them with the dignity, compassion, and courtesy we would expect for ourselves. We will treat our co-workers and colleagues as friends and professionals in the process of serving our patients. We will always strive to enjoy what we do.

YOUR MISSION LIGHTS THE WAY TO THE FUTURE

It's been said that vision is "the art of seeing things invisible." When you define your vision by creating a mission statement, you turn on the light in a darkened room. You make visible and tangible the future of your practice. And since that's where you are likely to spend the rest of your professional life, it helps not only to see the future but to know you took charge of getting yourself and those you are responsible for into it.

When you've created a mission statement that you and other physicians and staff in the practice truly believe in, don't file it away in a manila folder. Use it. Live it. Print it on the back of your business card, as did several practices we encountered. Frame it and hang it in the reception area where patients can see it (and hold you to it). If it's brief, consider putting it on the bottom of your letterhead. Include it in your practice brochure, office policy manual, and employee handbook. Have new employees sign a copy as a personal quality pledge. You could even print it on a small card and use the back side as an appointment card. Your mission statement gives direction and purpose to everyone in the practice. It lights the way to the future.

A mission statement serves as the foundation for practice objectives. Objectives form a more specific expression of what you intend to accomplish, thus helping remove uncertainty about the focus of the practice or your intended purpose. Whereas the mission statement says "This is what we are about," the objectives say "Here's how we intend to go about it." Objectives are goals: specific, achievable, and measurable and preferably with a time frame or date attached. To be effective, objectives should stretch the practice and get employees **and** physicians out of "in-a-rut" thinking and behaving.

Defining objectives is far from easy. It takes time, commitment, and planning, just as developing a mission statement does. Many practices and businesses function without any commonly accepted objectives or with conflicting objectives. For example, a nurse with a small multispecialty practice said, "Our objective is to satisfy the customer." At the same practice, the business manager informed us, "Our objective is to grow 10% a year and earn a minimum of 10% after-tax profit." How would staff members know what they are working toward and how they should behave given these two objectives?

DO YOU *REALLY* NEED A VISION?

Is it necessary for a practice to have a vision or a mission statement and objectives? Are these really critical to achieving patient satisfaction and ensuring quality service? In answer to these questions, we suggest that you look at it from a clinical perspective. Do you need to know the preferred outcome to treat a patient with asthma? The preferred outcome would be cessation of symptoms, and with that goal in mind you would prescribe medications, exercise, and environmental adjustment accordingly. The patient's physiology, environmental limitations, and other conditions may prevent a complete achievement of the goal you've set. Nevertheless, having a target helps you and your patient create a treatment plan that can be modified with time and changing conditions. Consider your practice objectives the "treatment plan" as you strive to reach the target you have created with your mission statement. ❧

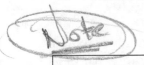

Action Steps for Creating a Vision

1. Define your own mission: Examine your beliefs, attitudes, and core values regarding the purpose of your practice, the role of your staff, and your personal and professional style.
2. Focus on the practice mission at an extended staff meeting:
   - Share your understanding of the mission.
   - Seek staff input.
   - Use brainstorming to encourage staff to share ideas fully.
   - Together, develop a mission statement in which everyone believes.
3. Make your mission statement highly visible in your practice.
4. Use your mission statement to define practice objectives.

—— 🙠 ——

8

Getting Ahead with Your Team beside You

"It's human nature. You want to go where people act like they want you to be there."

—Margaret Dieckhoner, Administrator,
Arthritis and Rheumatism Associates,
Silver Spring, Maryland

If you've ever played tug-of-war, you know that when everyone on one side pulls together in the same direction, enthusiastically cheering each other on, they are more likely to win than the other team, whose members are pulling in different directions or without enthusiasm. Not only is the energetic group likely to win, they'll have more fun pulling together.

In a medical practice, patients are better served and more satisfied when they're cared for by people who are part of a cohesive team. On a team, there are others with whom to share frustrations, burdens, successes, and ideas. But most important, teamwork is one of the most significant factors in ensuring quality service to your patients, day in and day out. Working together, the members of a team get things done efficiently and effectively, conveying confidence and competence to your patients.

What exactly is a team? Look at your practice and you may see several teams at work. There's the whole team: everyone in the practice—physicians, front office, and back office employees—

pooling their knowledge and skills to satisfy patients. There are functional teams—the billing team, the clinical team, the business office team, the cleaning team. There are informal teams as well as formal teams. Some teams form and dissolve when their task or assignment is completed, while others endure. You may create a "special purpose" team to solve a particular problem, such as planning the holiday party or redecorating the office.

WHAT HAPPENS WHEN A TEAM WORKS?

A quality team knows, understands, and **believes in** the practice vision or mission statement. The values of the practice may be framed and hung on the wall, printed in policy manuals, and even read aloud each day, but until these values burn within each individual, and unless each person is an apostle of the practice creed, sharing it with others and demonstrating it in action, there is no team.

Forming a team from a diverse group of individuals with distinct personalities, values, abilities, experiences, likes, and dislikes can be a complex and sometimes frustrating process. Just ask the coach of a major league expansion team. But look at what happens when a great team comes together—Super Bowl victories, World Series championships, practice success, professional fulfillment, and patient satisfaction!

DO AS WINNERS DO TO CREATE A GREAT TEAM

To form a quality team in your practice, do what the major leaguers do:

- Carefully scout potential players. This is a critical step in implementing quality service. Thorough, in-depth interviews of potential candidates can reveal much about a person's attitude, values, work ethic, and belief system. When the Four Seasons hotel chain opened its Los Angeles hotel, 14,000 candidates were interviewed for 350 slots. To find friendly, team-oriented people, hiring staff grilled final candidates in a

WHAT HAPPENS
WHEN A TEAM WORKS?

During a team-building staff meeting, the eight employees of a Southwestern Eye Center satellite office in Arizona were asked to name the benefits of working as a team. Here's the list they came up with:

- ☑ *Growth leads to success*
- ☑ *Quality work*
- ☑ *Practice growth*
- ☑ *Acceptance of change*
- ☑ *Increased satisfaction*
- ☑ *Decreased staff*
- ☑ *More positive atmosphere*
- ☑ *Jobs get done better/easier*
- ☑ *Learn from each other*
- ☑ *Staff happier about working*
- ☑ *Cross-training*
- ☑ *Sharing burdens*
- ☑ *Greater flexibility*
- ☑ *Happy doctors*
- ☑ *Happier patients*
- ☑ *Smoother schedule*
- ☑ *Peer review (second opinion)*
- ☑ *Better decision-making*
- ☑ *Results are more accurate*
- ☑ *Better physical health*
- ☑ *Dependability among team members*
- ☑ *Good morale/good attitude*
- ☑ *Increased efficiency*
- ☑ *Increased revenues*
- ☑ *Appearances*
- ☑ *More versatile staff*
- ☑ *Decreased down time*
- ☑ *Improved work skills*
- ☑ *Trust that work gets done*
- ☑ *Share "dump jobs"*
- ☑ *Quality patient care*
- ☑ *Sharing the glory*
- ☑ *Harmony*
- ☑ *Better/more productive help*
- ☑ *Ability to stay up to date*
- ☑ *More empathetic employees*
- ☑ *Better organization*
- ☑ *Better communication*
- ☑ *Everyone improves*
- ☑ *Creativity*
- ☑ *Assisting others lessens their burden*
- ☑ *Patients can tell if there's harmony or discord*

Source: Southwestern Eye Center, Mesa, Arizona.

round of four or five interviews.[1] You'll find techniques and forms to help in selecting candidates who are service-oriented in Chapter 9.

- Instill the practice values early and often. Team members won't reflect your patient-centered philosophy unless they know it and believe in it. For employees to understand the values of the practice, they must be thoroughly trained in them, then see them lived day to day. Acknowledge and reward team and individual actions that reflect organizational values; this reinforces with your team what is meant by "the customer comes first." Kathy Mosciski, office manager of Dr. Abrams' practice, says, "I try to observe our staff doing or saying things that show their concern for patients and let them know I've noticed, but it's especially appreciated when the doctors notice and say something."
- Work at building your team. You can't emphasize teamwork and team building enough, says office manager Margaret Dieckhoner of Arthritis and Rheumatism Associates: "Team building is like ground beef. There are a thousand ways to serve it, and you have to keep serving it up over and over—hamburgers, meatloaf, shepherd's pie—you can never feed enough team building to your staff."
- Don't skimp on quality people. No team ever climbed out of the cellar by settling for ninth-round draft picks. They spend money to trade for the best players on other teams and to get first-round picks. When your practice becomes known as a great place to work because you offer a higher salary, better benefits, and a pleasant work environment, you can select from the best office staff candidates available.

GET TEAM INVOLVEMENT BY ASKING FOR PARTICIPATION

Get staff input and participation when you are developing the practice mission, goals, and policies. Employees who understand how their jobs relate to the overall goals of the practice are more effective. During performance reviews, have individual staff members set personal and professional goals that relate to practice goals and values.

Cross-train employees whenever possible. Granted, there are limitations to how practical complete cross-training is, but employees who occasionally perform the jobs of other staff members are more likely to cooperate with one another. A Dallas, Texas hospital found that nursing staffs that worked one shift were quick to blame another shift for problems. Once the staffs started rotating shifts, even if it was briefly and only occasionally, cooperation improved. Said one nurse who primarily worked the day shift, "Until I worked some night shifts, I thought the night crew sat around and drank coffee. I didn't have much tolerance when I would come on in the morning and find things not done. After working some nights, I know their shifts can be as hectic as any I've worked during the day."

Phoenix, Arizona family physician Ray Hughes, MD, has a completely cross-trained staff of eight. Everyone can do general patient check-ins (weight, temperature, blood pressure, etc.) as well as EKGs and chest X-rays—basic tasks that require no certification. They're also trained to look for and point out "overlooks," errors (an abnormal Pap smear or a transposed Medicare code) that may have been missed. Patients, productivity, and efficiency all benefit from this cross-training. If you can't truly rotate employees, try to free them to "shadow" another employee or even you for at least part of a day. Strong alliances may be forged by such an experience.

Share business issues and clinical issues with all your staff. Too often, business issues stay in the front office, and clinical problems stay in the back office. The entire practice is affected by both sides of the house, and employees will work as a team more effectively if they understand this. Ophthalmologist Joseph Noreika, MD, holds quarterly "state-of-the-practice" meetings during which revenues, expenses, and other financial issues are shared with all 14 staff members. This regular financial review was begun at the request of the staff, he said.

Identify barriers that prevent working as a service-oriented team. Are there bottlenecks to work flow? Are some staffers unhappy, improperly trained, or simply uncommitted to your mission? Apple Computer calls the infection that radiates negativism and a bad attitude "Bozo cancer." Bozo cancer spreads fast; if it appears incurable (that is, if counseling and other treatments have failed); it's best to cut it out before it invades others.[2] Sometimes unhappy employees can be helped by your listening to their problems or perspective (perhaps serious issues at home are invading their work attitude and behavior), clarifying their role in team goals and expectations, or supplying positive reinforcement of their useful contributions. If none of this works, releasing the staffer may be the best option for all concerned.

Provide a threat-free atmosphere in which your staff can work. Threat-free doesn't mean "without consequences." It means a positive atmosphere in which employees aren't punished for taking risks and doing their jobs right. A threat-free environment encourages disclosure and discussion of embarrassing or sensitive behaviors, even (or especially) on the part of the physicians. It also encourages innovation because mistakes, the natural consequence of creative thinking, are not punished. They're regarded as growth bumps!

Provide resources—time as well as materials—when you provide problems to be solved or when you ask for staff involvement. Dr. Noreika turns over the monthly staff development sessions to his staff. It's their responsibility to plan and coordinate them. They are given a budget for "fun" outings; otherwise, all decisions are made by the team.

INCREASE PRODUCTIVITY AND MORALE WITH FUN

Take time for fun. Dr. Noreika closes his two offices one afternoon a month from 1 to 5 p.m. This time is used for staff meetings, in-services, and motivational talks, and every fourth session is reserved for fun. They've had bowling tournaments, gone to a comedy club (an evening event), and even held a staff golf tournament. Weather wasn't a problem for the golf tournament because the tees and greens were set up right in the office, with tape, boxes, and an assortment of furniture and supplies employed to create bunkers, fairways, and rough. It was a goofy game that gave staffers just the break they needed.

If there's a problem, acknowledge it and fix it. Turn appropriate problems over to the practice team, or to an ad hoc team, to analyze and solve. Even sticky problems need to be addressed.

One physician calls this "Your fly is open" problem solving: "Somebody needs to tell you, even if it's embarrassing to do so." For example, in another practice, a physician who prided himself on his "get-it-done" style often usurped the team process by jumping in and making decisions about office operations that were the staff's responsibility. No one would tell him that his decisions sometimes were disruptive and inappropriate; after all, he was "the boss." It finally came out in a staff meeting when the physician said he would take care of purchasing a new microwave oven for the employee lounge. "You don't even use the microwave!" a staffer blurted. The ensuing discussion revealed the staff's frustration with the physician's impulsiveness, and he agreed to try to curb his take-over tendencies in the future. Had the practice had a candid approach to problem solving, the situation might not have festered for as long as it did.

Show your commitment to patient satisfaction and quality service by showing your commitment to your staff. Host seminars and in-services at the office, and send employees to outside conferences when these would be beneficial. Staffers themselves, drug company representatives, hospital employees, and other local people may be undiscovered treasures waiting for an opportunity to share information. Educating and informing your staff tells them that you value them. We were impressed with the number of staff development opportunities offered by the practices we visited. Many devote at least one afternoon a month to formal educational programs in addition to short in-services, breakfast and lunchtime sessions, and other "feed the brain" get-togethers. A practice administrator said, "It kills us to close the office, but our staff really thrives on these meetings, and other practices are envious. And we see it returned in improved productivity and a renewed sense of teamwork." The physician said simply, "The patients I don't see when we close the office will come another day."

Encourage ongoing learning by circulating books, articles, audiotapes, and videotapes to staff members and by including a discussion of hot topics and meaty articles in meetings. One large practice has a book club for managers. Each month they select a new business or management book to read; during their discussion meeting, they analyze the points made in the book and look for ways to apply concepts and ideas in their departments or practicewide. Childress Buick in Phoenix, Arizona has an employee resource library with 400 books and tapes. When employees check out a book or tape, they fill out a card that's included with it, saying how they plan to apply the information they gain. The card goes in their personnel file and is considered during the annual performance evaluation.

ENCOURAGE AND REWARD ACCOUNTABILITY

Insist on individual responsibility and accountability, then reward it when it occurs. Tell your staff, "If you see a better way of doing something, tell us." Neil Baum, MD, a urologist in New Orleans, Louisiana, uses instant bonuses to reward good suggestions.

Please Make Me Feel Important

Remember This Principle: Please Make Me Feel Important. People want to feel valued, a part of the team. Seek a balance between recognizing and rewarding team accomplishments and individual accomplishments. Everyone wants to be a part of a group—a team—but each person also wants acknowledgment for his or her individual uniqueness. When recognizing team successes, point out individual contributions as well. Baseball selects the best team via the World Series, but outstanding individuals are also singled out with awards for the Most Valuable Player, lowest earned run average, most runs batted in, etc. Honor your team's outstanding effort, but also honor contributions by members who deserve it.

Some practices name an Employee of the Month or similar outstanding staffer. Although official recognitions are important, be careful about setting a precedent for a regular award, especially if you have a small staff. You'll soon be faced with the dilemma of what to do when one employee keeps winning the award, to the detriment of the rest of the staff's morale. It's usually better to make awards official but to keep them ad hoc. When you see an opportunity to recognize an achievement, do it. There's more on this subject in Chapter 11.

Support your employees. If you ask them to come up with a solution to a problem, give their idea a try. The Hunkeler Eye

Clinic's teams have come up with standardized dictation reports, a workable daily scheduling system, and a method for efficiently performing radial keratotomy eye surgery in the clinic. If you ask your staff to handle a problem with a patient, trust them to do so. They will sometimes make mistakes, and you must be willing to allow that.

Value the similarities as well as the differences among your staff. The common thread among all the unique members of your team should be a striving to achieve the practice goals through a commitment to the practice philosophy. You will enjoy some of your staff members more than others. Some will be more like you, and others will be different. If they all have the same strengths and weaknesses, you may have a staff of 20 but no one who can figure out the new copier. In *Team Players and Teamwork: The New Competitive Business Strategy*, author Glenn Parker describes four types of players on a team: contributors, collaborators, communicators, and challengers.[3] Each is an equally important team member but with unique personality traits. Understanding these types can aid in enhancing team productivity and building consensus. In Exhibit 8-1, the qualities of these team members are depicted.

Communication fosters teamwork. Schedule regular staff meetings, and assign different team members to run them. (This may take time. Dr. Noreika comments, "We've tried rotating responsibility for leadership, but sometimes people are fearful to make decisions, although they are given the right to.") The most effective practices with the most active teams hold regular staff meetings no matter how busy they are. Consider holding "stand-up meetings" to start the day. Everybody participates, and the purpose is to share the day's activities. ("Dr. A. will be in surgery all day, Dr. B. is at a conference, and Dr. C. will be here. The front office is swamped because two people are out sick—let's call and tell them hi, maybe send flowers—and the back office has a new nurse starting today—welcome! Does anybody have a special project or need help today? Let's all stay in close touch with the front office staff's workload; if there's a way we can help while you're short staffed, let us know.")

When you ask for employee input and involvement, follow through on it. There's no quicker way to demoralize someone than to ask for advice and then summarily disregard it. If you can't use a suggestion, explain why.

Exhibit 8-1

Who's on Your Team?

Contributor

A task-oriented person who enjoys providing the team with good technical information and data, does his or her homework and pushes the team to set high performance standards and use resources wisely. Seen as dependable, although he or she sometimes gets bogged down in details and data, may not see the big picture or the need for a positive team climate. Viewed as responsible, authoritative, reliable, proficient, and organized.

Collaborator

A goal-directed person who sees the mission or goal of the team as paramount but is flexible and open to new ideas, willing to pitch in and work outside his or her defined role, and able to share the limelight with other team members. While able to see the big picture, this individual sometimes fails periodically to revisit the mission, give enough attention to basic team tasks, or consider the needs of other team members. The collaborator is forward-looking, accommodating, flexible, and imaginative.

Communicator

A process-oriented person who is an effective listener and facilitator of involvement, conflict resolution, consensus building, feedback, and the creation of an informal, relaxed climate. A positive "people person," the communicator at times may see the process as an end in itself, may be unwilling to confront other team members or may not give enough emphasis to completing task assignments and making progress toward team goals. Considered supportive, considerate, relaxed, enthusiastic, and tactful.

Challenger

A person who questions the goals, methods, and even the ethics of the team, is willing to disagree with the leader or higher authority, and encourages the team to take well-conceived risks. The challenger's candor and openness is appreciated, but at times he or she does not know when to back off an issue and may become self-righteous and try to push the team too far. Viewed as honest, outspoken, principled, ethical, and adventurous.

Source: Copyright 1991 by Xicom, Inc., RR #2, Woods Road, Tuxedo, NY 10987. Reprinted with permission.

PUT THE TEAM TO WORK SOLVING PROBLEMS

Problem? Clearly identify it so that all parties agree on its parameters. Brainstorm about how to solve it. Eliminate the unworkable ideas. Prioritize the workable ones. Try out the best choice, give it time, and evaluate the results.

Don't send a message you don't mean. A family practice physician remembers his early days in practice:

> I was fresh out of a brutal residency program, in which competition was fierce and people were treated badly. I was determined to run my office as a democracy, where we were all equal. I didn't want a hierarchy in my office. About 2 years and a host of personnel problems later, it finally occurred to me: We're not all equal. And this was a medical practice, not a democracy. I'm the physician, and I have a lot at risk here if things aren't done right. I'm the bottom line. I'm the one with the liability, and I'm the one entitled to the greater rewards from my risks and efforts. There's nothing wrong with this. Employees understand and respect it, and they're relieved when somebody takes a strong leadership role. My problem was that I wanted to believe we all had the same risks and were entitled to the same rewards. Employees saw the fallacy in this rationale before I did. Now I'm more realistic. I recognize that employees all have their strengths, and they all contribute greatly to the success of this practice. I treat them with the respect they deserve, but every effort needs a leader, a boss, a captain of the ship who's willing to take responsibility for everything that goes on. In this practice, that somebody is me.

TEAMS TAKE PRACTICE AND LEADERSHIP TO WORK WELL

The message? It takes teamwork to have a practice that functions effectively and efficiently, but it also takes leadership. Don't be afraid to lead your team.

What's the bottom line in all this? Strong teams don't spring to life overnight. They grow and mature together with plenty of coaching and nurturing. There are days when the team members seem to pull against one another, but those days are far outnumbered by the days when the team members support and strengthen each other's efforts. Provide the right environment, resources, and rewards, and you'll be surprised at what your team can accomplish for you and your patients. ❧

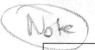

Action Steps for Making a Team Work

1. Hire quality people who demonstrate a service-oriented attitude.
2. Clearly communicate the value you place on a team approach. Reward actions that reflect team values as well as individual responsibility and accountability.
3. Work at team building. Encourage communication through regular staff meetings.
4. Seek staff input, and follow up on suggestions.
5. Cross-train employees.
6. Share business and clinical issues with all staff.
7. Identify barriers to working effectively as a team.
8. Address problems by creating teams and providing necessary resources.
9. Provide a threat-free work environment and staff development opportunities.
10. Take time for fun!

References

1. L. Armstrong and W.C. Symonds, Beyond "May I help you," *Business Week* (October 25, 1991): 100–103.
2. D. Armstrong, *Managing by Storying Around: A New Method of Leadership* (New York, N.Y.: Doubleday, 1992): 98.
3. G.M. Parker, *Team Players and Teamwork: The New Competitive Business Strategy* (San Francisco, Calif.: Jossey-Bass Publishers, 1990): 164.

9

Recruiting a High-Performance Team

You call the office of a referring physician, and her telephone is answered on the second ring. The receptionist is pleasant and warm and sounds genuinely interested in your problem. You hang up, pleased that your call has been handled with competence and even a smile.

Then you call your own office. You call the "front number," the one patients and other physicians call. You do it with a vague sense of dread because you're afraid of what you'll hear. Sadly, you're not surprised at the contrast. Your receptionist answers on the fifth ring, blurts "Please hold" before you can tell her who you are, and you listen to 2 minutes of a rock music station that isn't quite tuned in. When she returns to the telephone, she asks, "Who are you holding for?" She is clearly not right for the job; she is easily rattled and irritated by interruptions.

This is the third receptionist you've had this year. The first two quit after working less than 4 months each. The turnover in the back office isn't much better. Your office nurse has been with you only about 6 months; his predecessor left after only a year. You specialize in the treatment of elderly patients, and your current nurse is chronically impatient with them, his attention wandering when they tell a longer-than-necessary story.

What's wrong with this picture? Plenty.

PATIENTS APPRECIATE A CARING, COMPETENT TEAM

You know that your patients appreciate a staff that is caring and competent, people who work as a team. You know your staff members reflect your practice, your medical quality, and your service. You hear the resignation in your patients' voices as they are introduced to yet another new nurse, and you know they're probably wondering why your employees don't stay with you. You're wondering the same thing. You see the cost of turnover in your practice: the direct costs of advertising to fill vacant positions, severance pay, and similar expenses. You don't even want to calculate the indirect costs: lost productivity due to vacancies and the need to yank an experienced staffer from her job to train the new person, the impact of poor morale on productivity and efficiency.

You know that your team says a lot about you, and right now you don't have much of a team. Your patients grumble; service is minimal at best (Let's not even talk about quality!). Your bottom line is hurting, and you're tired of trying to fix it with bandages, quick hires who fill a vacancy but don't fill the bill.

So you ask around. Some of your colleagues admit to having the same problems. Others are more than a little smug about their wonderful employees, citing their longevity with the practice as proof that "something is right." Those same colleagues may be protective of their success, afraid that you will steal their employees. As one surgeon lamented, "I don't want to raid anybody else's staff; I just want to know where they find good people!"

She explained further:

> *Another surgeon here in town has an absolutely dynamite nurse working for her. She's bright, motivated, and organized. And patients love her! She and her employer have been together nearly 8 years—they work together like partners in a good marriage. The nurse could leave her current position and work for anybody in town; we all know she'd be an asset to our offices. In fact, I know a few people have tried to hire her away. But, for all her attributes, her strongest one is loyalty. She sticks with her employer through thick and thin. How does that kind of magic happen?*

Although there may be a touch of magic in the situation that brings, and keeps, the right people together, most of the success stories rely on common sense and hard work. Finding and hiring the right members for your team is the first step; without it, there is no team. How do you put that team together? Like everything else, it takes planning and specifics. In this chapter, we'll help you (or the person designated to put the team together) define the characteristics of individual jobs and team members. In the following pages, *you* refers to the person charged with selecting and managing the team.

PICTURE THE PERFECT PRACTICE

Before you start looking for the right people for your practice, spend some time defining the jobs they will do. Many practices hire good people but quickly discourage and demoralize them by simply asking them to do impossible tasks or poorly defined jobs or otherwise mismanaging them.

If you're starting a new practice or even if you're working within an established organization, start by listing the tasks that need to be accomplished daily, weekly, monthly, and yearly. (Note to office managers or practice administrators: This should be done together with the physicians in the practice.) Be brave. Be bold. Don't let yourself (or anybody else) yank you back to reality just yet. Assume, just for a moment, that you're living in a perfect world where you wield a magic wand.

Make a list of the things that make the perfect practice. Do you want somebody answering the telephone for 12 hours a day, including lunch? Put it on the list. Do you want your patients called the day after discharge from the hospital? Put it on the list. Do you want your patients to receive their lab results within 24 hours if at all possible? Put it on the list. Do you want to collect 90% of your billings? Put it on the list. You get the idea. If it's important to you, write it down.

Now take a look at your list. Free your brain of the "But . . ." phrase, and think of possibilities. How could you accomplish what's on the list? Do you need 2 more front office people instead of a nurse? Do you need a physician's assistant in addition to or rather than a nurse? Do you need to change your work patterns?

Let your "wish list" define the skills or positions needed to help you accomplish it. When defining positions, list the personality traits required. For example, if yours is a particularly hectic front office and you'd like the atmosphere to be more calm, list "patient, cheerful, quiet, and calm" as attributes you value in that area. Next, define the job and the nuts and bolts of getting the job done. Be honest. Include the negatives as well as the positives. If there is a way to turn the negatives into positives, by all means, do it!

HIRE ATTITUDE, NOT JUST SKILLS

Many hiring experts say that the successful hire is a result of emphasis on attitude, not simply skills. Says one family practice physician, "We can teach someone how to code billing properly. We can't teach them to care about our financial status as if it were their own. That must come from within."

You're looking for several attributes when you hire an employee. As a Manhattan oral surgeon put it:

> The best office assistant I ever had was one who had minimal experience in a doctor's office but who had a lot of experience with people. She was street smart. She had raised a house full of kids, had worked in community organizations for 15 years, and knew how to work with all types of people. She didn't know how to handle our telephones or book an appointment when she came to work here. But she picked that up quickly. She had the foundation to do a great job here. She worked here for 10 years, until her husband retired and they went off to travel together. I'm hoping she'll get tired of that and come back to work!

Dr. Hales, the New Orleans pediatrician, staffs his office differently from most offices. He has no nurse, preferring to do all patient care himself. He has no full-time office staff, preferring instead to hire part-time workers. He says:

> When I staffed this office, I hired the nicest people I knew. They are sharp, bright, wonderful women who are

*overqualified for what they are doing. We have 8 or 10
women now who share 3 or 4 full-time jobs. Working this
schedule gives them total flexibility in how they come and
go. Because they're not working full time, I think they bring
a freshness and an energy that is nice. They take a lot of
pride in what goes on here. I get as many nice comments
about my office people as I do about me, and that makes me
very glad.*

Some employers equate part-time workers with short tenure. Dr. Hales hasn't found that to be true. "I have had people here since I started 12 years ago. I also have some who have been here only a year. They all work together as a team."

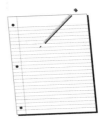

Steps in Recruiting and Hiring Patient-Pleasing Employees

1. Define the job.
2. Determine personality attributes as well as skills needed.
3. Look inside the practice first, then go outside.
4. Spread the word!
5. Screen applicants with resumé and cover letter.
6. Interview carefully, candidly, thoroughly.
7. Check references!
8. Make the offer and confirm the terms.
9. Don't forget on-the-job training, continual education, and frequent assessment and feedback.

FINDING PEOPLE WITH THE RIGHT STUFF

Where do you find people with the right stuff? First, look within your own organization. Is there a billing clerk whose people skills are strong enough that he or she would shine on the front desk? Is your front office person more comfortable with a computer than he or she is with a waiting room full of whining kids? Even if it means losing a superior secretary, if this person indicates interest in your marketing coordinator position, he or she should have an opportunity to apply.

In an article in *Harvard Business Review,* award-winning hospital administrator Tom Chapman said that 55% of the employees hired at his facility are recommended by current employees. "We have people who have already bought into the mission recommending people who they think will fit into the system, and it is a natural marriage. Another 29% applied because they were in this hospital, either visiting patients or receiving services themselves. So over 80% of our employees have some knowledge about us before coming here, and once we've infected them with our spirit, we try not to let them go."[1(p.94)] And they don't go; the turnover rate is as low as 4.5% in the hospital's nursing department, traditionally an unstable area.[2]

If you need to look outside, put the word out that you're looking for an employee, and define exactly what kind of person you need. Post notices at the local junior colleges, universities, and trade schools, in the medical staff office at the hospital, and with the medical society. You might run a classified advertisement, but be ready for an avalanche of telephone calls, letters, and walk-in applicants. Tell your pharmaceutical sales representatives that you're hiring. If you know of a particularly promising employee who happens to work for someone else, be careful. You don't need conflict with a colleague because you raided his or her staff. Only the rarest of employees would be worth the grief.

KEEP AN EYE OUT FOR POTENTIAL TEAM MEMBERS

Don't wait until you need to fill a position to start looking. Always be on the lookout for a bright, caring employee. When the right one is available, it may make sense to hire him or her, even if the timing isn't perfect for you. Exceptional people are worth their weight in gold, and they won't always be available on your timetable.

What about hiring spouses, children, and other relatives? In some cases it works, in others it's a disaster. One of the happiest arrangements we know of involved a physician's mother, who had retired from a local university as an executive secretary. She worked part time in his practice, answering the telephone and doing clerical work. A new employee attending her first staff meeting saw that the physician referred to this older employee as "Mom." The younger woman was incensed on behalf of her older colleague, feeling that the physician was calling her "Mom" because of her age. Later, she shared her indignation with a colleague: "Just because Mary is older than the rest of us gives him no excuse to call her 'Mom.'" The new employee did not realize, even after 2 weeks of working in the office, that Mary was indeed the physician's mother. Such a professional relationship among family members is probably rare; the family that works together doesn't always put others at ease!

Your best approach to recruiting and hiring employees will vary with the size, structure, and style of your practice. If you're solo, you're obviously the boss. If you're working within a partnership or a larger group practice, you'll need to work with your partners to develop a plan that fits the needs of the practice as well as your own.

IS AN EMPLOYMENT SERVICE WORTH IT? MAYBE.

Some employers say it's worth the money to use an employment service or even a temporary staffing service. If you use a staffing service, you'll see the employee in action on the job without any obligation to hire. Before you enter such an arrangement, however, be sure that you can hire employees away from the staffing agency. Expect to pay a premium fee for the privilege. But the pain of paying a premium fee may pale compared to the hassles of hiring the wrong person for the job.

No matter how desperate you are, don't hurry the process. If you hire the wrong person, you will be forced to take time to work through the mistake, possibly firing this person and hiring a replacement. It just makes more sense to do it right the first time. Your patients (and your patience) will benefit from time invested in finding and hiring the best people for the job.

Ask for resumés, knowing that people will present themselves in the best possible light. Look for gaps in experience. If the person was at home with a small child or an invalid parent, you want to know that. If he or she was serving time in prison, you'd like to know that, too. Also ask for a cover letter with the resumé. Some resumés will arrive without a cover letter despite this request. Obviously the applicant can't follow instructions. Is the letter literate? Misspelled? Friendly? A form letter? Clean and neat? Use the letter to evaluate the candidate.

Develop a job description, but don't use it to restrict or restrain a potential go-getter applicant. Developing the job description can be a good assignment for the person currently in the position or for other team members who are familiar with the job. List tasks, responsibilities, authority, and personality traits and attitudes required (for example, "Team-player, flexible, innovative, organized, customer-first approach). See Exhibit 9-1 for a sample form for creating a

Exhibit 9-1 Create a Job Description That Works

Job Description
Fill out this form listing the qualifications, tasks, and responsibilities actually performed in the job.

Job Title_____   ❏ EXEMPT   ❏ NONEXEMPT

Qualifications:
Education/Training: _____
Licensure: _____
Experience: _____
Job Summary (principal functions): _____
_____

Specific Duties and Responsibilities:
Technical: _____
Clerical: _____
Patient care: _____
Administrative/Managerial: _____
_____

Characteristics and Attitudes:
_____
_____

flexible yet specific job description. Don't oversell the job; if you do, you'll regret it as soon as your employee starts to see the real picture. Every applicant should see the job description.

Plan your interviews. You're not obliged to interview every applicant, and time constraints may not allow you to do so. A trusted staffer may be helpful in screening the first "tier" of applicants, with only the top contenders scheduled for interviews. When you do invest the time to interview someone, do it with a plan. It's tempting to interview after hours, when there are fewer demands on your time. But every candidate should have the opportunity to see the true atmosphere of his or her potential workplace. If the place is a zoo, you'll be better served if your applicant sees that. A Houston, Texas pediatrician explains:

> *I made the mistake of interviewing for an office nurse on a Sunday afternoon. This place was quiet and peaceful. The poor woman I hired was a nervous wreck by the end of her second day; she had no idea of the noise level of an office that cares for sick babies. Now I interview during business hours, taking them for a tour of the office and watching how they react to the chaos. I then take them to my office, shut the door and talk. We get some privacy, yet I don't misrepresent the job, either.*

SPECIFIC QUESTIONS TELL YOU MUCH ABOUT THE CANDIDATE

Review the candidate's resumé before the interview, formulating some specific questions. "I try to set up situations that occur in our practice and ask the candidate how he or she would handle it," says Margaret Dieckhoner of Arthritis and Rheumatism Associates. Tony Demetracopoulos, administrator of the 48-employee Heart Center in Manchester, New Hampshire, gives job applicants scenarios that are unrelated to the job and asks them what they would do. Their responses show their flexibility and adaptability, he said. You'll find a list of questions that will guide an effective interview in Exhibit 9-2.

Don't lead the candidate to the answer you want to hear. Give him or her just enough information to build a response. Listen to

Exhibit 9-2 Interview Questions That Tell You More

Exploring Questions

► Tell me about your education.

► What are your career goals?

► How would you rate the quality of the training you received at (school)?

► What did you like best about your last (or current) job?

► What did you like least about your last (or current) job?

► What strengths did you bring to your last job that made you effective?

► Which of your job skills need improvement? How will you improve them?

► How did you handle resubmission of Medicare claims?

► What procedure do you recommend for dealing with denied claims?

► Are you familiar with Medicare's prevailing fee schedule? Describe your experiences with it.

Probing Questions

► How could your last job have been improved?

► What do you consider the most important idea you contributed in your last job?

► What was your greatest accomplishment at your last job?

► Describe a typical day at your last (or current) job.

► Describe the best colleague you ever worked with.

► What would you do if (*describe a typical situation in your practice*)?

► What do you think is the key to a successful practice?

► Why do you think I should hire you?

► Are you a good team player?

► What do you think distinguishes you from other candidates for this job?

► How would you handle a patient who presented with (*describe symptoms*)?

► How do you feel about working with older people (or children)?

what the candidate says. Pick up on nonverbal clues. While you're looking for skills and attributes, convey the values and beliefs of the practice to the employee. Potential hires need to know what to expect so that they can determine whether they will fit in. If your practice is hectic and fastpaced and everyone has a workaholic mentality, that should be made clear. Some people will choose to eliminate themselves, and you will be better off if they recognize ahead of time that they don't fit. "We're a very interdependent group of people. We don't want anyone with a 'union' mentality, a 'not my job' attitude," says the Heart Center's administrator, "and we make this clear in the interview by the situations we present and the questions we ask." When you convey organizational values in the interview, you end up with a team of employees like this one described by Margaret Dieckhoner of Arthritis and Rheumatism Associates:

> *The receptionist, Sara, approached the manager. She did so with some trepidation because, even at this early hour of the morning, the manager was embroiled in a crisis. Apologizing for the interruption, Sara advised her boss that the troubled patient on the phone needed her intervention.*
>
> *Giving her an incredulous look that said, "Can't you see I'm in the midst of ten things?" the office manager asked Sara to find someone else to deal with the patient.*
>
> *Sara gently but firmly explained why the manager needed to take the patient's call. Her explanation, and the look that accompanied it said, "From the day I was hired, you told me the patient comes first. I believe it. Do you?"*
>
> *Initially annoyed at the disruption, the manager realized she had reason to be pleased. She knew that her constant reinforcement of the values and goals of the practice—to care for the patient every day in every way—had gotten through. Her team was feeding her message back to her.*

If you have a large staff, or if you will be interviewing a number of people for a single position, it's wise to have a "rating guide" to assist in comparing candidates after the interview. A sample form can be found in Exhibit 9-3. Adapt the form to your own practice and the positions for which you're hiring.

STATE THE PURPOSE; STAY IN CONTROL

Let the candidate talk about himself or herself, but stay in control of the interview. State the purpose of the interview up front (e.g., "I want to learn not only what your skills are but what your attitudes are so that we can select someone who will fit on

Exhibit 9-3 Job Applicant Rating Sheet

Interview Rating Sheet

Applicant's Name: _____

Date Interviewed: _____ Position: _____

Rating Scale

	No evidence of skill			Evidence of superior skill

Skill/Quality

Ability to prioritize projects	0	1	2	3	4
Ability to work with the team	0	1	2	3	4
Computer skills	0	1	2	3	4
Concern for patients	0	1	2	3	4
Detail orientation	0	1	2	3	4
Flexibility	0	1	2	3	4
Interest in learning new skills	0	1	2	3	4
Knowledge of HMO/PPO insurance	0	1	2	3	4
Knowledge of Medicare	0	1	2	3	4
Professional appearance and demeanor	0	1	2	3	4
Typing/word processing skills	0	1	2	3	4

Overall Impression

Confidence	0	1	2	3	4
Creativity	0	1	2	3	4
Industriousness	0	1	2	3	4
Intelligence	0	1	2	3	4
Motivation	0	1	2	3	4
Temperament	0	1	2	3	4

Describe applicant's other skills and experiences that would be beneficial to the practice: _____

_____

_____

Summary of references checked: _____

_____

_____

Reason for leaving last job: _____

_____

our team"). There are a few questions that are illegal to ask. Stay away from these topics:

- religion
- sexual orientation
- arrest record
- family matters
- ethnic background
- age
- disabilities

You can, however, ask about work history, educational background, and job-related skills. Your "radar" will help pick up information about personality and attitude. Does the applicant smile frequently during the interview? If not, he or she may be likely to exhibit the same dour countenance to patients and co-workers. "We look for someone who's friendly, not moody," says office manager Kathy Mosciski. "We want someone who is outgoing, but not abrasive or pushy. We look for personality characteristics because we can train someone to pull a file or check someone in."

You're looking for a good fit, someone who will meld with your team. You may wish to have the top candidates interviewed by staff members in the department or area in which they will work. This makes the team members feel that they had a voice in the decision and can hasten the new person's welcome into the group.

SUMMARIZE ATTRIBUTES AND NEGATIVES OF ALL CANDIDATES

If you're interviewing several people for a job, write a quick summary of each candidate shortly after he or she leaves your office. Some employers ask the candidates to write them a letter after the interview, explaining why they believe they're right for the job and the team. Says a Phoenix, Arizona employer:

> *It's surprising what people will tell you in a letter. I was really sold on one woman for my back office, but in her letter, she thanked me for the interview but said she didn't really want to work with infectious disease patients all day. Since that's the*

bulk of my practice, I was relieved that she realized that and was honest enough to tell me. I wonder what would have happened if I had offered her the job. I get the feeling she would have taken it against her better judgment.

How do you set salaries? Ask colleagues and your medical society for pay ranges. Some employers feel it's important to pay good employees better than marketplace rates. In many of the practices we visited, employees are paid at the upper level of the range. Conversely, these practices also have low turnover and high morale. As Dr. Hales explained, "My staff members are very well compensated; it's worth it to me to pay them well." The Heart Center likes to use frequent cash rewards as incentives in addition to salaries and profit sharing. "We give instant bonuses as a way to generate constant ideas and recognize employees," said administrator Demetracopoulos. These perks help set your practice above others and can make it a desirable place to work. Then you have the pleasant dilemma that Swagel Wootton Eye Care in Arizona does: people knocking at the door wanting to work there. The practice doesn't advertise for its rare job openings; it has plenty of applicants eager to join its cohesive, upbeat team.

Before you hire anyone, check references. Common sense tells you that your applicants will only supply you with positive references. Even references who might have a negative thought or two will be hesitant to share it; the liability of doing so isn't worth the risk. Sometimes people will be more honest verbally than in a letter. Ask questions such as, "Would you rehire? What were this person's strengths? Any weaknesses?" Do some digging on your own. First tell your applicant that you will be doing a thorough background check, and then do so. Call former employers and those within your personal network who may have known the applicant. Some employers perform credit checks on applicants, feeling that an employee with a shaky credit history will be a poor risk, especially if he or she will be handling money in the practice. If you will be requesting a credit check, always inform applicants of this fact.

After the candidate has been offered and accepted the position and a starting date has been determined, notify the remaining applicants. Be certain you've got a firm acceptance, or you may end up in the pickle one practice did. The physicians agreed on the perfect candidate for the office manager opening and promptly notified those they did not select. **Then** they offered the job to the top candidate, who began to dicker and dither about hours, salary, working conditions, and issues not mentioned during the interview. Ultimately they decided she would not be the best choice after all, and then they had to go back to candidate Number 2 and rescind their turndown. (Their second choice turned out to be tops, they reported with delight.)

Regardless of whom you hire, write all applicants a personal letter thanking them for their interest and their time. If you will honestly keep their resumé on file and consider them for future positions, tell them that. You want to leave every applicant with a professional impression of the practice.

TRAINING: A CRITICAL STEP IN BUILDING YOUR TEAM

Once you find, interview, and hire the very best employee, provide thorough training. Too often, someone with potential is hired and tossed into a new environment with people he or she doesn't know, policies that are never spelled out, and rules that are never quite clear. What happens? The new employee selects another staffer as the example to follow. If that staff member is not a stellar example, you now have not one but two less-than-super employees. A better approach? Make the new person feel welcome by assigning him or her a "buddy"—someone familiar with the practice, policies, and people—who can act as a mentor and get him or her off on the right foot; this will make **and** maintain a favorable impression of the practice in the new employee's mind. Follow these basic guidelines for orienting new staffers:

- Welcome new employees graciously. They should be introduced to everyone in the practice (or in their department, if it's a large practice).
- Establish the ground rules for office behavior. An employee policy manual is helpful for letting staff know what's expected as far as dress, professional behavior, confidentiality, and so forth. It doesn't have to be long and stuffy or crammed

with legalese. Make the policies friendly but clear. In today's employment environment in which it can be difficult to discharge an employee, the office policy manual can serve as a framework for expectations. A physician told us of his experience with an employee who was undermining staff morale, providing less than optimum patient service, and performing at sub-par level, yet circumstances prevented discharging her. When annual staff bonuses were given out, the employee called co-workers to ask how much they had received. "We had clearly spelled out in our employee manual that any discussion of salary or compensation would be cause for termination, and we were able to legitimately terminate her for her action," the physician said. Of course, the flip side of this is that anything that is included in the policy manual can be viewed by employees as contractually binding, so it's wise to have your policies reviewed by a personnel expert, labor attorney, or similar expert.

- Develop a manual of office instructions and protocols. Starting a new job is overwhelming, and a procedure manual can be helpful as a reference. It's also a great tool for cross-training, which not only improves staff productivity but enhances patient satisfaction (for example, when Mrs. Cruz asks John a routine billing question, he can give her an answer even though he works in the lab).
- Assign new staff members a mentor or a series of mentors, a "buddy" to show them around and acquaint them with everything from where the soda machine is located to where you earned your medical degree and residency training.
- Use a written checklist of orientation and training tasks. This ensures that nothing is forgotten.
- Spend a few moments at the end of the day talking with new employees and emphasizing their importance in providing the best service your patients have ever encountered, no matter what department they work in.

So now your new employee is oriented, trained, and settled in. What do you do if you discover you've made a mistake, that you've put a left-brain person into a right-brain job? Fix it fast. Don't wait for the problem to fix itself. It won't happen. If you're convinced that you have a winning employee in a poorly described or ill-matched job, change the job, the tasks, or the responsibilities. If you've made a really big mistake, acknowledge it and terminate the relationship. But before you fire anybody, document the problems, and use the job description to outline your expectations. Talk to the employee. Be sure that he or she has a chance to correct the problem. Many practices set up a 90-day probationary period for each new employee, making it clear that this is a time to get acquainted and to learn whether a longer relationship is advisable.

THERE'S NO MAGIC, JUST ATTENTION TO DETAIL

There's no magic to finding and hiring the right office staff. Like any good relationship, it only looks easy from the outside. Those involved know it means lots of hard work, common sense, and attention to detail every day. But for patient satisfaction, your satisfaction, and bottom line success, it's critical.

One 20-year veteran of a cardiologist's office sums it up:

> *We're family here, but we're family with a business to run.*
> *Sometimes we're happy to be here, sometimes we'd rather be*
> *driving a bus. That's the way it is with any job. It's on those*
> *"bus-drivin' days," as we call them, that we really need a*
> *sense of humor, a strong network of support, and a system*
> *to get things done well and keep everyone happy.*

Every organization has an occasional bus-driving day, but with a super team your patients will never know. And if they do, they'll think there's nothing you and your staff would rather be doing than driving that bus! ❧

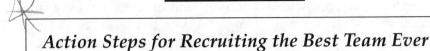

Action Steps for Recruiting the Best Team Ever

1. Write accurate, realistic job descriptions based on the tasks that need to be accomplished in your practice.
2. Look inside as well as outside your practice to fill open positions.
3. Hire attitudes as well as skills.
4. Conduct interviews during business hours. Ask candidates how they would handle typical practice situations.
5. State the purpose of the interview, and stay in control.
6. Set salaries to reflect your commitment to quality.
7. Check references thoroughly.
8. Make sure your top candidate has accepted before you notify the remaining candidates.
9. Provide comprehensive training, including manuals of office rules, policies, instructions, and protocols, and a new-employee mentor.

References

1. N. A. Nichols, Profits with a purpose: An interview with Tom Chapman, *Harvard Business Review* (November/December 1992): 86–95.
2. Nichols, Profits with a purpose, 86–95.

10

Empowerment: "I'll Take Care of That!"

"It's not my job."
"We don't do it that way here."
"I'll have to ask . . . ."
"We've always done it this way!"

The only thing worse than these lame, hollow excuses is the message they send to your patients and colleagues: You don't trust your employees' judgment (i.e., they are not qualified for the job they're doing), they don't trust themselves to make good decisions, or they don't trust you to stand behind them when they do make a decision. These problems clog your practice with indecision and send a negative message to the world and, especially, to your patients.

How to change the negative to a positive? The "can't do it" to "can do it"? How do you create team members who not only are committed to patient satisfaction but have the knowledge **and** the authority to see that it happens? You encourage independence and autonomy, also known as empowerment. Here's how:

- You build confidence in your employees and your team by giving them information, ongoing educational opportunities, and organizational values and standards.
- You set forth clear expectations. Your staff perform better when they know what is expected of them.
- You train people thoroughly, give them the resources they need, then hold them accountable for their areas of responsibilities and actions.

- You set limits so that people are comfortable making decisions within certain parameters. Employees of urologist Neil Baum, MD, can take any necessary customer-pleasing or service recovery action with an expense limit up to $100: "If a patient is unhappy about the wait for a $35 office visit, my front office staff can waive the fee, and they alert me, so I can write a personal note apologizing for the inconvenience. If a piece of equipment breaks down and the repair or replacement is less than $100, they can get it fixed without needing a bunch of authorization forms and approvals."

- You stand behind employees who do their jobs well. The physicians and office managers we interviewed follow this philosophy: Praise people in public, and correct them in private. They compliment exceptional actions liberally and frequently—verbally, in writing, and with occasional rewards such as bonuses or gifts. One office manager told of a staff meeting at which she called up each employee one by one to receive an "Employee of the Quarter" award with a check attached to it. She concluded the surprise presentation with the comment, "I couldn't pick just one of you; you've all gone above and beyond, and you all deserve recognition."

Michael LeBouef, author of *How To Win Customers and Keep Them for Life*, says, "The things that get rewarded get done."[1(p.149)] He calls it the world's greatest management principle: People behave as the reward system teaches them to behave.

- You give staff immediate and concrete feedback. When they have made an error in judgment, tell them so in private, chastising the action but not the individual. Then together come up with better options for similar situations in the future. When employees have made a good call, especially one that involved some risk on their part, recognize their good work.

- You treat your staff as a team, letting your patients and colleagues know you value your employees by the respect you show them. This gives their actions credibility in the eyes of others; they are viewed as acting on your behalf. The result? Your time is leveraged effectively, and your "reach" is extended.

EMPOWERED EMPLOYEES YIELD LASTING BENEFITS

Although empowerment requires an investment of trust, its benefits are specific and lasting. In an article in *Sloan Management Review,* Bowen and Lawler list these outcomes[2]:

- Quicker on-line responses to customer needs during service *delivery*
- Quicker on-line responses to dissatisfied customers during service *recovery*
- Employees who feel better about their jobs and themselves
- Employees who interact with customers with more warmth and enthusiasm. Research, the authors point out, supports the view that customers' perceptions of service quality are shaped by the courtesy, empathy, and responsiveness of staff. But we didn't need to tell you that. You see it every day in the interactions your patients have with your staff.
- Employees who are a source of ideas about how best to serve the customer
- Employees who provide word-of-mouth advertising and customer retention.

Empowerment improves practice productivity, physician and staff efficiency and effectiveness, and patient satisfaction. Think of the patient's reaction to "Sure, I can fix that billing error" compared to "I'm sorry, I'll have to check with my supervisor, and he's out for a week. Check back with us later." Learning to empower employees wisely is a delicate skill, requiring balance between too much and not enough. The overloaded, harried practitioner may be tempted to delegate tasks wholesale without training or follow-up. The result can vary from excellent to something as drastic and disappointing as embezzlement and fraud. And anyone who has had a taste of the latter is more than a little hesitant to turn loose of even the keys to the coffee maker, much less the keys to the front door. Then there's the other end of the spectrum, in which employees are viewed as having extremely limited capabilities. An administrator of a large Philadelphia ophthalmic practice with several locations told us, "Our philosophy about staff is the same as a fast-food restaurant. My job is to make sure the machines know what they're doing." Then he added, "We try to make this a place where people want to work." Who would want to work in an environment in which the employees received the same high regard as the equipment and machines?

EMPOWERMENT STARTS WITH GOOD PEOPLE

Hiring the right people is the critical first step in feeling **comfortable** with empowering people to perform to their maximum abilities. But even the most skilled, conscientious employee needs guidance, coaching, and plenty of cheerleading along the way. (If this sounds like Parenting 101, you're beginning to get the idea. Employees aren't children, but there are more than a few similarities between effective parenting and effective leadership.) And then they need to be let loose to do what you hired them to do—Give service. Satisfy patients. Build a successful practice.

There are some risks to empowering employees to do their jobs and a little more. What if they overreach? They will do so occasionally. And when they do, the mistake should be pointed out in private, along with the reason it is a mistake. Example: Your new partner is less empathic than patients (or you) would like. You're working with her, trying to realign her thinking and behavior. In the meantime, however, patients don't like to see her. Your staff are frequently caught in the middle, trying to schedule appointments for her but hearing patients complain about her manner. You overhear a receptionist telling a patient, "We know she's awfully blunt and doesn't always understand, but Dr. Sims says she's a good doctor. Would you please see her just one more time?" What do you do? You've encouraged your employees to empathize with patients, to act as their advocates. You've also asked them to work with the new physician. Your receptionist is doing what you've asked, but she could have phrased her message more diplomatically. How do you handle this effectively without cutting off future decision making in the employee?

Take her aside immediately if possible, and calmly and without judgment tell her that her words could have been chosen more carefully. Suggest that she tell patients, "Dr. Byrne is an excellent doctor and she is interested in what her patients have to say. Sometimes her style is more straightforward than some people are used to. Why not explain to her yourself that you have a hard time with that approach?"

TAKE THE RISK, BUT FIRST, TRAIN WELL

There's the risk that employees will do too much (the manager's fear that they'll give away the store). But there's also the risk that they'll draw the line very restrictively. In *The Service Edge: 101 Companies that Profit from Customer Care,* Zemke and Schaaf tell of a bank in which line employees were given authority to make the check-cashing decisions traditionally reserved for branch management. The tellers wrote check-cashing regulations so restrictive that even the bank president had to show three forms of identification just to deposit his paycheck.[3] The problem here may have been a lack of thorough training of the tellers in the bank's customer service philosophy, and an environment that was not threat-free.

Empowerment gives individuals (or teams) the ability and the authority to act in the best interest of the customer and the organization, particularly when unusual or unpredictable events or activities occur that require an immediate response. When you empower your staff, you give them autonomy. You credit them with intelligence. You permit and encourage them to act with some degree of independence in making decisions that may extend beyond the normal realm of their authority, as a team as well as individually.

In any organization, each member has certain tasks and responsibilities that are clearly spelled out. Each also has restrictions and limitations, usually clear boundaries beyond which he or she isn't authorized to go or act under any circumstances. The area beyond the normal daily tasks and limitations is where autonomy is conferred in the empowered employee or the empowered organization when unusual situations occur. In empowered organizations, individuals and teams have the authority—even the requirement—to act when atypical events arise, sometimes taking action that goes beyond the boundaries of their usual restrictions and limitations. What scares many managers, and even some employees, is the fuzziness of autonomy, the fact that appropriate actions, responsibilities, authority, and limits are not always clear.[4]

To define and clarify the scope of actions acceptable when unusual events occur that don't fit into the daily tasks or individual limitations, you must allow the employee to act when these events arise. It helps if you've discussed general guidelines (i.e. "Use your best judgment to solve problems;" "Write off a charge up to $___ under these circumstances"). How far and how quickly you extend the individual's authority depends on the judgment shown in taking action. Thus, it's wise in the early stages of empowerment to review the action mutually according to the outcome, patient needs, and organizational values to determine whether the employee went far enough or too far, or whether it was entirely appropriate to the situation, the customer, and the practice goals. Figure 10-1 illustrates what empowerment might look like in a practice that gradually increases individual and team authority and autonomy.

Figure 10-1 What Empowerment Looks Like

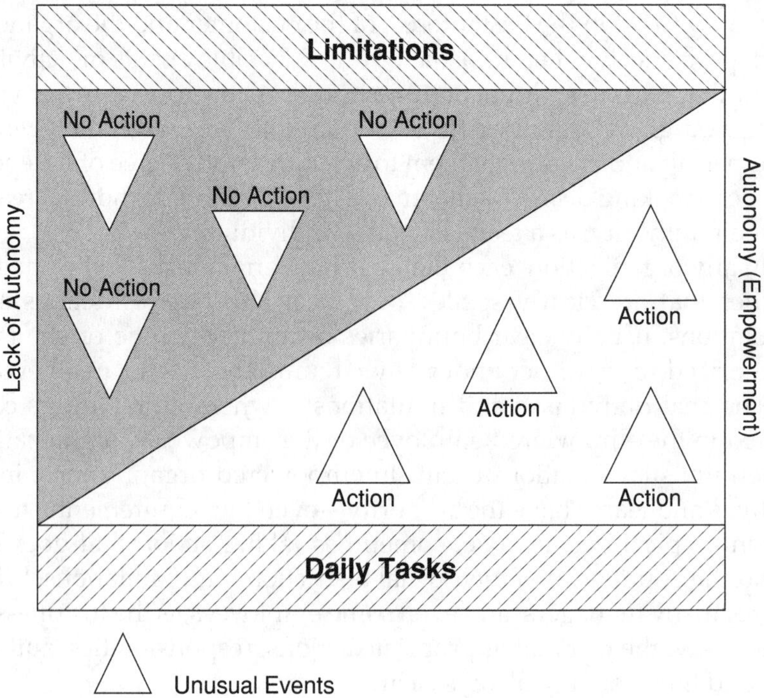

EMPOWERMENT CONVEYS TRUST AND GIVES CONTROL

Empowerment tells your employees, "I trust you. I have confidence in you." It gives them control, and control can be very powerful. A psychology experiment was once performed in which two groups of adults were given a similar assortment of tasks requiring physical and mental dexterity. In the background was playing a loud, distracting, cacophonous noise. The individuals in one group had an "off" switch by which they could turn the noise off any time they wished. The group given control (via the "off" switch) completed more tasks more accurately than the group without the switch. Yet they never used the switch to turn the noise off. The mere awareness that they *could* increased their productivity.

Bowen and Lawler argue that when service delivery involves managing a relationship, especially an enduring relationship, empowerment is a better approach than "production line" management.[5] (That's the "keep the machines working" theory of the Philadelphia practice administrator.)

For empowerment to work effectively and to provide the results you want (satisfied patients), these factors need to exist:

- Leaders and managers who believe in the ability of their staff to exercise judgment and self-control
- Employees who have strong needs to grow and test their personal competencies on the job. Not everyone wants autonomy, challenge, and responsibility, Bowen and Lawler point out.[6] Through skillful interviewing of job applicants, you can avoid bringing these rigid machine-people into your practice.
- A group of employees who function as a team, caring about each other as well as the customer
- Employee understanding of the practice philosophy as well as their tasks, and how employees support the entire organization in expressing the philosophy
- Employee problem-solving and teamwork skills
- An atmosphere of confidence in individuals and teams
- A nonpunitive attitude toward mistakes
- Accepted practice service standards that guide behaviors and decisions

- Ongoing staff education for personal and professional development and more informed decision making
- Encouragement, implementation, and recognition of internally generated ideas and suggestions from employees at all levels
- A stake in the success and growth of the practice through profit sharing, advancement opportunities, rewards, and recognition

RITZ-CARLTON EMPLOYEES CAN "MOVE HEAVEN AND EARTH" TO SOLVE PROBLEMS

Does empowerment yield results? It depends on the kind of results you seek in your practice. If your goal is a patient-centered practice, take a look at organizations with highly empowered employees: Nordstrom, The Ritz-Carlton Hotel Company, Marriott, and Federal Express. All are companies renowned for their service quality. Ritz-Carlton, a 1992 National Baldridge Quality Award winner, for example, says, "Employees are empowered to 'move heaven and earth' to resolve the problems of a guest." Intensive and ongoing training provides the hotel's staff with the ability to make these heaven-and-earth decisions. In addition to a 3-day orientation of new staff, Ritz-Carlton has "daily line-ups" in each department, during which information is passed from one shift to another and the organization's Gold Standard is reinforced (the Gold Standard refers to the organization's credo, motto, and 20 basic expectations for employees; see Exhibit 10-1).

"Good Idea" boards in each department encourage charting and logging of ideas suggested by employees or teams for improving service. Problem-solving teams are formed to analyze and resolve a service hang-up in any area. Empowered staff are rewarded with instant recognition, such as the Lightning Strikes Award, which can be given to any employee who goes above and beyond the call of duty in service to a guest or a co-worker. The Five-Star Award is a formal, much-cherished award given quarterly and annually to employees at each hotel. It's based on exemplary attitude, performance, attendance, dependability, and service.

Exhibit 10-1

The Ritz-Carlton® Credo

The Ritz-Carlton® Hotel is a place where the genuine care and comfort of our guests is our highest mission.

We pledge to provide the finest personal service and facilities for our guests who will always enjoy a warm, relaxed, yet refined ambience.

The Ritz-Carlton® experience enlivens the senses, instills well-being, and fulfills even the unexpressed wishes and needs of our guests.

The Ritz-Carlton® Basics

1. The Credo will be known, owned, and energized by all employees.
2. Our motto is: "We are Ladies and Gentlemen serving Ladies and Gentlemen." Practice teamwork and "lateral service" to create a positive work environment.
3. The three steps of service shall be practiced by all employees.
4. All employees will successfully complete Training Certification to ensure they understand how to perform to The Ritz-Carlton® standards in their position.
5. Each employee will understand their work area and Hotel goals as established in each strategic plan.
6. All employees will know the needs of their internal and external customers (guests and employees) so that we may deliver the products and services they expect. Use guest preference pads to record specific needs.
7. Each employee will continuously identify defects (Mr. BIV) throughout the Hotel.
8. Any employee who receives a customer complaint "owns" the complaint.
9. Instant guest pacification will be ensured by all. React quickly to correct the problem immediately. Follow-up with a telephone call within twenty minutes to verify the problem has been resolved to the customer's satisfaction. Do everything you possibly can to never lose a guest.
10. Guest incident action forms are used to record and communicate every incident of guest dissatisfaction. Every employee is empowered to resolve the problem and to prevent a repeat occurrence.
11. Uncompromising levels of cleanliness are the responsibility of every employee.
12. "Smile—We are on stage." Always maintain positive eye contact. Use the proper vocabulary with our guests. (Use words like—"Good Morning," "Certainly," "I'll be happy to" and "My pleasure").

(continues)

Exhibit 10-1 continued

13. Be an ambassador of your Hotel in and outside of the work place. Always talk positively. No negative comments.
14. Escort guests rather than pointing out directions to another area of the Hotel.
15. Be knowledgeable of Hotel information (hours of operation, etc.) to answer guest inquiries. Always recommend the Hotel's retail and food and beverage outlets prior to outside facilities.
16. Use proper telephone etiquette. Answer within three rings and with a "smile." When necessary, ask the caller, "May I place you on hold." Do not screen calls. Eliminate call transfers when possible.
17. Uniforms are to be immaculate: Wear proper and safe footwear (clean and polished), and your correct name tag. Take pride and care in your personal appearance (adhering to all grooming standards).
18. Ensure all employees know their roles during emergency situations and are aware of fire and life safety response processes.
19. Notify your supervisor immediately of hazards, injuries, equipment or assistance that you need. Practice energy conservation and proper maintenance and repair of Hotel property and equipment.
20. Protecting the assets of a Ritz-Carlton® hotel is the responsibility of every employee.

The Three Steps of Service

1. A warm and sincere greeting: Use the guest's name, if and when possible.
2. Anticipation and compliance with guest needs.
3. Fond farewell: Give them a warm goodbye, and use their names if and when possible.

Source: © The Ritz-Carlton Hotel Company, 1983. Ritz-Carlton® materials were provided by The Ritz-Carlton Hotel Company. The Ritz-Carlton® is a federally registered trademark of The Ritz-Carlton Hotel Company.

As practices escalate their service quality, the demands on employees will escalate. One way to help staff learn appropriate ways to deal with situations and problems is to review situations as soon after they occur as possible, and discuss a variety of ways to handle them. This is common in patient-centered practices. In these staff meetings and small group meetings, role playing and situation analysis give employees specific, hands-on understanding of acceptable responses.

PRACTICE GOALS TELL EVERYONE WHAT YOU'RE WORKING TOWARD

Administrator Dieckhoner says that empowerment requires "establishing what you're working toward. In our practice, our purpose is excellence—to give patients the best care we can. We know we've gotten our message through when our employees repeat it back to us as the reason for a decision they've made."

Empowerment also requires clearly defined expectations, she agrees: "You hire good people, let them know what's expected of them, then let them do their job, and recognize them when they go above and beyond." It's just as important for the physician(s) to acknowledge good work, perhaps even more important than for the supervisor or manager to do so. It may be difficult for you and your practice partners to catch staff in the act of doing good, so you must make an effort to be observant. Look for little things—the receptionist assisting an elderly patient to a seat in the reception area—and also ask your manager and supervisors to inform you of acts that deserve recognition.

Employees will understand the limits and responsibilities of empowerment when they observe **you** consistently acting out a patient-centered service philosophy. (Remember what we said about leadership in Chapter 5?) Richard Abrams, MD, the Denver internist, believes "Everything that happens in our practice comes back to me—the way the patient is greeted, scheduling, the appearance of the office, the medical quality. I have to set the tenor for everything in order to direct it."

He adds, "I want my staff to know their role in the practice. At the end of the day, I try to give specific feedback." One day a staff member was doing an oximetry on a patient and, noticing that the man's pulse seemed slow, notified Dr. Abrams. The patient was found to have a heart blockage. "I acknowledged her observant and caring attitude."

Dr. Abrams is absolutely correct in his understanding that "more important than parties or bonuses, employees want to know that what they do has value." His staff are encouraged to handle situations when they can, but they also know they're free to hand the problem or the patient to him or the office manager if they feel it's out of their reach or ability.

INVEST IN SUCCESS BY INVESTING IN YOUR TEAM

You must select, hire, and train employees very carefully to give them responsibility and authority. But this initial investment in the selection saves in the long run; you'll have less turnover when staffers truly fit their assignments and feel comfortable carrying out the practice philosophy. Labor costs may be higher: Rather than paying minimum wage (and getting a minimum wage mentality and attitude), you must pay more for intelligent, personable people, but over time, these higher-salary employees pay their way in productivity.

Changing the "Not my job" attitude to "I'll take care of it" isn't without a few potholes into which you and your employees may occasionally stumble. But if you've hired the right people, given them the best foundation, and kept up the coaching, you may hear from your patients what one physician told us he often hears: "Doctor, you've got such a great bunch of people. I feel like I can ask them anything!" And you and your patients will hear this sweet-sounding phrase a lot more often: "Sure, I can take care of it!" ❧

Action Steps for Empowering Your Staff

1. Build employee confidence with information, educational opportunities, and organizational values and standards.
2. Set forth clear expectations.
3. Hold people accountable for areas of responsibility and actions.
4. Set limits and decision-making parameters.
5. Praise in public, and criticize in private.
6. Believe in your employees' abilities, and reward good work.
7. Review "empowered" employee actions according to outcome, patient needs, and organizational values.
8. Chart and act on ideas suggested by employees for improving service.

References

1. M. LeBouef, *How To Win Customers and Keep Them for Life* (New York, N.Y.: The Berkley Publishing Group, 1987): 149.
2. D.E. Bowen and E.E. Lawler III, The empowerment of service workers: What, why, how, and when, *Sloan Management Review, 33*(3) (Spring 1992): 31–39.
3. R. Zemke and D. Schaaf, *The Service Edge: 101 Companies that Profit from Customer Care* (New York, N.Y.: New American Library, 1989): 66–67.
4. C. Handy, Balancing corporate power: A new Federalist Paper, *Harvard Business Review* (November/December 1992): 59–72.
5. Bowen and Lawler, The empowerment of service workers, 39.
6. Bowen and Lawler, The empowerment of service workers, 38.

11

Staff Satisfaction: It's More Than a Paycheck

Texaco Refining and Marketing, Inc., in El Dorado, Kan[sas], continues to find ways to improve by increasing employee involvement, improving communication, and refining its reward and recognition systems. . . . Teams created note pads featuring the Texaco star logo, designed so anyone in the plant could thank a peer for contributions. "I didn't recognize the power of something so simple until I put a note on an exceptionally good piece of work someone had done," [Richard] Masica says, "and a few weeks later, when I had forgotten about it, I saw it pinned up on his bulletin board."[1(p.4)]

"How do you get people to do what you want them to?" physicians and practice administrators often ask.

You don't. People do what they want, not what you want.

Your task is to get your team members to want the same things you do: To aim for the same goals—quality service and satisfied patients—and to seek the success you want in your practice. Getting people to work willingly toward achieving a common objective is what motivation is all about.

HOW *DO* YOU GET PEOPLE TO DO WHAT YOU WANT?

But how do you do this? How do you motivate people? With money? If you are using money as the primary motivator in your practice, you probably are wondering why your employees don't stay or don't care or why they're always angling for bigger raises or better bonuses.

People **do** work for money—it's an extrinsic reward for their effort—but they also work for intrinsic rewards such as recognition and personal satisfaction. Money becomes important as a motivator when salaries are at the low end of the wage scale or not competitive with those of similar jobs in the marketplace.

Think back to your Psychology 101 class and Maslow's hierarchy of needs. According to Maslow, once a person's basic physical needs (food, air, shelter, and safety) are met, then the social needs (belonging, esteem, and recognition) become more important. If you meet your staff's basic needs with competitive salaries, good benefits, and a pleasant work environment, you'll find that intrinsic rewards are powerful motivators. Still not convinced? Check your beliefs against those of your employees. Take a look at the list of motivators in Exhibit 11-1. Rank them in order according to what you think your staff respond to most, then give the same list to your employees and ask each person to rank the items in order of what's most important to him or her. You can use this exercise as an excellent discussion topic for staff meetings; it's also a good means of determining what motivates individual employees.

Although a few people are self-motivated—they have an internal drive that propels them to do their best no matter what's going on around them—the dilemma facing many office managers and/or physician leaders is this: What works most consistently to keep people motivated?

The broad answer: recognition, appreciation, and participation. The detailed answer: Every type of motivator works for someone, sometime. Usually it takes a mix of motivators—some financial, some verbal, and some tangible—to keep people excited and enthusiastic about continually stretching to reach the target. But no reward will work unless it is tied to personal and practice goals and service standards. People need to know what success looks like, what the reward is for. For example, if patient satisfaction is the practice goal, individual and team rewards should be related to staff participation in measurable patient satisfaction results.

Exhibit 11-1

WHAT MOTIVATES EMPLOYEES

☑ Appreciation for work performed

☑ Participation in workplace information and decisions

☑ Understanding attitude by supervisor

☑ Job security

☑ Good wages

☑ Interesting work

☑ Promotion opportunities

☑ Loyalty from management

☑ Good working conditions

☑ Tactful discipline

FOR MOTIVATION, CHECK FOR THESE PRACTICE CHARACTERISTICS

Before setting up individual rewards, however, take a look at the overall atmosphere in your practice. The following organizational characteristics must exist for people to become and remain motivated to work toward practice goals:

- **Communication**: Keep communication flowing up, down, and across all lines and levels in the practice. Use formal communication methods—staff meetings, memos, newsletters, and one-on-one discussions—as well as informal methods. The physician's failure to listen is the number one gripe of medical practice employees, according to surveys.[2] This doesn't mean you must have heart-to-heart chats with every staff member. Your practice administrator, office manager, and supervisors are your surrogates. Their responsibility should be to listen and respond to specific staff concerns. Through communication, give people an understanding of the organization's mission and philosophy in general and *their roles and importance* as individuals and team members in helping the organization achieve quality service.

- **Participation**: Involve staff in practice decision making, goal setting, planning, and problem solving whenever possible. People own what they create. If members of a practice staff feel a sense of ownership and participation in the practice, they will be motivated to improve their skills and service continually because they realize that the success of the practice reflects on them.
- **Values**: Make the practice philosophy of patient-centered service known through your actions and words as well as those of other leaders and managers in the practice. The practice values and philosophy should be reinforced continually through recognition of actions that exemplify it and constructive, private correction of actions that diminish it.
- **Personal power**: As you learned in Chapter 10, organizations large and small are discovering that giving people the authority to make decisions on their own makes them more productive and more committed; their morale improves as well.
- **Challenge:** Provide challenging work, and encourage career development with information, added responsibilities, and training.

MAKE PRACTICE GOALS AND VALUES CLEAR

Let's say you're doing all the above. You have regular staff meetings, you listen to your office manager and he or she listens to supervisors and staff, you offer plenty of opportunities for learning and growth, and people solve problems independently every day.

How do you keep people motivated, excited about their work, interested in providing the highest level of service, and constantly looking for ways to do things better? How do you get them to do what you want? How do you get them to strive for top-quality service and satisfied patients as much as you do?

First, you make it clear what the goal is, what the practice values are. You give them information about the practice. You educate them and encourage them to seek education; knowledge is power in more ways than one. You give people jobs that allow them to demonstrate responsibility, that make them feel in control and allow them to grow. When you see people acting out the values and doing things that move them, and the practice, toward the goals, you encourage, recognize, and reward it. The reward will depend on the situation and the individual, but some assumptions can be made about workplace motivators, according to management expert Frederick Herzberg.[3] He says that the factors that contribute to job satisfaction fall into the following categories:

- achievement
- recognition
- the work itself
- responsibility
- advancement
- growth

On the other hand, Herzberg says, certain factors contribute highly to job dissatisfaction.[4] He characterized these as "hygiene" factors. They include company policy, supervision, work conditions, salary, relationship with peers and subordinates, personal life, status, and security. Want staff to be satisfied with their jobs and motivated to perform? Concentrate on enhancing the motivators—achievement, recognition, responsibility, advancement, and growth—and diminishing the impact of the "dissatisfiers"—the rules and regulations, unpleasant working conditions, and supervisor-employee stress.

To keep employees motivated, enrich their jobs. Job enrichment means making work meaningful. Don't simplify the receptionist's tasks; add responsibility, such as the reception area refreshment cart. This means that the receptionist is completely responsible for this task, including selecting, ordering, and maintaining the refreshments in addition to offering them to waiting patients. Herzberg calls this "vertical job loading."[5] In Exhibit 11-2, there is a depiction of how the principles of vertical job loading can be adopted in an individual's job and the motivator involved.

BEST MOTIVATOR: GET PEOPLE INVOLVED

According to Herzberg, the best form of motivation is the kind that gets people involved with what they do, making them feel that their efforts result in worthwhile contributions to the organization.[6] Does this sound a great deal like empowerment? It does. And it is. It's putting real responsibility on the individual's shoulders and holding the individual accountable for what happens. It's giving them control. When people feel a sense of control, productivity soars and errors decline.

Exhibit 11-2 Principles of Vertical Job Loading

Principle		Motivator
Remove controls/retain accountability	☞	Responsibility/personal achievement
Increase individual accountability	☞	Responsibility/recognition
Give individual complete work unit (e.g., module, division, area, etc.)	☞	Responsibility/achievement/recognition
Grant additional authority, job freedom	☞	Responsibility/achievement/recognition
Make periodic reports available to worker rather than to supervisor	☞	Internal recognition
Introduce new/more difficult tasks	☞	Growth/learning
Assign specific/specialized tasks to encourage expertise	☞	Responsibility/growth/advancement

Source: Reprinted by permission of *Harvard Business Review.* An exhibit from "One More Time: How Do You Motivate Employees?" by Frederick Herzberg, Reprint no. 87507. Copyright by the President and Fellows of Harvard College. All rights reserved.

Physicians and office managers in practices with "enriched" jobs contend, however, that recognition and rewards also play a role in motivation. And we agree. As LeBouef said in *How To Win Customers and Keep Them for Life*, "You get more of the behavior you reward. You don't get what you hope for, ask for, wish for or beg for. You get what you reward."[7(p.149)] What forms of recognition and rewards work best for your team? We suggest that you choose from the following options the motivators that best fit the needs of your practice and your employees:

- Are your salaries competitive? As noted in previous chapters, offering wages that are slightly higher than normal allows "skimming the cream," choosing the absolute best of the job pool. It also assures you that the needs on the "bottom rung" of Maslow's hierarchy are satisfied, so that you can concentrate on the social motivators. Equally important, wages say a great deal about how much you value the responsibilities of a job. For example, if your practice philosophy is patient satisfaction through quality service and quality care but your receptionist and other front line staff are paid minimum level wages, your message is clear: "We don't really mean it!"
- Look at your benefits package. Does it really provide what employees want? Could you offer personal days off in some reasonable ratio to unused sick time? Would a "cafeteria plan" of benefits meet a greater variety of employee needs?
- Specify expectations. Every staff member should have written standards and expectations for his or her position, and each person should be evaluated at least annually, and preferably quarterly, to determine where he or she is meeting or exceeding expectations and where improvements are needed. The best way to accomplish this is through a performance appraisal in which the employee has the opportunity to evaluate his or her own performance with the same form that the supervisor uses. During the performance evaluation, the employee and supervisor appraisals should be compared. The appraisal form should include written job-related goals for the employee to achieve in the coming 3, 6, or 12 months. These goals should relate to the practice mission directly and

indirectly. This gives both employee and supervisor specific measures of change and improvement. The Sansum Clinic in Santa Barbara, California measures all its employees during their annual reviews in terms of their service attitude. Those who don't have direct patient contact are evaluated according to the service they provide to fellow employees. This approach helps convey that patient satisfaction is up to every individual in the organization. A sample performance appraisal can be found in Exhibit 11-3.

PEOPLE OWN WHAT THEY CREATE, SO ENCOURAGE STAFF INPUT

Encourage and use employee input and ideas. This is a strong motivator; people own what they create. A gynecologist intent on increasing his office efficiency and billings met with his staff and asked what they would do to improve the practice. The ideas ran the gamut. The nurses suggested upgrading their ultrasound skills; the office assistants not only wanted to streamline collections but also advocated a practice brochure and new Yellow Pages ads; and the front office staff asked to sign up for management and computer seminars. Coupled with a profit-sharing program, the practice experienced a 10% increase in earnings by year end, with no increase in patients. Three years later, the practice reported expenses down and profits up, with a $100,000 bulge in the bottom line over the 3 years, a revenue increase in which employees shared. The kicker: The physician said, "Employees have renewed pride in their work [and] I've never had as much fun as I'm having now."[8]

When an employee's action saves the practice money or brings in extra income, give the employee an "instant bonus" commensurate with the savings or action. Include a personal note of thanks. When reinforcement occurs simultaneously with the behavior, as psychologist B.F. Skinner discovered with his research many years ago, the behavior continues. See additional tangible incentive ideas in Exhibit 11-4.

Encourage staff members to recognize each other's efforts. At Childress Buick, employees fill in a "Round of Applause" form to acknowledge a co-worker's good work. The notice is then posted

Exhibit 11-3 Performance Appraisal Form

Performance Evaluation

Employee _____ Evaluator _____
Supervisor_____ Date of review _____
Date of hire _____ Date of last review _____
Performance scale: (0) poor; (1) below average; (2) average; (3) above average;
(4) superior

Performance on the job   **Individual characteristics**

Punctuality   _____   Appearance   _____
Initiative   _____   Service attitude   _____
Dependability   _____   Enthusiasm   _____
Accuracy   _____   Diplomacy   _____
Ability to assume   Flexibility   _____
  responsibility   _____   Cooperation with other
Knowledge of procedures   _____   team members   _____
Exercise of judgment   _____   Verbal and written
Organizational skills   _____   communication skills _____
Ability to solve problems _____   Ability to follow directions _____
Quality of service to patients _____ Ability to learn   _____
Professional goals to be pursued in the next year: _____
_____
_____
_____

Other comments: _____
_____
_____

_____   _____
Employee's signature   Date

_____   _____
Evaluator's signature   Date

---

on a central bulletin board; the employee also receives a personal note of thanks from the company's general manager. In Dr. Neil Baum's practice, the "ABCD" award signifies efforts "Above and Beyond the Call of Duty" by a staffer. The employee receives a "Golden Attitude" pin at a staff meeting. Dr. Baum recalled an

Exhibit 11-4 Staff Recognition and Rewards

Incentives That Motivate

- Immediate, sincere, verbal compliment or recognition from physician(s)
- Letter of thanks or appreciation mailed to employee's home, copy in personnel file, and copy posted on bulletin board
- Business cards for every staff member

Instant Rewards

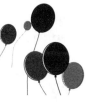

- Flowers or green plant
- Books
- Gift certificates
- Goofy gifts
- $1 or $5 bill handed out to show appreciation spontaneously
- Certificates ("Thank You-Grams," "You Did It!" award, etc.)

Success Celebrations

- Lunch or dinner gift certificates for employee and spouse (with baby sitter money)
- Department store shopping spree
- Half-day off with pay
- Ice cream social
- Pot luck: everyone brings their specialty dish (doctors, too!)

Team Incentives

- Regular staff meetings
- Close office for in-service or educational seminar
- Lunch paid for by the practice
- Parties and special events
- Open house planned by staff for other office staffs
- Strategic planning session or staff retreat
- Casual day once a week
- Educational opportunities paid for by the practice

Financial Rewards

- Salary increase
- Benefits increase
- Reduced work-week hours
- Interim bonuses for specific outstanding achievement (e.g., $25 check)
- Bonus plan tied to specific goals or practice goals

employee who earned a pin for going to a patient's home to fix a catheter when the patient was unable to come to the office. In appreciation, the patient sent a $1,000 check to the hospital in honor of the staff. Dr. Baum also has a "Thanks a Million" award, a certificate that looks like a check. Employees receive it when they deserve more than a verbal "thank you." See Exhibit 11-5.

SOCIAL ACTIVITIES FOSTER TEAM SPIRIT

Buy lunch. Some physicians do it every day, making it part of the staff's benefits. The practice of Arthritis and Rheumatism Associates in Silver Spring, Maryland, buys lunch for biweekly staff meetings. The staff is also paid for these mandatory meetings because they are working through lunch. In another practice, a surgeon takes his staff of six out to lunch once a month and bans business talk during the meal to enhance camaraderie.

Host socializing activities for you and your staff. Include families in some, and reserve some for staff only. Remember that families and individuals vary in how comfortable they are with after-hours activities; be sensitive to all your staff when planning outings. Make social activities optional to avoid liabilities that are

Exhibit 11-5 "Thanks a Million" Award

NEIL BAUM, MD
3525 Prytania St., Suite 614
New Orleans, LA 70115
(504) 891-8454   _____ 19____

PAY TO THE
ORDER OF .... $ THANKS
                    THANKS A MILLION   _____

Baum's Bank of Gratitude
    Wiz's Branch   ....signature...................

Source: Courtesy of Neil Baum, MD, New Orleans, Louisiana.

incurred when you require employees to participate in more than their job responsibilities.

Create a special award to recognize outstanding employees. Southwestern Eye Care in Mesa, Arizona has the "PLUS" Award, which can be given by employees or patients. The "PLUS" Award criteria and description are in Exhibit 11-6.

Watch for actions that show an employee's commitment to and understanding of the practice philosophy. Said Margaret Dieckhoner of Arthritis and Rheumatism Associates, "Doctors have so much power, and so little awareness of what an impact it makes when they notice good work. Something simple like telling a staff member, 'You were great with Mr. Needham this morning. He was not very pleasant, and you were as calm and nice as could be. Thanks.' Doctors need to say thank you to staff. It makes a big impression." Ask managers and supervisors to let you know when an employee should be recognized.

Use bonuses to reward achievement of practice goals and personal job-related achievements, such as when your surgical nurse earns her RN First Assistant certification.

Share customer compliments about the practice and/or individual employees with the person mentioned **and** the whole staff. Post letters of praise in a central place, and put a copy in the employee's personnel file. Send a copy to the employee's home, along with your own note of thanks, so that the individual can share the glory with family members.

Use financial incentive programs to encourage and reward achievement of practice goals. Goals to shoot for might include reduction in accounts receivable, reduction in denied Medicare claims, a monthly or quarterly revenue target, and scheduling of new patient appointments or surgeries. If it's important to the practice, make it important to staff, and reward them for their part in reaching the goal. (If you set targets and don't reach them, don't chastise; bring staff together to review the goal and to strategize how it can be reached.) Incentive rewards should be distributed frequently enough to motivate (at least quarterly). Here's a system used by some practices: Dedicate a portion of the practice revenue—say, 25%—to a staff incentive pool. Every 6 months, the account is reconciled with actual expenses; employees receive a bonus if staff salary expenses are lower than 25% of rev-

Exhibit 11-6 The "PLUS" Award

The PLUS
Above & Beyond Club

Service excellence in all aspects of patient care is an organization-wide commitment at Southwestern Eye Center. Our physicians and staff strive to demonstrate this philosophy in each and every patient encounter.

However, sometimes a member of our staff gives that little "extra effort" from the heart or performs a task that goes "above and beyond" their normal job requirements. The **PLUS** *Above & Beyond Award* was developed to recognize just such special individual efforts.

We invite you our patient, to help us recognize an act of distinction by nominating anyone in our organization that you feel has provided exemplary service "above & beyond" their job requirements. By filling out the attached **PLUS** *Above & Beyond* ballot, you can nominate a deserving Southwestern Eye Center staff member. Simply fill out the form and drop it in the **PLUS** box in our reception area, or mail it back to our office at your earliest convenience.

Above & Beyond Award recipients will receive an award certificate and a special bonus.

This we believe
at Southwestern Eye Center

The physicians and staff at Southwestern Eye Center are committed to a mission of service excellence. Our goal is to provide personalized, quality care to our patients; to develop and maintain positive relationships with our associates; to assure job satisfaction for all professionals and staff; and to be responsive and sensitive to the communities we serve.

To successfully achieve this goal, we have made a corporate-wide commitment to providing care **PLUS . . .** *to* **Promote, Listen, Understand and Serve** *our patient community to the best of our abilities.*

In every encounter, with every person, in every part of our organization, we want our patients to feel . . . **Pampered, Loved, Unique and Special.** *We know that respect, concern and sensitivity to each individual is the basis of service excellence.*

We feel that every person and every job has equal value toward the realization of our group goal. The individuals on our staff are **. . . Proficient, Loyal, Understanding and Successful.** *An organization of vision values the unique qualities of each individual, while recognizing the interdependence of employees, physicians and patients in achieving a successful health outcome.*

Above & Beyond Club BALLOT

I would like to nominate _____
for exemplary service at Southwestern Eye Center

I am pleased to make this nomination because: _____

_____

_____

Signature _____ Date _____

Source: Courtesy of the Southwestern Eye Center, Mesa, Arizona.

enues. This encourages efforts toward patient satisfaction (which encourages referrals) and a strong desire for efficiency. If desired, half the bonus can be given immediately and half at the end of the year, and employees who leave before year end forfeit their bonus.

CELEBRATE BIG DAYS AND SMALL VICTORIES

Throw a spontaneous celebration occasionally. Recognize the significance of small wins: They line the path leading to the big ones. One infertility specialist keeps a bottle of sparkling cider in the refrigerator and opens it to celebrate when a particularly hard-fought battle is won. "When one of our long-standing patients delivers a healthy baby, we break out the cider and pass it around, even to patients in the waiting room. We want everybody to enjoy the good news." When the staff stay late without complaint on a particularly frenetic day, order a basket of fresh muffins to greet them the next morning, along with a note that says simply "Thanks for yesterday—and for coming back this morning!"

Buy gift certificates for manicures, a round of golf, a dinner for two, an afternoon at the zoo, or an evening at the movies. Keep them on hand and present them to employees when they need or deserve a little boost.

When employees are ill, call and check on them personally. Avoid sounding as if you're calling to see if they're really sick. Show your concern, and see if they need anything. Are they getting good medical care? If not, offer to get them in to see someone you trust.

Hospital staff need recognition too; when a job is well done, send a note to the employee with a copy to his or her supervisor. Send pizza to the night shift—nobody ever remembers them! Look around the nurses' station and lounge; is there anything you could do to make their workplace more pleasant? Talk with the nursing supervisor before you do anything, but you might buy a stereo system, a microwave oven, a coffee pot, a popcorn popper, or a lounge chair. Whatever you do, affix your gift with a tasteful brass plate saying something like "Thanks for all your hard work—Dr. Zane and Staff." Not only does this form of recognition make the hospital staff, and you, feel good, it's a subtle but wonderfully effective form of marketing for your practice. Hospital nursing staff can be superb referral sources for physicians and practices they respect.

Build fun into the workplace. We talked to a great many physicians, office managers, and employees in a lot of very busy practices. In all of them, the focus was constantly "making our patients feel at home and happy with us." These physicians and staff work hard. They also take time to play. They incorporate games and humor into their staff meetings; they schedule bowling, comedy club, and other outings; and they plan birthday, St. Patrick's Day, Hanukkah, and "TGIF" celebrations for the middle or end of a busy day. The Orlando (Florida) Regional Magnetic Resonance Center finds that patients enjoy occasional frivolity. At Halloween, employees participated in a pumpkin decorating contest; staff members created their versions of the practice mascot, Mortimer the Magnetic Moose, which then were judged by patients. Celebrating and laughing together reinforce the team's togetherness for team members **and** patients.

"TRAINING IS CHEAP R&D"

Use training and education as a motivator. "Education is cheap R&D," says Judy McDonald, office manager of McDonald Eye Clinic in Fayetteville, Arkansas. The practice holds monthly educational sessions for staff on clinical, personal, and team-building topics. Emphasizing a variety of educational topics acknowledges to your staff that you regard them as complete and complex individuals, not just "workers." ServiceMaster, the "housekeeping" company for business, allows employees to attend classes on company time in personal finance, stress management, and other subjects. The company's janitors and boiler operators attend seminars in communication and customer service; sometimes these are conducted by hospital administrators or physicians. According to a ServiceMaster vice president, "Our root motivator for committing so much time, money and effort to training is the company's second corporate objective: To use our business as a tool to help people grow and develop." The company has found that education motivates low-level employees to move up to high-level, even managerial, openings.[9] Education enhances participation and self-esteem for everyone, not to mention increasing your staff's knowledge and ability to make decisions!

Last, and equally important, share some of the profits with your employees. Give them a reason to perform their very best. Although money itself is not a primary motivator, the ownership that profit sharing conveys is. If your employees have a stake in the practice's success, you will see them fired with an almost missionary zeal for efficiency and profitability. This accountability will translate into personal satisfaction when they see the results from their efforts. A surgeon who implemented a profit-sharing system said, "Employees who had worked here for years suddenly began taking an interest in maximizing collections."

REWARD FAIRLY, CONSISTENTLY, AND OFTEN

Your office staff's "culture" will determine much of what's right for your employees. Some practices are run like a big family, and others take a more businesslike approach. The atmosphere in your practice will depend on how you and your colleagues view yourself and your employees as well as the size and type of practice. Regardless of the culture in your office, reward your employees with a fair, consistent hand, and do it frequently. Show no favoritism, and be clear about what you're doing: You're saying "thank you" for a job well done.

The rewards **you** earn for motivating your staff with recognition and rewards? There are many: Lower worker's compensation costs, greater retention, easier recruitment, higher morale, greater trust, improved productivity, and better service to customers.[10]

Sounds rewarding, doesn't it? ⚘

Action Items for Staff Motivation

1. Talk with each of your employees to understand what motivates each one to perform effectively.
2. Provide ongoing recognition, appreciation, and participation in decision making.
3. Keep communication flowing, formally and informally.
4. Make your patient-centered practice philosophy visible through your words and actions.
5. Empower staff to make decisions and to contribute to the practice in meaningful ways.
6. Provide challenging work, and encourage career development.
7. Offer competitive salaries and benefits that meet your employees' needs.
8. Specify expectations, and reward results.

References

1. Involving workers, gainsharing lift plant from its doldrums, *Total Quality Newsletter* 3, no. 11 (November 1992): 4. Reprinted with permission of *Total Quality Newsletter*, Lakewood Publications, 50 S. Ninth Street, Minneapolis, Minnesota 55402.
2. F. Herzberg, One more time, how do you motivate employees? *Harvard Business Review* reprint no. 87507.
3. Herzberg, One more time.
4. Herzberg, One more time.
5. Herzberg, One more time.
6. Herzberg, One more time.
7. M. LeBouef, *How To Win Customers and Keep Them for Life.* (New York, N.Y.: The Berkley Publishing Group, 1987): 149.
8. Encourage your staff members to speak up by listening to them, *Physician's Marketing and Management* (December 1988): 8.
9. Focus on . . . ServiceMaster, *Service Edge* (February 1992): 3.
10. L.R. Brecker, Circles style management creates committed employees, *Advance for Physical Therapists* (July 6, 1992): 9–12.

12

For Practice Administrators and Managers Only: Gaining Physician Participation

Throughout this book, we talk about leadership, commitment, vision, goals, and objectives for achieving "super service" and patient satisfaction. We've offered concepts and suggestions with the understanding that the physician is our primary audience, for he or she is the person with the greatest potential influence in the practice.

But we are pragmatists. We deal in reality and so do you. We know there are practices in which the administrator, office manager, or staff members are the driving force behind quality service and patient satisfaction. So this chapter is written to help you, the administrator, manager, and staff member(s). Because we know that in some practices the office manager or staff must encourage the physician(s) to communicate with patients, to educate them about their conditions, to spend an appropriate amount of time with them, and to meet their needs. We've been in practices where most of the innovative ideas are developed and put in place by the receptionist, bookkeeper, medical assistant, office manager, secretary, or nurse.

IT TAKES MORE THAN QUALITY MEDICAL CARE

We know there are practices in which the physician is focused on quality medical care but not necessarily on the customer. As a result, the practice may be drifting. Patients come for their appointments not because they are committed to the practice and impressed with the level of caring attention they get but because it's too much trouble to change. Or they like the office staff. Or because their health plan offers few other options. Or because it's convenient. (Our physician friend is still amazed, after 15 years in practice, that people will **choose** a doctor based solely on the fact that "the office was nearby and I saw the sign.")

Some patients will continue to come to practices in which service is secondary because they are healthy and the interaction with the practice or physician is infrequent. Given a medical emergency or health care crisis, however, their views of the practice and the physician might change significantly. Meanwhile, **you** know that they're not giving favorable recommendations to their friends, co-workers, or anyone else they encounter. So the practice isn't growing. You're frustrated because you know Dr. Michaels is a good physician. You know that he cares. You know that, if you could just **get him motivated,** get him to understand how important it is to patients and to the practice to provide excellent service, his attitude would change. The practice would be a better place for everyone: the physician, the staff, and especially the patients.

But how do you motivate the physician, or several of them, to focus on patient satisfaction? How do you get physicians to become committed to providing excellent service along with excellent medical care?

We can't work miracles. There are some physicians who are simply burned out. Their fire is gone. They are limping toward retirement in a few years or drifting along until an employment position presents itself where they believe they no longer will have to deal with the frustrations of private practice. But that's not a description of your physicians. The physicians in your practice **can** be motivated. You're sure of it. You just need some assistance in helping them understand the benefits that will accrue to everyone in the practice if they will commit to patient satisfaction through quality service.

WHAT TO DO?

Here's what you need to do. Read (or reread) the previous chapter on motivating staff. The guidelines for getting staff motivated and enthusiastic apply to anyone, including physicians. Keep the following principles in mind as you plan your strategy for motivating the physicians in your practice:

- People do what **they** want to. You can't make people want something; what they want (what they respond to and are motivated by) must be consistent with their internal values and goals. You must provide reasons for the physicians to **want** to improve patient satisfaction. Find a time to engage each of them individually in conversation. Ask why they went into medicine. Their responses are quite likely to be similar to the reason given by our friend: "I wanted to help people. I admired the dedication of doctors I encountered when I was young. I wanted to be able to do something for people and feel good about it." If the physicians say that their reason for entering medicine was to give to others, you've found a motivator. The desire to satisfy patients relates strongly to the "giving" value.
- People are inspired and motivated by those who are passionate and show conviction. Actively demonstrate your strong belief in quality service; be enthusiastic no matter what the attitude or reaction of others.
- People respond to positive feedback no matter who they are or what their position or status. When you observe a physician meeting or exceeding a patient's expectations (and you hear or observe the patient's favorable reaction), casually mention to the physician how pleased the patient was. Put it in writing if appropriate.
- People follow leaders. In Chapter 5 we said that the physician is the natural leader of the practice, but managers, administrators, and even line staff can provide quality leadership by example if the physician is uninterested or reluctant. Demonstrate leadership through subtle (**not** subversive or deceitful) action.

Determine what the physician responds to. If you have to persuade more than one physician, you may need a variety of approaches. Most physicians respond to facts and data. They're oriented to research because of their background in medical education and clinical training. Seldom do they prescribe a drug or hospitalize a patient on the basis of a hunch. They do tests, take X-rays, perform biopsies, and review the medical history before they make a decision. They gather and rely on facts and data, then interpret them.

ROUND UP FACTS AND DATA TO SUPPORT YOUR POSITION

So you need to do the same. Arm yourself with facts and data. Prove with detailed information why a practice focus on patient satisfaction through superior service will yield tangible benefits. The practice may already have evidence in patient survey results, patient record transfer requests, percentage of patient referrals, and the like. Some of the facts and data are included in this book. Chapter 2 has statistics and testimonials on the bottom line benefits of patient satisfaction. Other chapters point out the unavoidable pressures being brought to bear by managed care organizations and the government. There are references and citations throughout this book that specifically demonstrate the advantages of striving to achieve satisfaction *from the patient's perspective* with every encounter and interaction.

One office manager in a practice of 20 physicians, most of whom are quality oriented, said that she presents recalcitrant physicians with the need to improve patient satisfaction by positioning it as a risk management issue. She cites research studies that show reduced malpractice liability in practices with good communication and a high level of patient satisfaction. "They need to hear it," she said.

Use the kind of data to which the physicians in your practice will respond. If you need dollars for the bottom-line doctor, use dollars. Use productivity improvement for the physician oriented toward productivity. Use professional pride and satisfaction for the physician seeking that ethic. Use whatever is appropriate, or a combination. Support your argument with the kind of results that will get attention from your audience.

Put persuasive information (your facts and data) in a format to which the physician will respond best. Some people respond to visual stimuli. If so, use slides, overheads, presentation boards, a flip chart, and plenty of diagrams, charts, and graphs. Some people are print oriented. Give them a report, but make sure you go over it with them personally.

Provide ongoing support for your argument. Clip or mark articles pertaining to the benefits of patient satisfaction and service quality, and circulate them to those you are trying to persuade. Make sure favorable notes and comments from patients about a positive interaction or experience in the practice go to the physician as well as staff. Call attention to these items during your regular meeting with the physician if you suspect they may end up buried unnoticed under a pile of reading material.

INFLUENCE HAS POWER: KNOW HOW TO USE IT

Use the power of influence. In his book *Influence: The New Psychology of Modern Persuasion*, Robert B. Cialdini, PhD, cites the following "weapons of influence" that can be used ethically to win someone over to your point of view.[1] Use these weapons as appropriate:

- **Reciprocation:** Make a deal with the physician: "I'll try this change in the schedule you've been asking for if you'll try these two communication techniques with your patients." When you give someone something, the recipient feels an obligation to reciprocate. Try starting with a bigger request, and if you get a "no," scale it down to something smaller. You may just get a "yes."
- **Commitment and consistency:** People tend to act consistent with previous behavior. If you can get Dr. Michaels to agree to try some small change in his service quality behavior (and you then document favorable or nonnegative results), you have a better chance of "upping the ante" when you suggest a related activity.
- **Social proof:** People want to do as their peer group does. Talk about and cite evidence of patient satisfaction efforts in other practices in your community or elsewhere. Check with specialty organizations, the American Medical Association, the American Osteopathic Association and similar groups for documentation, examples, and specifics. Denver, Colorado surgeon Donald Par-

sons, MD, says it's the "implicit value-sharing" of group pressure that encourages change in physicians who are outliers, whether it's clinically, in their relationships with patients, or in other ways. The Noran Clinic, a 15-physician neurology group in Minneapolis, Minnesota, uses a form of social proof to show individual physicians where they are weak. Quarterly patient surveys that identify physicians by name establish a physician group mean and range for patient satisfaction with waiting time, sensitivity, listening skills, and other areas. Results comparing an individual physician with the "bell curve" are reviewed with the physician by the practice administrator, and then a plan for improvement is developed. In 6 months, survey results are reviewed again to see if patient satisfaction has increased in the target areas.

- **Liking:** People want to do things their friends and colleagues do. This "influence weapon" is a further example of social proof. Point to examples of patient satisfaction efforts by professional colleagues. (Make certain that your physician respects the colleague you name and that this individual truly supports the quality service effort, however, and isn't just going along with it because his or her partners have applied pressure.) Watch for medical staff meetings, committees, and other gatherings where service quality or patient satisfaction is the discussion topic, and if possible encourage the physician to attend "to see what kind of results the Westside Medical Group is having."
- **Authority:** People tend to respond to authority figures, so you can try citing evidence from medical leadership: the Surgeon General, the medical staff president, or any other individual or group respected by your physician.
- **Scarcity:** When there are two people and only one cookie in the cookie jar, the cookie becomes far more desirable. People want what they can't have. Use the scarcity principle to influence physicians to learn more about patient satisfaction. For example, a seminar or meeting that features patient satisfaction as a discussion topic might be of greater interest if Dr. Michaels were to learn that there is space for only a very few additional registrants (i.e., this is a **hot** topic, and if you don't participate, Doctor, you're going to miss out on knowing what all your friends know).

CREATE A SATISFYING SYMPHONY WITH COMMITTED PHYSICIANS AND STAFF

Patient satisfaction is not an option in medical practice. The commitment and participation of the physicians is a vital component of a successful, lasting, quality service process that results in satisfied patients and economic, professional success and fulfillment. When physicians and staff members work together in concert to make every patient's experience as positive as possible, the effect is harmonious and lasting. Compare this concordant, cooperative approach to that of one person playing Beethoven's Fifth Symphony on the piano. The pianist can make beautiful, uplifting music, but when the whole orchestra—strings, woodwinds, and percussion instruments—joins in, following the lead of the conductor, the effect is stirring, satisfying, and memorable for performers and audience alike. ❧

Action Items for Office Managers and Administrators

1. Talk with the physician to discover his or her personal motivators.
2. Actively demonstrate your enthusiastic belief in quality service.
3. Share comments from satisfied patients with the physician.
4. Assemble facts and data about the tangible benefits of a practice focus on patient satisfaction, and share the information in a format suited to the physician's style.
5. Provide ongoing evidence of the benefits of patient satisfaction.
6. Use the "weapons of influence" to convince the physician of the advantages of a patient-centered practice.

Reference

1. R. B. Cialdini, *Influence: The New Psychology of Modern Persuasion* (New York, N.Y.: Quill Publishing, 1984).

Part 3

Expectations: What Do Your Patients Want?

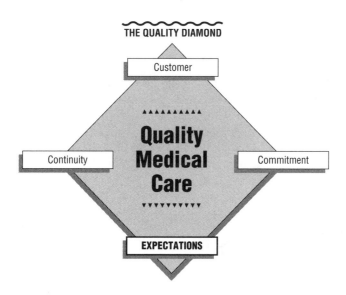

THE QUALITY DIAMOND

Customer

Quality Medical Care

Continuity

Commitment

EXPECTATIONS

What *do* patients want? It's a legitimate question, and not always an easy one to answer. Sometimes what they want isn't possible; economics, managed care, or Medicare restrictions may limit or prevent providing what they, or even you, believe is best.

Yet knowing what your patients want is the key to quality service; it paves the path to satisfaction. In this section, you'll learn the role of patient expectations and perceptions and why it's important to understand, monitor, and manage them. You'll also learn more about topics already familiar to you: creating "the tie that bonds" in the physician-patient relationship, why patients put such tremendous weight on your communication (and ways you might improve yours), what patients think of waiting time, partnerships that lead to good medicine, and other fundamental elements of quality service. ❧

---·&·---

13

Patient Expectations: More Reasonable Than You Might Think

Patients want a sense of caring, an individual relationship, a feeling that the doctor is sensitive to them and their needs. Scientific excellence is a given. Patients expect it.
                    James McNamara, MD, The Sansum Clinic,
                                        Santa Barbara, California

Patients want what everyone really wants an old fashioned family doctor who holds their hands and specializes in their problem.
                        Saul Schreiber, MD, Phoenix, Arizona

I want my doctor to show concern for me, an interest in me and not only the doctor, but his staff. I like it when he asks about my health, gives me advice and tries to help me stay healthy.

I want to get in promptly without waiting.

I want to be treated as an individual.

                                                    A patient

---

In Chapter 3 we said that patient satisfaction hinges on expectations. And because one of the purposes of this book is to help practices improve patient satisfaction through better service, it would certainly simplify matters if we could give you a Comprehensive Patient Expectations Inventory (Form B6921RS) that would allow you to predict exactly what questions or concerns you could anticipate simply by matching column A with category B.

But we can't give you a comprehensive list. The reason? Individual patient expectations vary according to:

- age
- sex
- problem
- day of the week
- time of the day
- mood
- attitude
- the breakfast cereal he or she ate that day

You get the picture. Patient expectations change, from one individual to another and even with the same patient from one visit to another. But this doesn't get you off the hook. You must know what your patients expect. What they need. What they're concerned about. You need to know this before you depart the exam room and move on to another patient, or how will you know if you have met or surpassed the patient's needs and expectations? How will you know if your patient's expectations are unreasonable or unachievable? (Patient satisfaction sometimes means managing expectations.)

In the next chapter, we'll give you ways to identify and monitor the expectations and needs that your patients have individually as well as collectively. But first, let's clarify why you need to know what your patients' expectations are.

WHY ARE PATIENT EXPECTATIONS IMPORTANT?

Expectations are the mental videotape mentioned in an earlier chapter. Your patient previews in his or her mind every "moment of truth" in the practice before the actual experience: the telephone appointment, the check-in at the front desk, the wait in the reception area, the greeting by the nurse or assistant, the interaction with the physician, and any physical treatment or procedure that occurs. Here's one person's "preview":

I went to a new doctor, checked in at the front desk, and sat down with a magazine, figuring I'd finish several articles if not the whole magazine. Ten minutes later, the receptionist came out and said, "Dr. Hastings has had a couple of emergencies. Your appointment will be delayed by about 30 minutes. Would you like to reschedule for another day, or would you prefer to wait?"

I was amazed. My previous doctor always kept me waiting an hour in the waiting room, then I'd spend up to an hour in the exam room. It was ludicrous, but I guess I'd grown to expect the long wait. It was a pleasant surprise to be asked if I minded waiting and to be given an option. And as it turned out, I was taken back to the exam room about 20 minutes later.

This patient anticipated a long wait; his past experience told him to expect it. He was pleasantly surprised when the "moment of truth" in the waiting room turned out to be a moment of triumph (especially for the practice). This practice obviously made an effort to stay on top of patient expectations regarding reasonable waiting time and had a recovery strategy for dealing with problems when they arose.

Knowing your patients' expectations individually and collectively helps you set standards—minimum daily service requirements—for the practice. The more you know about your patients' expectations, the more appropriately you can respond to them, proactively rather than retroactively. Otherwise, you could find yourself in the same situation as a major food company a few years ago whose research and development staff spent a great deal of time and effort developing an instant frozen breakfast. The company's food scientists toiled in the kitchen to overcome rubbery English muffins, blueberries that bled in the pancakes, and other unacceptable taste and consistency problems. Finally, the "successful" frozen breakfast was shipped to supermarket freezers. It flopped. Consumers didn't buy it. No one had taken the time to find out what consumer expectations and needs for frozen breakfast foods were. Had customers been consulted appropriately, the firm might have learned that their expectations for breakfast food items were significantly different than those for other meals. The company might have discarded the whole concept of frozen breakfasts.

The message applies to service as well. Know your patients. Learn what they want and what they **don't** want. Then act accordingly.

HOW ARE EXPECTATIONS AND SERVICE QUALITY LINKED?

When you go to a coffee shop, you expect speedy, friendly service, a meal that's tasty, and an accurate check, but you probably don't expect a picture-perfect presentation and sorbet between your ham on rye and apple pie. On the other hand, if you go to a fine restaurant, you may expect to be warmly greeted by name by the maitre d' and escorted to a table set with stemware, tablecloth, flowers, and fine china. You would be disappointed if servers did not hover attentively, refilling water glasses, brushing crumbs from the table after the meal, and presenting the final "cheque" unobtrusively on the table in a padded leatherette case. If you were to switch these "expectation videotapes"—if you mentally previewed the fine dining scene before walking into Benny's Diner—you would be sorely disappointed by the service and setting. Expectations escalate or diminish satisfaction.

WHAT CAN YOU DO ABOUT PATIENT EXPECTATIONS?

First, understand these two critical factors about expectations:

1. Your patients' collective expectations form the platform on which you build standards of service quality for your practice.
2. If your patients have unrealistic expectations and you do not gently realign them through education, they are likely to be disappointed when the Academy Award–winning mental movie they've created is overlaid with reality. This may affect their confidence in you and their willingness to follow prescribed treatment, to return for follow-up visits, and to recommend others to your practice.

"Aha!" you say. "I get your point—I need to know what my patients want. Well, that's easy. Hundreds of surveys and studies say what consumers expect of their doctors. I'll just refer to those surveys."

Good idea. But don't stop there. Those thousands of consumers are not patients in **your** practice. What each of your individual patients wants and expects from **you** and your staff is all that counts, no matter how many pollsters with their pencils come knocking at the door.

This doesn't mean that national surveys have no value. They provide trend information and a general sense of what consumers as a group want from the health care system. For example, our physician friend believes that patients today are more demanding. They expect more, he says. He's right. Patients have raised their standards as they've experienced the seemingly miraculous benefits of technological changes such as endoscopic surgery and lasers. They switch doctors, sometimes because their health plans change and sometimes because they've not experienced the caring that they seek. In 1968, only 38% of patients said that they had ever left a physician because of dissatisfaction. By 1989, 59% said that they had walked out of a physician's office never to return.[1]

Although national surveys are helpful to gain the broad perspective, it's important for you to know on a personal level what *each* of your patients wants and expects from you so that you and your staff can meet or manage these expectations.

What we're saying is that quality care and service are not collective but personal. Your knowledge and experience allow you to make some general assumptions about diabetic patients, but to treat 42-year-old Sidney Burns, a brittle diabetic, you must ask specific questions about his medical and family history, insulin requirements, diet, and other matters. This research requirement applies to Sidney Burns' expectations of his health care encounter as well. Your 22 years in medical practice allow you to make some generalizations about what patients expect; nevertheless, Sidney Burns has specific expectations that you need to understand if you and your staff are to provide optimum service. For example, Sidney may expect to be called Mr. Burns. He may expect a detailed explanation of your treatment protocol for diabetes. He may expect that you will lecture him about diet. He may expect your office to be open early in the morning or late in the day to accommodate people who work. By knowing these expectations, you and your staff can strive to achieve them or discuss with Mr. Burns alternative ways to satisfy his needs.

BUT FIRST, A FEW GENERALIZATIONS

Now that we've agreed that patient expectations are personal, let's take a look at some generalizations that can be made about the expectations of most patients:

- **Generalization 1:** People expect you to honor their appointment times. If an emergency disrupts the schedule, however, they appreciate being informed about the estimated delay and to be given options if they can't or don't want to wait.
- **Generalization 2:** Patients want you to communicate with them in everyday language (no medical jargon; or, if medical terms are necessary, translate them).
- **Generalization 3:** Your patients want a role in the interaction. They want you to ask them for their opinion and then to give them time to voice it. They want time to ask questions and to have their questions answered.
- **Generalization 4:** Patients want personal concern. Each wants to feel that during the time you spend with him or her, he or she is the only person who matters to you.
- **Generalization 5:** Your patients want information about their condition and treatment. They want it personally from you and your staff, and they also want something to review with family members.
- **Generalization 6:** Your patients expect care, concern, and courtesy from your staff, and they will evaluate you and your practice accordingly.

Patients want to have their needs met. With appropriate questioning, probing, and other techniques, you and your staff can determine what each individual wants and needs. As you do, you'll note some similarities among age groups, among men compared with women, and among patients with certain diseases or medical problems. You'll also find disparities. Althea Littner and Eleanor Ruby may both be overweight women in their late 60s, but their experiences, medical history, current personal situation, and word-of-mouth communication may add up to very different needs and expectations regarding treatment and service. The more you learn about each of their needs, the better the care you can provide.

LOTS OF THINGS INFLUENCE EXPECTATIONS

Your patient's "expectation videotape" is a montage of his or her previous health care experiences (good or bad), descriptions of your practice from other patients, medical encounters told in lurid detail by friends and families, and media coverage ranging from *USA Today* to Dr. Dean Edell's syndicated television program. The videotape may create expectations of a superb experience, or it may be the basis for anxiety and concern.

Listen to how a 29-year-old woman described her visit to an oral surgeon:

> *After 10 years of procrastination, I finally made an appointment to see about having my wisdom teeth extracted. Armed with a bevy of irrational fears, I anxiously awaited my consultation. After reviewing my X-rays and the clear need for removal of my wisdom teeth, the surgeon addressed each one of my concerns. Nevertheless, I scheduled surgery with great reluctance and trepidation.*

> *The dreaded event turned out to be a pleasant experience at every turn, with an exceptional level of service. On the first visit, I received a sheet of presurgery instructions (complete with parking information) and a patient education handbook—at no charge! The office manager handled the paperwork to ensure precertification from my insurance company. I received a letter from the insurance company and the practice confirming coverage several weeks before surgery. The surgery went as planned; I followed the postsurgery instructions handed to my husband as we left. Three hours after arriving home, the surgeon called to check on my progress.*

> *What professionals! I survived. No complications. No hassles. No side effects from the anesthesia. What a pleasure!*

Your reaction to this woman's description of a fairly routine surgery may be that the surgeon and his staff didn't do anything extraordinary except make a follow-up phone call. That's the point. Creating a favorable set of expectations for your patient requires communication to understand his or her needs and wants followed by consistency of service in addressing the needs you've identified and **shaping** or **managing** of those needs or wishes that are unrealizable.

ASK PATIENTS WHAT THEY WANT

David Silverman, MD, a Connecticut gerontologist, says, "You have to ask patients, 'What is it you want from this visit?'" How patients spell relief for what ails them varies according to individual needs, concerns, status, education, and other factors. You can't standardize patient expectations. That's why you need to bring patient wants and needs down to the personal level—a Gallup poll of one patient.

Lana Holstein, MD, does this routinely, posing an open-ended question sometime during the visit, no matter how mundane the purpose of the appointment. For example, her patient is a middle-aged man. He's complaining of a dry cough at night and a wheezing cough with exercise. The problem has lasted for 3 weeks. After a few pleasantries and a physical exam, Dr. Holstein reviews with the patient previous discussions they have had regarding this recurring problem. She then suggests medication options. After the two have agreed on a treatment plan and she has noted the symptoms and treatment in his chart, she says to the patient, "What else do we need to talk about today?" She asks this question of every patient she sees that morning.

Get personal with your patients. As one physician commented, "We have a real advantage as doctors. Our customers expect us to get personal. They're disappointed if we don't. We should use this advantage to learn everything we can to provide the best diagnosis and treatment." And to meet, manage, or exceed their expectations, need we add? ❧

Action Steps for Understanding Patient Expectations

1. Understand that patient expectations change. Maintain a flexible attitude.
2. Find out what *your* patients want and what they don't want. Ask questions, and listen attentively to their answers.
3. Address the needs you identify through consistent service.
4. Gently manage unrealistic expectations through patient education.

Reference

1. L. Farber, ed., *Medical Economics Encyclopedia of Practice and Financial Management* (Oradel, N.J.: Medical Economics Company, Inc., 1985): 303.

14

Essential Tools for Measuring Your Patients' Expectations

When a Dell computer salesperson takes an order from a customer, he or she gathers details about the desired features (larger disk drive, built-in modem), and then sends the order with detailed specifications to the manufacturing facility. The product is custom-produced and shipped to the customer within five days. By selling direct to end users through its sales staff rather than through dealers, Dell learns firsthand about customer needs, interests and problems. "We use service to build loyalty," a Dell spokesman says, "and the information we get as a result helps to make improvements."[1(pp.1–2)]

*   *   *

"My knee had been bothering me for some time, so I finally made an appointment with a doctor. She came into the room, and there was no eye contact at all, even when she shook my hand very perfunctorily. I felt like a body part, not a person. She examined me, then gave me several options—'You could do this, you could do that, it's up to you.' I wanted to feel like the doctor was decisive, in control. I wasn't expecting a Dr. Milquetoast. She might have been a great diagnostician, but she didn't meet my needs. I'd never go back."

—A patient

*   *   *

"My experience as a patient has heightened my awareness of certain things that patients expect. For example, I discovered that as a patient, when I called my doctor for information, I wanted him to call back as quickly as possible. I realized that when patients call me, they're often sitting by the phone waiting for my return call."

—Marvin Korengold, MD

Medical care is an intimate business. Consider the typical interaction: The physician asks personal, detailed, probing questions of the patient, who is often a complete stranger. After answering these questions, the patient may then partially or fully disrobe to be subjected to physical prodding, prying, and probing.

This intimacy imposed by the medical care process makes establishing a "relationship" (rather than merely an "interaction") simpler, yet the process of nurturing and maintaining the relationship then becomes more critical. Prepared for what will happen by previous health care experiences, hearsay evidence, observation of your office decor, and evaluation of your staff's behavior and interaction, your patient waits in the exam room or consultation room. He or she expects you to ask personal questions, questions that might not even be asked by a spouse or close family member, and usually is prepared to answer them. In return, he or she seeks a connection, an emotional bonding at some level. He or she expects that in return for your personal probing you will show compassion and caring. Expectations are perhaps higher than they might be for other service encounters. That's the tradeoff: "If you're going to pry, Doctor, this had better be worth it."

YOUR PATIENTS EXPECT YOU TO GET PERSONAL

Because your patient expects you to get personal, you have an advantage: You have the opportunity to learn exactly what his or her needs and expectations are at that moment.

This one-on-one "expectations analysis" isn't the only time or technique for determining expectations, however. Remember, we said that expectations change from person to person and from one day to the next. So it's a good idea to use as many ways as possible to find out what your patients want, individually and collectively. That's what this chapter is all about. It's about determining hopes and needs, and especially it's about **anticipating** expectations, because staying a step ahead of the customer is what superior service is all about. By paying attention to the information you and your staff gain from observing and listening to what patients tell you they want or need, you can find out what people like about the service you're providing and what services, information, or assistance they wish you would provide. By determining patient expectations, you can anticipate what they may want or need in the future. And in the process, you create a personal bond, evidence that you view this person **as** a person, not merely as a patient.

Customer-focused practices that continually strive to improve the level of service they offer know that anticipating patient expectations is critical, that measuring and monitoring wants, needs, and satisfaction with results determine continued success. Peters and Waterman point this out in *In Search of Excellence*.[2] They say that effective service organizations have a remarkable people orientation, active involvement of senior management, and a high intensity of measurement and feedback. It's the good news–bad news story: The better you are, the better you must strive to be. Patients expect something "a little better" each time they visit a practice that's outstanding.

INCORPORATE INCREMENTAL IMPROVEMENTS

This means not only that you must continue to provide superior service in every aspect of your practice but that you and your staff must continually look for ways to incorporate service "booster shots," incremental improvements that subtly tell your patients you're paying attention to them and their needs. Because they are paying attention to you.

Service mistakes, even small ones, are the thorns in a practice that has grown and attracted patients with a philosophy of service excellence. These careless errors, like the thorns on roses, don't affect quality of care. You may not even notice them, but if your patient gets pricked by a thorn—a slip in service—he or she may become wary. Patient expectations are high because experience with your practice has led them to believe there are no thorns.

To avoid breeding too many thorny roses in your practice (or to find them before they grow large and bushy), continually look for ways to improve. Radiologist Lawrence Cohen, MD, of the Washington, D.C. Imaging Center, does it with staff get-togethers every few weeks. There's always a topic for discussion, but one week, Dr. Cohen said, "The office manager told me we didn't have any topics or problems and so we didn't need to have a meeting. I said yes we did, and we talked about how to look for problems and how to fix them when we find them."

You must continually measure and monitor patient expectations to learn how they're changing and whether you're meeting them. In this chapter we're going to give you 16 techniques for evaluating patient expectations. Some of the techniques help you determine in advance what your patients' needs and hopes are. Some are after the fact—they measure a patient's evaluation of the experience after it occurred—but this postinteraction feedback is helpful for determining future expectations.

TECHNIQUES FOR MEASURING EXPECTATIONS AND SATISFACTION

One, some, or all of the techniques that follow can help you and your staff discern patient needs and concerns on an immediate, "this visit" basis as well as over the long term. At the same time, by determining expectations you're conveying personal concern to your patients. You're letting them know, "I care about you, it's important to me that we know what you want and need." Just remember that patients may escalate their expectations as service performance escalates, so that measurement (and improvement) must be continuous and never ending.

Pre-Appointment "Prying"

Prying usually doesn't have a favorable connotation, but in this case it's positive. At Forest Rim Family Medicine in Flagstaff,

Arizona, the telephone receptionist is trained to ask specific, detailed questions about the patient's complaint or reason for the appointment. The office manager says, "We pry in order to make sure we know what patients need to see the doctor for, so they get the right amount of time allotted." In return, the practice lets patients know what to expect by sending an information sheet before the first appointment that explains the practice philosophy.

New Patient Information Form

Include a question on your new patient information sheet that probes expectations such as, "What do you hope to gain from your appointment today?" or "What can Dr. Goodhealth and her staff do to meet your health care needs?" Open-ended questions such as these solicit the patient's own opinion, but you can also provide a checklist of responses to these or similar questions, if you wish.

Reception Area Clipboard

The Heart Center in Manchester, New Hampshire provides a clipboard with a notepad in the reception area so that patients can write down their questions or concerns, which often tend to be forgotten in the sometimes stressful setting of the exam room. A question card handed to patients by the receptionist can also accomplish this. Printed on the card could be, "Doctor: This is a question or concern I'd like you to address today." The patient then fills in the blank card and hands it back to the receptionist, who puts it in the patient's chart for the physician to refer to during the appointment.

Staff Screening

The Heart Center uses a "set-up" person to gather demographic data and other information about what's going on in the patient's life. For example, Alan Kaplan, MD, says, "The set-up person found out that a patient who was not supposed to be exerting herself at home wasn't getting any help with housework from her husband. So I knew that was something to discuss with the patient and her husband." Some patients are also seen by a nurse practitioner or physician's assistant, who performs a physical examination and gathers additional information. The physician then reviews the data and conclusions in the chart with the patient, giving the patient the chance to concur with or correct the assumptions.

The Direct Approach

It sounds too simple. The physician asks the patient, "What would you like to come away from this visit with?" It's an approach used by Heart Center cardiologists. (Do you get the feeling that they know the importance of understanding patient expectations?) "The need is different with each patient. Some want information; some want to feel better," Dr. Kaplan says.

Introductory Visit

Several practices encourage no-charge introductory visits, during which the patient can size up the physician and the physician can size up the patient. Many physicians we interviewed believe that it's best to determine physician-patient compatibility early in the relationship and to acknowledge openly if it's not there, before the seed of mistrust is planted and lack of confidence begins to bloom.

Medical History Questionnaire

Denver, Colorado internist Carol Gilmore, MD, spends an hour with each new patient, going over a detailed six-page medical questionnaire that the patient completes before the appointment. The form covers the patient's personal history, medical history, and lifestyle issues. "We go over it line by line. By the time the patient leaves, they tell me they've never had anyone ask these questions before. I get to know the patient personally, and follow-up visits are much simpler. I know everything about this person, what they need and expect medically and otherwise. It makes follow-up visits much easier," Dr. Gilmore explains. Arlan Cohn, MD, uses the General Health History Questionnaire from Bibbero Systems, Inc. This questionnaire asks detailed lifestyle as well as medical questions of the patient (a sample page from the Bibbero questionnaire can be found in Exhibit 14-1). He supplements it with questions such as, "What's the worst thing going on in your life right now? The best thing?" to get qualitative perspectives from his patients.

Staff Discussions

At the end of each day, Robert Bright, MD, gathers his staff to go over the next day's schedule. They discuss certain patients, for example Mrs. Keith, who had a fractured hip and a subsequent implant. "We'll show the X-ray to the staff and discuss how her condition may be affecting her life." Involving the staff more intimately with patients allows them to obtain lifestyle information and to pass it on to Dr. Bright, who can use it to determine patient expectations and needs. Dell Computer Corp. holds weekly customer advocate meetings, at which employees identify all the issues that customers have brought up during the previous week. This information is used to make improvements in products or processes. The company also uses surveys to measure customer satisfaction, not only with its computers but with the whole experience of acquiring and using them: sales visits, service calls, telephone conversations, and product quality.

Post-Visit Card

It's only the size of a postcard, but it can pack a wallop, telling you what went right, what didn't, and what you need to change or rectify to meet patient expectations. This brief 5- or 6-question survey card can be handed to patients by the doctor (for best

Exhibit 14-1 Sample Page from General Health History Questionnaire

Chart No._____

ANDRUS/CLINI-REC® HEALTH HISTORY QUESTIONNAIRE

Identification Information   Today's Date_____

Name _____ Date of Birth _____

Occupation _____ Marital Status _____

PART A—PRESENT HEALTH HISTORY

I. CURRENT MEDICAL PROBLEMS

Please list the medical problems for which you came to see the doctor. About when did they begin?

<u>Problems</u>   <u>Date Began</u>

_____   _____
_____   _____
_____   _____

What concerns you the most about these problems?

_____
_____

If you are being treated for any other illnesses or medical problems by another physician, please describe the problems and write the name of the physician or medical facility treating you.

Illness or Medical Problem   Physician or Medical Facility   City

_____   _____   _____
_____   _____   _____

II. MEDICATIONS

Please list all medications you are now taking, including those you buy without a doctor's prescription (such as aspirin, cold tablets or vitamin supplements)

_____   _____   _____   _____
_____   _____   _____   _____

III. ALLERGIES AND SENSITIVITIES

List anything that you are allergic to such as certain foods, medications, dust, chemicals, or soaps, household items, pollens, bee stings, etc., and indicate how each affects you.

<u>Allergic To:</u>   <u>Effect</u>   <u>Allergic To:</u>   <u>Effect</u>

_____   _____   _____   _____
_____   _____   _____   _____

IV. GENERAL HEALTH, ATTITUDE AND HABITS

How is you overall <u>health now</u>? ... Health now: Poor___ Fair___ Good___ Excellent___

How has it been <u>most of your life</u>? . Health has been   Poor___ Fair___ Good___ Excellent___

In the past year:

    Has your <u>appetite changed</u>? .... Appetite: Decreased___Increased___Stayed same___

    Has your <u>weight changed</u>? ..... Weight: Lost___lbs. Gained___lbs. No change___

    Are you <u>thirsty much of the time</u>? Thirsty: No___ Yes___

    Has your overall 'pep' changed?. Pep: Decreased___Increased___Stayed same___

Do you usually have <u>trouble</u>

    sleeping</u>?.................. Trouble sleeping: No___ Yes___

(continues)

Exhibit 14-1 continued

How much do you <u>exercise</u>? . . . . . . Exercise:	Little or none___ Less than I need___ All I need___
Do you <u>smoke</u>? . . . . Smokes:	No___ Yes___ If yes, how many years?___
How many each day?	___Cigarettes ___Cigars ___Pipesfull
Have you ever smoked? . . . . Smoked	No___ Yes___ If Yes, how many years?___
How many each day?	___Cigarettes ___Cigars ___Pipesfull
Do you <u>drink alcoholic beverages</u>? . Alcohol:	No___ Yes___
. . . .	I drink ___Beers ___Glasses of Wine
. . . .	___Drinks of hard liquor - per day
Have you ever had a <u>problem</u> with alcohol? . . . . Prior problem:	No___ Yes___
How much <u>coffee or tea</u> do you usually drink? . . . . Coffee/Tea:	___cups of coffee or tea a day.
Do you regularly wear <u>seatbelts</u>? . . Seatbelts:	No___ Yes___

DO YOU:	Rarely/Never	Occasionally	Frequently
Feel nervous?	_____	_____	_____
Feel depressed?	_____	_____	_____
Find it hard to make decisions?	_____	_____	_____
Lose your temper?	_____	_____	_____
Worry a lot?	_____	_____	_____
Tire easily?	_____	_____	_____
Have trouble relaxing?	_____	_____	_____
Have any sexual problems?	_____	_____	_____
Ever feel like committing suicide?	_____	_____	_____
Feel bored with your life?	_____	_____	_____
Use marijuana?	_____	_____	_____
Use "hard drugs"?	_____	_____	_____
Do you want to talk to the doctor about a personal matter?	No___ Yes___		

response rate) or by the billing desk employees after the visit; patients can be encouraged to complete it in the office and then drop it in a **sealed** box in the reception area. Or prestamp the card, and let the patient fill it out at home and mail it back. The Noran Clinic in Minneapolis, Minnesota uses this minisurvey technique along with regular quarterly patient questionnaires. A sample card is seen in Exhibit 14-2.

Exhibit 14-2 Post-Visit Survey Card

1. How long did you wait in the reception area? _____ minutes
2. Did you consider the waiting time: ❏ Brief ❏ Reasonable ❏ Excessive
3. Were you treated courteously by **all** staff members? ❏ Yes ❏ No
4. Was the doctor knowledgeable? ❏ Yes ❏ No
5. Was the doctor friendly? ❏ Yes ❏ No
6. Did the doctor spend enough time with you? ❏ Yes ❏ No
7. Would you recommend this practice to others? ❏ Yes ❏ No
8. Do you have any suggestions or comments for improving our practice?
   _____
   _____
   _____

Follow-Up Phone Calls

After a patient's first visit, designate a nurse or other staff member—or, ideally, the physician—to call the patient at home. This informal, friendly call might go something like this: "Mr. Smith? This is Dr. Goodhealth. I was just calling to see if any questions or concerns came to you after you left our practice today. And I wanted to know if you felt there was anything we could have done better or differently during your visit today." Gregory Darrow, MD, a family physician in Janesville, Wisconsin, described in *Medical Economics* how he personally calls patients who ask to have their records transferred.[3] This tactic has led to changes in office policies and staff and occasionally has retrieved an unhappy departing patient. Denver, Colorado internist Richard Abrams, MD, said that unsolicited follow-up phone calls to patients have built his practice: "I do it first thing in the morning. It takes less than 60 seconds. I can't begin to tell you how many patients I've gotten referred as a result of these phone calls."

Suggestion Box

It's an ancient idea, but it still works. Put a suggestion box in your reception area, put one in each exam room, and put cards nearby. Post a sign or print on the cards, "Please tell us what we're doing right and what we can do better." Act on every suggestion, and when patients sign their name respond personally to thank them and let them know what you've done. The Heart Center has a patient suggestion box. "Patients use it when there's something they don't feel comfortable addressing with the doctor or staff member—miscommunication, misunderstandings, things we could do better," according to Dr. Kaplan. So does the Sansum Clinic in Santa Barbara, California; an employee group evaluates and makes recommendations on the suggestions.

Focus Groups and Patient Councils

The focus group, once the domain of high-powered, high-cost market research firms, has taken seats in the medical practice. Although formal market research calls for a precise and structured method of conducting a focus group, you can use the concept less formally in your practice to determine what patients need and want. For many years, Marvin Belsky, MD, a New York internist, used to hold patient meetings twice a month in his office. He and half a dozen patients would meet from 7 to 10 p.m. to discuss "what most of them have never dared verbalize before: their fears, uncertainties, grievances, needs."[4(p.20)] During these sessions, "patients' expectations and understanding of their responsibilities [were] interchanged and heightened." Dr. Belsky's leadership role was only to ask questions: "What do you feel makes a good doctor?" and "How do you feel about me as your doctor?" Otherwise, he would "listen, listen, listen, and interrupt as infrequently as possible."

Your practice focus groups need not be held twice a month. Try bringing together a random group of patients twice yearly. You'll be enlightened, even amazed, at what you may learn. Stew Leonard's Dairy in Norwalk, Connecticut, regularly assembles 10 or 15 customers to find out what they like and don't like about the store's products and service. Leonard says, "Customers are our advisors and consultants."

Another option is to form a patient council, a group of patients who present ideas, complaints, concerns, and suggestions for improvement. The council meets three or four times a year; discussion topics can be random or specific (particularly if an issue has been identified in the practice as affecting service quality). Wilmington Health Associates, a North Carolina group practice of 21 physicians, has a patient advisory council that meets monthly. The only problem, says the office manager, is that "at this point, everyone says everything is great." Nice problem! He makes the point, however, that council membership needs to be rotated more frequently to ensure an infusion of new perspectives.

Should the physician participate in focus group or patient council discussions? It depends. Some physicians may be uncomfortable listening to their patients tell them that they come across as uncaring. Their discomfort is likely to inhibit discussion. Also, some patients may be reluctant to voice criticism directly to their doctor. Some physicians, such as Dr. Belsky, can handle negative comments easily, using them to move the discussion along. You know your style and your ability as a facilitator best; use this judgment to decide whether you should participate in patient council discussions. An alternative is to have an office manager or even an impartial outsider facilitate the discussion; the physician can observe and occasionally ask for clarification but not be actively involved. Still a third option: Let the office manager or third party lead the focus group, but videotape it for later review by physicians and even staff members. A videotape can be compelling evidence of the need for change in attitude or behavior within the practice.

If you conduct focus groups or form a patient council, remember this unbreakable rule: Implement recommendations when you can, and follow up with the patient(s) on those you can't. You will lose credibility (and patients) if no action results from their input.

Breakfast or Lunch Review Meetings

In several practices we encountered, the physicians, nurses, physicians' assistants, receptionists, and other staff members get together in small interdepartmental or intradepartmental groups at breakfast or lunch to share ideas and observations about individual patients and patients in general. The purpose of these discussions is to bring up patient attitudes, concerns, complaints, and compliments and to come up with ways that physicians and staff can better understand and meet patient needs.

Patient Questionnaire

This is a means of determining patient expectations on a collective basis; it's also a way to monitor satisfaction, problems, concerns, and trends. You'll find a sample patient survey in Chapter 27, Appendix 27-A. Meanwhile, here's a tip from the Noran Clinic: Include a question on your patient survey, such as the following one, for revealing insights into patient expectations: "Would you want to see this physician again in the future? Why or why not?"

Referral Physician Survey

You may wonder, "What can a referral physician survey tell me about patient expectations?" You might be surprised. Patients often report back to the physician who referred them (and the savvy referring physician solicits feedback) to say, "Dr. Gottlieb really knew his stuff. But I wish he had given me a pamphlet or something about the surgery. I didn't really understand some of what he was saying, so I couldn't explain it to my wife." Referring physicians file these nuggets away, and if they accumulate, they may influence future referrals. Find out what referral sources and their patients say about you with a well-structured survey. Knowing referral source opinions and needs is also a way to reassure patients that there is continuity of care and communication among all their providers. It's a satisfying thought.

Summary

There you have it—an assortment of techniques for determining, anticipating, and monitoring your patients' expectations. You can't satisfy your patients if you don't know what they're after. Talking to and **listening** to your patients in a variety of ways is the only means of understanding and meeting their needs and, ultimately, surprising them by surpassing their expectations. ❧

Action Steps for Measuring Patient Expectations

1. Recognize that patients expect a personal relationship that shows compassion and caring.
2. Incorporate service "booster shots" in your practice, continual improvements that tell your patients that you're responding to their needs.
3. Train your receptionist to identify effectively why each patient needs an appointment so that the correct amount of time can be allotted.
4. Send a practice philosophy information sheet before a new patient's first appointment.
5. Seek information about patient expectations on your new patient information form.
6. Provide a note pad or question card in the reception area to encourage patients to write down questions.
7. Use your staff to help you uncover things going on in a patient's life. Encourage staff to verbalize their observations and ideas.
8. *Ask* your patients, directly, what they want.
9. Obtain patient feedback with confidential post-visit survey cards, follow-up phone calls, a suggestion box, focus groups, patient councils, and patient questionnaires.
10. Conduct a referral physician survey.

References

1. Taking on the "big boys" with service, *For the President's Eyes Only*, 14, no. 7 (April 14, 1991): 1–2. Copyrighted material reprinted with permission of *For the President's Eyes Only* and the Bureau of Business Practice, 24 Rope Ferry Road, Waterford, Connecticut 06836.

2. T. J. Peters and R. H. Waterman, Jr., *In Search of Excellence: Lessons From America's Best-Run Companies* (New York, N.Y.: Harper & Row, 1982): 249.

3. G. L. Darrow, I learn a lot from patients who leave me, *Medical Economics* (April 22, 1992): 116–125.

4. Marvin Belsky, *How To Choose and Use Your Doctor* (New York, N.Y.: Arbor House, 1975): 20.

15

Quality Service Is Clinical Mastery

"Despite His Patients' Pleas, Eye Doctor Still Can't Practice"

Denying passionate pleas on behalf of two patients who say they are desperate for a suspended eye doctor's services, an administrative law judge refused Thursday to modify the suspension to allow the doctor to treat them.

The patients instead will have to find other physicians to care for them while the state proceeds with its allegations that the physician, Dr.___, performed unnecessary and questionable eye surgeries and procedures.

. . . petitions were filed by Jack Okun, 72, of Los Angeles, who said __ is the only doctor in Southern California who can perform the no-stitch cataract surgery he desperately needs.[1(p.1)]

"What about the role of *medical expertise* in quality care and patient satisfaction?" asked a friend while we were writing this book. This individual is a health care professional who works with physicians. The question was insightful and appropriate.

At first blush, the answer seems simple: Quality service can't compensate for less-than-expert care. Yet, although this is certainly true, there are cases in which the surrogates of medical care—soothing staff, a seemingly empathic physician, plush of-

173

fice furnishings, fancy brochures, and flowery words—obscure poor-quality medical care. As we discussed in Chapter 3, most patients judge expertise according to nontechnical characteristics, the surrogate indicators. Thus a pleasing demeanor and a pleasant environment can mask a lack of knowledge or skill.

It's unfortunate but true: Warmth, an attitude of concern, and personal service are the means by which quacks and charlatans survive and sometimes get rich. An exemplary focus on patient satisfaction can allow mediocre physicians and those with limited diagnostic or surgical skills to have thriving medical practices. You may know of a physician who is personable, affable, and brilliant when it comes to the business side of medical practice. He or she probably has a successful, growing practice. Yet his or her surgical skills may leave much to be desired; a routine procedure is complex and difficult. But patients don't know it; this physician is warm and friendly, and his or her staff members reinforce the positive impression that he or she makes.

CHARM CREATES RAPPORT, BUT IT'S NOT ENOUGH

These physicians build trust around a smile and a warm touch, creating rapport one by one with a less-than-knowledgeable public. Some of those who are most likely to trust these individuals are older patients, who grew up in an era in which "the doctor knew best" and physicians were never doubted or questioned. Some patients accept the superficial security of a friendly face because they simply don't know the right questions to ask to determine a physician's expertise or where to find the resources that will give them the information they need regarding medical competence.

David M. Eddy, MD, PhD, professor of health policy and management at Duke University, referred to public and professional reliance on nonclinical indicators as "decisions without information," pointing out that patients, payers, and even physicians often must select a provider in this fashion. He described this dilemma as "an intellectual crisis in medicine" and decried the lack of an organized database of clinical outcomes information for many medical procedures and treatments.[2]

PARAMETERS AND STANDARDS ARE CLARIFYING SELECTION

This blind approach to physician selection is slowly eroding. Governmental policymakers, professional medical societies, and third party payers are gathering data, stockpiling statistics, and cross-tabulating inputs and outcomes. All this detailed information pours into databases that determine practice parameters and clinical standards to guide medical decisions. One of the most recent and innovative efforts is Medicare's Health Care Quality Improvement Initiative, which searches for patterns of consistently substandard care by using treatment and outcome profiles for physicians and hospitals to establish benchmarks. The pilot began in late 1992 with four test sites, starting with cardiac care.[3]

Researchers are going beyond the data and the statistics to search for subjective evidence of favorable outcomes. Increasingly, patient "quality of life" indicators are measured along with lab tests, X-rays, blood counts, and other clinical statistics.[4] This approach acknowledges that evaluating quality of care depends on what the patient thinks and feels as well as what the statistics say. The surveys seek to define what a positive outcome is. Yes, the patient was cured according to the clinical parameters, but how did the hip implant surgery affect her life? Can she shop, go for a walk, and sit comfortably? This multipronged approach to outcome assessment, involving objective data as well as subjective perceptions, is being used by business and industry as well as governmental agencies to guide and evaluate physicians collectively and individually. It may well become valuable information to physicians in determining their own limitations and areas in which additional education or training is needed.

Organizations such as the American Association of Retired Persons (AARP) recognize that their members sometimes need help in selecting quality physicians. The AARP has launched a campaign to reform medical licensing boards and has developed a manual for consumers to get them involved in safeguarding medical quality.

BUT DECISIONS WITHOUT INFORMATION ARE STILL MADE

Despite this trend to "quantify" quality, decisions without information are still made routinely by your patients and others when they call your office for a first-time appointment. They choose you and other physicians on the recommendation of a family member, a friend, or a co-worker. Some rely on Yellow Pages advertising, a brochure mailed to the home, or an impression gained after hearing you speak to an organization. Sometimes they have the benefit of a referral from their own primary care physician. But the decision frequently is made on the basis of the surrogate indicators: friendliness, a show of concern, or even a convenient office location. Physician competence is assumed.

Fortunately, research suggests that consumers are becoming more aware that physician competence levels may vary, and some consumers are seeking information that will help them evaluate physicians. The *Keckley Report* noted as early as 1989 that consumers will "lap up data about clinical outcomes . . . they are cautiously becoming receptive to comparative data, and are strategically oriented toward finding 'the best.'" The Keckley organization predicted that "payors, hospitals and physicians will find themselves doing battle on the field of quality, playing to a packed house of turned-on consumers."[5(p.2)]

But let's face it: Physicians sometimes assume that the colleagues to whom they refer patients are competent. Most physicians couldn't go into the OR or exam room with every one of their consulting physicians to observe their technique or apparent knowledge. And even if they could, it might be difficult for them to evaluate the level of competence or knowledge in a particular procedure, condition, or treatment with which they are unfamiliar. (That's why they made the referral in the first place.) So they rely instead on what they hear from others, what they are able to observe, and the feedback their patients give them about the providers they send them to.

Alan Kaplan, MD, medical director of the Manchester, New Hampshire Heart Center, is keenly aware of the gap that can exist between competence and quality service. He believes that physicians have a responsibility to educate patients in selecting a quality provider. "The three As (availability, affability, and ability) still determine physician quality, but most patients rely solely on the first two As. The only way they can get guidance on ability is within the medical system," he says.

"When we have patients who need certain kinds of cardiac surgery," Dr. Kaplan says, "we'll refer them to Boston or some other center because they'll get better surgical treatment there, even though we'll lose revenues because we can't follow the patient. We tell these patients, 'You won't be as comfortable because you're not in your home town, but you're there to get the best care, and that's what counts.'

"Does this affect referrals?" he continues. "I think the referral physicians know there are certain cases we don't send to them. We know their strengths and capabilities and those are the cases we refer. I don't refer a patient to any surgeon I haven't scrubbed with."

Dr. Kaplan adds, "Too many doctors get in a corner. They're asked by their colleagues to do something they're not skilled at. They're afraid of losing business if they don't do the procedure, but the person who loses is the patient. He's getting less than excellent care."

USE OUTCOMES INFORMATION AND CLINICAL PARAMETERS WISELY

As outcomes measurement and clinical parameters become more common and more commonly shared, a responsibility is placed on physicians individually and collectively to use the information on a personal basis as a yardstick and, whenever possible, to consider it to make informed referral recommendations to patients or colleagues.

We believe that the vast majority of physicians are competent, concerned, and caring. This book is offered as an adjunct to the medical expertise you possess. By implementing the suggested strategies for increasing patient satisfaction, you can conceivably improve clinical outcomes while reaping the rewards of practice growth. Nevertheless, patient satisfaction strategies—a pleasant reception area, minimal waiting time, thorough and friendly staff, a warm smile, eye contact, and a follow-up phone call—should never take the place of optimal technical skills in diagnosis and treatment. Most of the physicians we talked with in writing this book pointed this out. Berkeley internist and humorist author Arlan Cohn, MD (*Kill as Few Patients as Possible*), responded in a serious vein when asked for his definition of patient satisfaction. "The first rule is always competence," he said. "Quality service begins with the intelligence and knowledge of the doctor. Personality, charm, communication, and friendliness are all secondary to diagnostic skills and ability."

One physician has recognized in writing the importance of competence and technical skill. Jerald L. Tennant, MD, of Duncanville, Texas, has developed a "Patient's Bill of Rights" that spells out what his patients can and should expect from him (Exhibit 15-1).

Carol Gilmore, MD, sometimes will refer patients to physicians who lack empathy and communication skills if she believes their medical skills are far superior to those of others. "I always tell my patients why I'm referring them to a certain doctor. I'll preface his shortcomings—for example, I frequently refer to a specialist who has a poor bedside manner; he's very blunt with his patients. I tell patients this up front, but I also explain that this doctor is the best person to give the quality of care the patient needs."

It's important to have "the candor to admit when we are beyond our capabilities and to possess the grace to direct the patient or problem to the appropriate individual. A corollary is that it is as or more important to know and admit what we don't know, as it is to act proficiently when we do know how to proceed," said Bruce E. Spivey, MD, past executive director of the American Academy of Ophthalmology.[6(p.1)]

MEASURE YOUR SKILLS; KNOW YOUR CAPABILITIES

We couldn't say it any better. Satisfy your patients by providing quality service in all areas of your practice, clinically as well as in the delivery mechanisms and processes, surrogate indicators, and service extras. Measure your technical skills against available guidelines and standards from medical societies, independent organizations, and agencies such as the National Institutes of Health.[7] Be aware of your limitations as well as your capabilities; improve your skills through continuing education, medical and professional journals, and collegial consultation and discussion. Know when you're not ready for a new procedure, when you don't know enough about a new drug, or when you've reached the outside limits of your knowledge of a certain condition. When necessary, refer your patients to the experts, and know who they are and what their skills as well as **their** limitations are.

Exhibit 15-1

Patient's Bill of Rights

In over twenty years of practice, I have often heard patients complain about doctors. I have tried to live by certain principles. I have decided to write them down for you.

A patient has the right to know what his or her illness is and what trouble it is likely to cause.

A patient has a right to have the illness explained in ordinary English, not medical terms.

A patient has the right to know the treatment options, the advantages and disadvantages of each, and what each will cost.

A patient has the right to know the doctor's qualifications and experience.

A patient has the right to consult other doctors without me being insulted or angry that the patient wants another opinion.

A patient has a right to understand my fees.

I have also tried to live by these standards:

I will spend a patient's money as wisely as possible as if I were spending my own money. I will look for and recommend the least expensive way of solving my patient's problems.

I will not recommend surgery unless the patient needs help that only surgery can provide.

If a patient feels I have not provided him or her with my best efforts, I will refund the money he or she paid me—no questions asked. I can't guarantee results of treatment, but I can guarantee you my best efforts to treat you honestly and fairly.

JERALD L. TENNANT, MD

Source: Courtesy of Jerald L. Tennant, MD, Dallas Eye Institute, 720 S. Cedar Ridge, Duncanville, TX 75137.

Be honest with yourself as well as with your patients. Charles Inlander, president of the People's Medical Society, points out, "The doctor has the information, tools, and the key to the rest of the system. Thus the doctor has enormous responsibility in providing information, advising candidly, and protecting the best interest of the patient.

"The physician has the advocacy role, and should use it," In-lander adds. You as the physician can be an advocate with your patients and the public for information as well as quality in all areas. Use the knowledge, influence, and educational opportuni-ties available through your status and position to ensure that you are informed about the best qualified providers, to maintain and upgrade your technical skills, and to inform your patients and the public about the range of providers and the benefits and risks of treatment options available to them.

Ultimately, this is the best way to satisfy patients and to pro-vide quality service. ❧

Action Steps for Proving Clinical Mastery

1. Recognize that patients are increasingly taking a "con-sumer approach" to evaluating medical care. Be pre-pared to provide them with information to help them evaluate your clinical expertise and that of other doctors.
2. Use outcome measurements and clinical parameters to make informed referral recommendations to patients or colleagues.
3. Manage your patients' expectations when making referrals to physicians who are technically excellent but fall short in patient interaction skills.
4. Evaluate your technical skills against available stan-dards and know your capabilities and limitations. Refer your patients to experts with appropriate skills when necessary.

References

1. B. Callahan, Despite his patients' pleas, eye doctor still can't practice, *San Diego Union* (August 14, 1992): 1.
2. D. M. Eddy, Decisions without information: The intellectual crisis in medicine, *People's Medical Society Newsletter* (December 1991): 1–6.
3. S. McIlrath, Quest for quality: Medicine cautiously optimistic about new PRO initiative on health care improvement, *American Medical News* (October 5, 1992): 1, 35–36.
4. R. Winslow, Questionnaire probes patients' quality of life, *Wall Street Journal* (July 7, 1992): B-1.
5. P. Keckley, ed., What is a high-quality physician? *Keckley Report on Health Care Market Research* (November 27, 1989): 2.
6. B.E. Spivey, Dr. Spivey calls for renewed principles of patient care, *Argus* (October 31, 1990): 1.
7. P.B. Ginsburg and G.T. Hammons, Competition and the quality of care: The importance of information, *Inquiry* (Spring 1988): 108–114.

16

Take a Walk in Your Patient's Shoes

You're sitting in a darkened theater, munching on popcorn with ersatz butter. The background music of the action-packed film swells and folds around you. You're enveloped in the turmoil and troubles of the characters. Suddenly, someone pipes up loudly, "Ha! Look at that car in the background! It's a 1949 Buick—and this movie is supposed to take place in 1943!" He continues to point out flaws until an usher shushes him.

Noticing the errors briefly diminishes your enjoyment of the film. But soon you're engrossed once again, the production glitches and outrageous script forgotten.

Next day your spouse talks you into going to another movie. You arrive late at the theater and discover that the only seats left are in the second row from the front. Your spouse insists on staying, adding that the movie has gotten four-star reviews. Twenty minutes into it, you wonder how anyone could rave about this witless, plotless movie. The longer you sit, the more you find to dislike, from the music (too raucous) to the humor (nonexistent) to the popcorn (stale).

The rating you give each movie contrasts dramatically. One had mistakes, but you overlooked them because the overall experience was favorable. "Two thumbs up!" you rhapsodize the next day to colleagues. In the second movie, every error in production, lighting, scripting, and theater ambience simply confirmed and compounded your opinion. "Trash!" you pronounce it.

We don't want to compare health care to movie making—one is real life and life giving, the other is fictional entertainment—but there are some similarities in how each experience is evaluated. Every health care experience is a compilation of expectations, personalities, and processes. Like the moviegoer rating a film, a patient's overall evaluation of his or her experience depends on the total picture, the accumulated moments of truth, not one individual frame. People aren't perfect, and processes have many parts, so mistakes will sometimes occur. From the highly trained staff and structured activities of the Mayo Clinic to the unpredictable pace of the one-physician, one-employee practice in rural America, service slip-ups occur. Even in the most tightly organized, customer-oriented practice, employees, doctors, and patients get short tempered, schedules get delayed, reports get misfiled, and phone calls get put on indefinite hold.

One incident is not likely to result in complete dissatisfaction. Patients who know you and your staff and who know that your normal practice style is efficient, friendly, and customer centered will forgive the noisy reception room—once. They will overlook having their phone call transferred to three different people if it seldom happens. They may ask more insistently for details about their scheduled laparoscopic cholecystectomy if they believe you haven't done your usual clear job of explaining things. They will call your bookkeeper with confusion, not anger, in their voice when the bill arrives showing a balance due that they've already paid if this is a rare occurrence.

MOMENTS OF TRUTH ADD UP

Your patients look at and judge their overall experience in your practice as an accumulation of *moments of truth*. If the accumulated moments weigh in on the favorable side of the scale with only one moment on the unfavorable side, the final assessment will probably be favorable. (We're assuming that the negative interaction is a small one and not one of major significance, of course.) Here's how a patient may subconsciously process the experience:

> *The doctor was friendly and informative; the staff were*
> *courteous; the office was clean and conveniently located; I*

only waited 10 minutes in the reception area; the practice is on my health plan. The check-out clerk seemed a little preoccupied, but that's the exception. The doctor gave me this videotape to look at because she figured out I needed more information, and she told me to call if my condition didn't clear up in a week. She seemed a little rushed, but the place was pretty busy, and usually she gives me her full attention.

Patients also tend to evaluate each visit to your practice from the perspective of their needs at the time, which may change from week to week. A secretary who is docked for every moment she is gone from work may put more priority on being seen on time today when she has taken time from her job for a routine Pap test. Two weeks ago, when she brought her son in for a fit-in appointment because of a high fever and an earache, getting full information about his condition and how to treat it was far more important than the dollars she lost from her paycheck because she had to wait an hour.

Look at your practice from the perspective of your patients, who on each visit evaluate the total experience. If you understand your patients' expectations collectively, and if you or your staff take a moment during the visit to identify each patient's specific needs, you're likely to get a thumbs up each and every time, even with the glitches and goof-ups that occur during a normal day in any practice.

A TYPICAL PATIENT VISIT, MOMENT BY MOMENT

In the following chapters, we'll look in detail at the typical office visit. We'll put a magnifying glass to it, helping you see your practice through your patients' eyes, so that you can whisk away the dust and clutter, eliminate the activities and processes that hinder productivity as well as satisfaction, and smooth the rough edges that irritate and diminish the professionalism of your office. By getting up close and personal, we'll help you see where a new approach, a better attitude, or a different way of doing things can make all the difference in the snapshot that patients have of your practice.

In Chapter 17, we'll take a look at the all important "first impression" created before your patients ever meet you—on the phone, in the reception area, and from the staff who greet them and take care of pre-exam essentials. Chapter 18 takes a close look at what happens when **you** enter the exam room—the actions and behaviors that create or diminish the doctor-patient relationship. Chapter 19 follows with follow-up: what happens when the doctor departs and the nurse, lab technician, check-out desk, billing/insurance clerk, surgical scheduler, and others take over to leave their lasting impressions with the patient.

Chapter 20 offers specifics on how to make the faceless telephone connection between staff and patients a positive interaction for patients. In Chapter 21, you'll learn why patients hate to wait and what other practices are doing to make sure their patients don't. Waiting time is such a critical service factor that we've devoted a separate chapter to developing a schedule that will help prevent or minimize excessive waiting time. The relationship between physician and patient is another critical aspect of patient satisfaction and practice success. Thus, several chapters are devoted to it, with tips on "the tie that bonds," communication, and partnership responsibilities.

Taking your patient's perspective will always be the surest way to give good service. Although prepaid health plans and third party payers are exerting more and more control over patient choice, a great deal of individual discretion remains. A 1990 *Medical Economics* survey found that two of five patients reported having switched doctors because they disliked something about the doctor or his or her methods or assistants.[1] By evaluating your practice as your patients do, you stand a better chance of making the numbers add up to a positive rating, even if an occasional negative shows up in the column.

ACCENTUATE THE POSITIVE AND DELETE THE NEGATIVES

It's an accumulation of negative numbers that leads to an unfavorable rating—of you as a physician, the care you provide, and your practice in total. A single bad "moment of truth" won't drive a patient away (unless it's associated with something of overwhelming importance to the patient), but a heap of them will. Here's how one woman described the sequence of events that led her to move her family of four from one physician to another:

> We had been very happy with the diagnostic and treatment care from the doctor we used, although we were not impressed with his office management. We always had to wait more than I considered reasonable, and once we were forgotten for almost 2 hours. On another occasion, I had taken my daughter in for a sore throat. The 2-minute strep screen tested negative, but I later learned the 3-day culture was positive for a staph infection. More than a week after the culture, I came home to find a phone message on our answering machine: "Mrs. R., please call the practice. Dr. L. wonders how Gina is doing." When I called, I was told they had been leaving messages on my home answering machine for a week. I hadn't gotten any of the messages. My daughter should have been put on antibiotics as soon as the lab report came back positive. I expressed anger that the office hadn't made a greater effort to contact me by calling my office, and I was told they never call people at work unless specifically asked to do so. Dr. L. has no policy brochure; how was I to know this? I insisted on speaking to the doctor about the possible consequences of the untreated infection and to express my dissatisfaction. He said he would check into the problem, but never got back to me.

> We belong to a PPO; only one doctor of this two-physician practice is a provider. Several times, we were led to believe that we would see the PPO physician, when in fact the partner was the only one in the office. We had to pay a higher deductible for seeing the nonprovider physician.

> The final straw occurred when my husband woke up one Sunday morning with severe vertigo. The answering service put us in touch with the doctor on call from another practice. He said he would phone in a prescription to the pharmacy and emphasized that my husband should be seen by our doctor the next day. It took almost 4 hours before the on-

call doctor phoned the prescription in to the pharmacy. The next day, my husband called Dr. L.'s office to request an appointment and mentioned the covering doctor's recommendation that he be seen that day. The receptionist said she didn't know if she could get him in. At that point, he said thank you, hung up, and called another doctor. We don't plan to go back to Dr. L.

As you review the next nine chapters as well as the rest of this book, take your patients' perspective. Play back a typical office visit like a videotape, and view it as your patient would. Walk in his or her shoes through your office; see and hear yourself and your staff through your patient's eyes and ears. Are your services customer oriented? Do you and your staff members sound compassionate and informative? Do your words and actions say that you care?

How would you rate yourself, your staff, and the accumulated "moments of truth" if **you** were the patient? ❧

Reference

1. H. Eisenberg, How your patients feel about you, *Medical Economics* (April 23, 1990): 49–80.

17

Your Practice and Your Patients: Love at First Sight?

The gynecologist had been highly recommended to the woman, who was new to the city and seeking to establish herself with a personal physician. She also needed a routine prescription refilled. Knowing that no reputable physician would renew a prescription without first seeing the patient, she called the office to request a brief initial visit:

> *The person I spoke with said that the doctor could not possibly do what I was asking, that I would need a full extensive exam and the cost would be $250; and how would I be paying for it? I once again explained my situation, pointing out that I was already scheduled by my new employer for a comprehensive physical, including Pap smear, and it seemed a wasteful duplication of service and expense. I asked if there wasn't some flexibility and was told in a very abrupt tone, "That's not the way the doctor practices medicine." The doctor may have been wonderful and caring, but her apparent inflexible approach lost her a new patient. I told the receptionist this; she did not seem sorry at all, and did not offer to have the doctor or anyone else on staff explain the policy further. The impression I got from the conversation was that **money** was the overriding factor in enforcing this policy.*

Just as Mom told you when you were growing up, you never get a second chance to make a good first impression. For your patients, that first impression sets the expectations for their encounter with your practice and sets the tone for your relationship. Dr. Gilmore, the Denver internist, knows this: "The first visit is important to patients. They're giving you a chance to get to know them, and they're measuring you. If I get to know them well on their first visit, follow-up visits are much simpler. They don't feel shortchanged." Dr. Gilmore gives her new patients a lasting, lengthy positive first impression with a 1-hour visit—a comprehensive lifestyle, medical, and personal overview. And she starts the appointment on time, every time.

Mark Allison, MD, of the multispecialty Springer Clinic in Tulsa, Oklahoma, discovered how important that first impression can be. An elderly man was referred to him for a possible cataract. In his usual lighthearted manner, Dr. Allison made several jokes during the exam, but realized at the conclusion of the visit that he had failed to establish rapport with the patient. Nevertheless, the man scheduled surgery. During his post-op visit, the patient confided in the nurse, "I think a doctor should be serious. My eyesight is a serious matter to me. But I decided I had confidence in Dr. Allison's surgical skill, and I liked the office staff a lot. That's why I scheduled the surgery." Although the first impression Dr. Allison made was not favorable, his patient gave him a second chance. The ophthalmologist has since worked to earn his patient's respect and to create a positive relationship with his patient—one that matches the favorable impression his staff had already made.

HOW DO YOU CREATE A GOOD FIRST IMPRESSION EVERY TIME?

Let's say you and your staff are committed to taking good care of your patients and that you'd like to start off on the right foot (or feet). You bring your front office and back office staff together regularly to talk about how to give the best possible service and the best possible medical care. How do you fulfill your patients' expectations? How do you make a good impression every time?

The first step is to look at your practice from your patients' perspective. Are your patients elderly and suffering from hearing or vision loss, arthritic changes, or possibly loss of a mate? Are your patients youngsters with parents who work full time? The idea is to walk, see, and listen from your patients' multiple perspectives. Think through every step they take in getting medical care in your office.

FIRST, PATIENTS MUST FIND YOU

Are you listed in the White Pages and the Yellow Pages of the telephone book? How are you listed? Patients might look under more than one category of the Yellow Pages for a physician in your specialty. Does your ad tell patients about your services, office hours, location(s), and other convenience features?

If you care for patients whose vision may be impaired, is the type in your ad or listing large enough for them to read? Is the sign in front of your office readable?

Do referring physicians, your medical society, the hospitals where you practice, and the managed care plans in which you participate have current information about you, your skills, and your practice?

PATIENTS MUST MAKE CONTACT WITH YOUR OFFICE

Are your telephones answered by staff rather than an answering service during hours when patients are likely to call? Many people need to make telephone calls before they start work themselves or on their lunch breaks. If your telephones are answered by a service during these times, you're making it difficult for patients to contact you. This is not the best way to start a relationship. An added benefit of making your staff available for longer periods of time instead of relying on an answering service is that your incoming calls will be spaced more manageably.

When your staff members answer the telephone, is their response quick, friendly, and efficient? Is the call answered without being immediately placed on hold? (You've had this happen: "Hello, doctor's office. Hold please.") If your staff frequently find it necessary to ask callers to hold, you may need more people answering the telephone, you may need more lines, or you may need to extend the hours your telephone is answered. Chapter 20 has detailed information about how you and your staff can make a positive first and continuing impression on the telephone.

When a new patient calls, it's important to find out about his or her insurance so that misunderstandings can be headed off early. But doing so without sounding offensive requires more than a little tact. One way to handle this important issue so that the staff person doesn't come across sounding as if money is the first priority of the practice is to use a phrase such as this: "So that we may have the proper paperwork ready for you, what insurance plan do you belong to?" If this question reveals that the patient is insured by a plan that you do not accept, or does not have any medical coverage, your staff can politely inform him or her of financial arrangements that are required. ("I'm sorry, but Dr. Internist doesn't participate in the ABC Plan. We'll be happy to schedule your appointment. You just need to know that your insurance won't pay us directly for your visit and the charge for a first visit is approximately $58. We'll provide all the paperwork for you to file your insurance.")

Do you make your fees known in advance to your patients? There is considerable controversy about this, but many physicians are finding that patients appreciate knowing approximate fees before services are rendered. One way to do this is to write a friendly "letter to my patients," stating that you too are concerned about rising medical costs, and to list your most common visits, procedures, and fees together with an invitation for patients to inquire about other fees through your office manager or a designated staff member. Place a stack of the letters in the reception area so that patients can take one. Although we don't necessarily recommend posting a "menu of services and prices" in your reception area, it is a good idea to have a policy, protocol, and designated staff person(s) who can discuss fees, payment options, and especially alternatives for uninsured patients or those with low incomes.

HOW DO YOU HANDLE DOCTOR SHOPPERS?

Do you have a way to accommodate patients who are "shopping" for a doctor? Allow time for get-acquainted interviews for potential patients. Many physicians charge a regular office visit for these interviews, but those who do them as a courtesy report that the marketing benefit far outweighs the fee they would earn. These interviews should be scheduled at a time when your office manager or nurse is available; allow 10- or 15-minute appointment slots to get acquainted with the potential patient.

When a new patient is scheduled and there is time to send information by mail before the appointment, send a personalized letter confirming the appointment, welcoming the patient to your practice, and explaining your office policies and procedures. This friendly letter can set the right tone so that you and your patients work effectively together. Take care that it doesn't come across like some letters we've seen, as a briefing on "rules of conduct for our patients." Consider enclosing a medical history form for the patient to fill out before he or she arrives for the first appointment, and enclose a business card. It's also a nice gesture to enclose a map showing patients how to locate your office and, in big medical complexes, where to park.

What's your method for scheduling patients? Do you leave plenty of room in your schedule for unexpected problems? If your sick patients can't get in to see you promptly, take a look at your scheduling system (you'll get help with this in Chapter 22).

Does your schedule make it possible to run your office on time? Does a 3 p.m. appointment mean 4:15 on a good day? When you are running chronically late, something is wrong. Do you have extended or weekend office hours? Evening and Saturday morning appointments are popular with many patients; parents with school-aged children especially appreciate the opportunity to see their pediatricians for well-child visits on Saturday mornings.

Chauncey McHargue, MD, a dermatologist in Culpepper, Virginia, opens his office two nights a week until 9 p.m. Although he and his staff work 12 hours on those days, the office is closed on Fridays. His patient satisfaction strategy has been very welcome to his semirural population. He says, "I can't go out during the day to see my dentist, so why should I expect my patients to take off from work to see me?" Working professionals and families with children especially appreciate the evening hours, he adds.

If a patient becomes ill on a holiday, how does he or she reach you? Is your answering service responsive? If you're not sure, have your spouse or a close friend place a call to you, posing as a patient. What kind of response does he or she get? How does your office staff respond to calls for medical advice? Does your office nurse or someone truly qualified screen your calls? Put yourself in your patients' shoes. Ask a family member or close friend to pose as a patient and make a call asking for medical advice.

In an attempt to cross-train his staff and broaden their opportunities for career growth, an Albuquerque pediatrician occasionally used the office receptionist to screen calls for medical advice. She had only minimal medical experience, and parents didn't feel comfortable that she was accurately relaying their questions to the physician or that she was accurately relaying his advice back to them.

Hesitant to complain about the friendly but less-than-competent receptionist upon whom they depended to gain access to the doctor, parents were increasingly uneasy. The pediatrician didn't immediately pick up on the problem. He was pleased that his receptionist was showing an interest in broadening her experience, and having an employee who was capable of doing more than just one job was really helpful. Finally, one of the doctor's close friends called for advice regarding an infant who showed signs of being allergic to an antibiotic. The receptionist, warm and friendly as ever, took the parent's question, discussed it with the doctor, and called the parent back with his advice. The parent, a former pediatric nurse, didn't feel that the response made sense. She asked to speak to the doctor personally and had to be firm and insistent to get past the receptionist. Once she did speak with the pediatrician, they discovered that his advice had not been relayed accurately. When the physician asked some of his patients how their calls were handled, he discovered, to his embarrassment, that the receptionist left many of them feeling that their concerns weren't dealt with appropriately.

A triage policy for handling phone calls could have avoided this ongoing problem. You'll find information about developing a telephone triage system in Chapter 20. (We tell this story not to discourage cross-training of staff but to encourage careful, accurate, and thorough training to avoid incidents such as this—and potential malpractice liability.)

DOCUMENT ALL CALLS AND PATIENT CONTACT

When you get a call at night or on weekends, how do you keep a record of it? Keep a log of every call, and have the information transcribed into the patient's chart. To keep transcription time to a minimum, use a separate sheet for each call, and have the sheet attached directly to the chart. This is critical for accurate, comprehensive documentation; it also conveys to patients that there is continuity in your care, no matter what time of day or night it occurs.

What's it like to park in your parking lot? Far too many practices still do as one Phoenix, Arizona pediatric practice did, which irritated its patients by providing covered parking clearly marked "for doctors only" immediately in front of the building while parents with sick children were forced to park in the blazing sun.

Is the location of your office convenient to patients? Do they feel safe coming and leaving? Can patients find directional signs and open doors? One rheumatology group was embarrassed to be told by a wheelchair-bound patient that the front door of the office building owned by the practice was so stiff and heavy that her elderly husband couldn't open it without help. The 1991 Americans with Disabilities Act mandates not only sensitivity to the needs of the disabled but accessibility as well. You can't afford to make your practice difficult to get around in, legally or from a patient satisfaction perspective.

WHAT KIND OF IMPRESSION DOES YOUR OFFICE MAKE?

When patients arrive, what do they see? Your entire office, including the entryway, should be immaculate. Keeping the fingerprints off the glass doors and keeping floors swept or vacuumed can be time consuming in a busy office, but a dirty or disheveled appearance sends a message you don't want to hear. In Dr. Stephen Hales' office, as soon as the last morning patient leaves at noon, a staff member heads for the reception area to straighten magazines, pick up toys, wipe up fingerprints, and make it "first-impression perfect." The selection of magazines at this practice, by the way, reflects diverse patient interests. It includes *Working Mother, Mirabella, Architectural Digest*, and the *New Yorker* as well as children's reading material.

Arlan Cohn, MD, the Berkeley, California internist, knows that attention to decorating and housekeeping details pays off: "I think a doctor's office should be like a home, with good magazines, good books, lighting that's bright but flattering, homey furniture. The exam room should be comfortable, not crowded and cluttered. It should give patients confidence. I try to lighten the atmosphere with color and paintings. Instruments should be kept out of sight. I once went to a proctologist's office and he had every kind of viewing instrument hanging on the examining room walls, like instruments of torture."

Housekeeping, Dr. Cohn believes, is important. "I look at my office every day as a patient would. There may be a discarded paper towel under the exam table that patients see, but I don't see it unless I look for it." What he says is good advice. View your office from your patient's vantage point, and you'll see things you don't see from your side of the examining table. He offers additional suggestions for making a good impression in his book *Kill as Few Patients as Possible*, a series of humorous essays about "how to be the world's best doctor." A few of these suggestions by Dr. Cohn (who writes under the pseudonym Oscar London, MD) are in Exhibit 17-1.[1(pp.5-6)]

COMFORT IS IMPORTANT

Gynecologists and other specialists whose patients are predominantly women know that comfort is a significant first-impression factor. For obstetrician/gynecologist Susan Northrup, MD, of Scottsdale, Arizona, patient comfort was a driving force in furnishing and equipping the office. Private changing areas, cloth gowns instead of paper, comfortable room temperature, and other "little things" mean a lot in Dr. Northrup's practice. New patients are seen first in the physician's office, not the exam room. (This matters! One woman, describing a visit to a new doctor, expressed favorable amazement that the visit did not begin with a request from the nurse to strip, put on a gown, and wait on the exam table for the physician's arrival.)

Is the front office configured so that waiting patients can easily overhear conversations that should be kept private? Please don't resort to the impersonal sliding glass window to solve this problem. Front desk staffers should be trained to speak in low tones

Exhibit 17-1 Excerpts from *Kill As Few Patients As Possible*

Rule 2. Have a Lovely Office

. . . A doctor's office should be decorated tastefully—but not expensively, unless he prefers a burglar over a janitor to clean up after hours.

. . . He must not pipe music into his waiting room. If he has a burning desire to inflict music on his patients, he should bring in a live string quartet and restrict them to Haydn . . . if he wants to destroy his practice, he might consider bringing in an accordion player. (One night at a restaurant, I reached out and plunged my dinner knife into the bellows of an approaching accordion; the stricken look on the player's face when the wind was knocked out of his "Lady of Spain" was well worth the price of damages.)

He should choose indoor plants for his waiting room carefully. That unseemly bulge in his Venus flytrap might have been his three o'clock appointment.

Source: Reprinted from *Kill As Few Patients As Possible, and 56 Other Essays on How To Be the World's Best Doctor* by O. London, pp. 5–6, with permission of Ten-Speed Press, © 1987.

and to adjourn to a private office when discussions with patients touch on personal and sensitive issues. The sliding glass window is a cold and outdated physical barrier that is seldom seen in a customer-oriented practice.

What happens at check-in? Is patient confidentiality respected? Gustavo Colon, MD, of New Orleans, Louisiana provides individual cards for patients to sign when they check in; there's no scribbled listing of patient names, addresses, and telephone numbers for every new arrival to scan (see Exhibit 17-2). The Heart Center sends new patients a "membership card" that immediately establishes a relationship with the practice and entitles them to discounts at local retailers (Exhibit 17-3).

MAKE A GOOD FIRST IMPRESSION WITH A PERSONAL INTRODUCTION

Physicians at the Sansum Clinic in Santa Barbara, California make a superb first impression. The patient's physician person-

Exhibit 17-2 Sample Check-In Card

Gustavo A. Colon, MD

A Medical Corporation

SIGN-IN CARD

Name _____

Date _____

Time _____

Source: Courtesy of Gustavo A. Colon, MD, New Orleans, Louisiana.

ally comes to the waiting room to introduce himself or herself and escorts the patient to the consultation office for a get-acquainted chat. A patient services representative who is a registered nurse is also available to handle patient concerns and requests. Throughout the clinic, attention to patient comfort and privacy is apparent in seating arrangements, use of color, and lighting that casts a warm glow.

Is your reception area comfortable for the patients you serve? Older persons, pregnant women, and patients with arthritis or orthopedic problems appreciate chairs that are easy to get in and out of. Do you have a wheelchair or walker available for patients who need them? (You'll find an exercise in Chapter 31 to help sensitize the whole practice team to the needs of the elderly as well as other suggestions for addressing special needs of patients.) Is the restroom well-marked, accessible, and nearby? Is there fresh drinking water available? Some practices provide light refreshments in the reception area; if you do this, choose food and drink that are healthy and easy to keep tidy.

Use your reception area as a place to educate your patients. Stock a rack with brochures and helpful articles that relate to your specialty. Add information about community services and agencies, special events, and programs relevant to your specialty or wellness in general. (Just call local agencies and organizations; they'll be happy to keep you stocked with information and up-

Exhibit 17-3 The Heart Center Membership Card

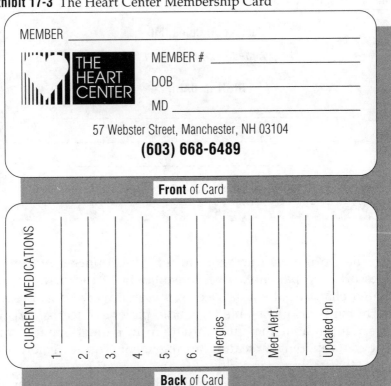

Source: Courtesy of The Heart Center, Manchester, New Hampshire.

dates.) Some practices have VCRs with tapes that relate to their specialty or bulletin boards with notices of interest to patients (support group meetings, safety recall notices of baby products, etc.). This sends a message that you're as interested in helping your patients stay healthy as you are in treating their illnesses.

PEOPLE TREAT OTHERS AS THEY ARE TREATED

Don't forget your internal customers: your staff. People treat others as they are treated. Just ask the CEO of a very successful company: William Marriott of Marriott hotels. He says that the key to his organization's success is creating satisfied customers

and satisfied employees. Marriott has found that happy, contented employees tend to treat customers better, thus increasing the customers' satisfaction with the hotels. Within your practice, do you provide an employee break room, restrooms, and a lunch room with microwave, refrigerator, table, and chairs? Are these areas attractively furnished, or are they equipped with cast-off items rejected by the local thrift store? Employees need to get away from the stress of the work environment during the day; give them a comfortable and pleasant place to do so, and they'll return to their jobs with a positive and patient-pleasing attitude. At Swagel Wootton Eye Care in Mesa, Arizona, the physicians join the staff in the lunch room, where they socialize, discuss what's happened during the day, and solidify working relationships.

Why are all these little details such a big deal? It's much easier to establish rapport with your patients if they are in a positive frame of mind. Your interaction with them is very important, but it is only a fraction of what they experience when they visit your practice. Leverage the time you spend with your patients by making sure that every contact with your practice is as positive as it can be. ❧

Action Steps To Make a Positive First Impression

1. Make sure a patient's first impression of your practice is a good one by communicating your values to front and back office staff.
2. Evaluate your Yellow Pages listing. Be sure listings are comprehensive and provide key information.
3. Train your staff to handle telephone calls in a friendly, efficient, and courteous manner.
4. Ensure that staff handle insurance and billing questions tactfully.
5. Make "get-acquainted" appointments available to new patients.
6. Send new patient information by mail before the first appointment.
7. Make patient-sensitive scheduling options available in your practice.
8. Check to be sure that your answering service is responsive to the needs of ill patients and that office staff handle calls for medical advice appropriately.
9. Document all calls and patient contact.
10. Assess your office environment, inside and out, for accessibility, convenience, and appearance.
11. Establish protocols to protect patient confidentiality and privacy.
12. Provide employees with a comfortable break/lunch room and restrooms.

Reference

1. O. London, *Kill As Few Patients As Possible and 56 Other Essays on How To Be the World's Best Doctor* (Berkeley, Calif.: Ten-Speed Press, 1987): 5–6.

18

Doctor, Take Your Hand Off the Doorknob!

Unable to tolerate his symptoms, the nagging worry, or his worried spouse any longer, Mr. Roth has decided to see a doctor. Asking around, he gets a favorable recommendation from two co-workers and makes an appointment with you. He has found your office building and has navigated the parking lot, the reception area, and the front desk.

Now he is ready to meet you and your staff for diagnosis, discussion, and treatment. His perception of this brief time spent with you and your office staff depends on everything he sees, hears, and senses in the practice: what the office itself looks like, how he is greeted, and the professionalism of the nurse who weighs him and takes his blood pressure. Once he is brought into the exam room, it's pretty much up to you. Mr. Roth will listen, observe, and evaluate. And like it or not, much of Mr. Roth's medical outcome depends on the rapport that develops between the two of you. If he has confidence in you, he's more likely to listen carefully to you, to ask questions, and to follow your advice. If he believes you are concerned about **him,** not just his prostate problem, Mr. Roth is likely to regard the medical care you provide as high quality. On the other hand, if doctor-patient rapport is limited, the patient is likely to evaluate the medical care as poor.

You like what you do, and you like your patients. You hope that your patients feel the same about you and your practice. You and the other physicians in your group, with the help of your staff, have formulated a philosophy for the practice. You've even put it in writing: Your mission statement says that patients always come first, and this means giving the best possible service and topnotch medical care. But you're faced with the practical question: *How to deliver on this pledge?*

WALK IN YOUR PATIENT'S SHOES

The answer is the same low-tech method advocated in the previous chapter: Put yourself in your patient's shoes.

A 55-year-old Tennessee woman told us, "I can't judge my doctor's clinical competence. But I am a good judge of people. I know when somebody is really listening to me, when he's distracted by other things, and when he's just plain not interested in working with me. I can tell when somebody cares. And caring is a big, big part of the relationship I have with my doctor."

This woman's views are not unique. They are reflected again and again in consumer surveys and one-on-one interviews. People want *personal interest* and *concern* from their physician, that is, caring.

We distributed questionnaires to patients in the practices we visited. One of the questions was, "What is the one thing you wish doctors would do to ensure a positive experience during your visit?" Here are a few of the responses:

- Treat you as an individual. Show personal interest. Act like they're really concerned about you.
- Look at a person as a total health care entity—not just a particular problem or disease.
- Some doctors seem not to be too concerned about the person as an individual (just one of the numbers). Treat **each** one and be genuinely concerned with their needs. **Listen.**

Dr. Arlan Cohn echoes these sentiments: "Medicine is not all that scientific. We doctors have information that a patient needs. The best way for me to convey that information is to make the patient feel I have nothing else to do during his time in my office."

BRING PATIENTS INTO YOUR "LIVING ROOM"

Easy to say, but how do you make the patient feel that he or she has your undivided, **caring** attention, especially in the typically hectic office? Dr. Cohn keeps his desk free of clutter and brings patients there for consultation before the exam. "It's like the 'living room' of my office. I can visit with patients and family members and give them my undivided attention."

Stepping into the patient's shoes and walking through an office visit reveals a lot about a practice. A practice that provides a little cupboard in the restroom for patients to leave urine samples discreetly sends a message to grateful patients: "Your dignity is important to us." Medical professionals who are accustomed to routinely handling urine samples forget that people come into their office from a world where no grown-up walks around in public with a container of bodily waste.

Weighing patients in a private area is important to the patient who dreads facing the numbers. Structuring an office visit so that new patients first meet the doctor with their clothes on says, "We know you're more than a sore throat." Escorting a patient to the exam room with the comment, "Dr. Appleby will be in to see you in about 5 minutes; here's the new *Reader's Digest* to fill those 5 minutes" demonstrates caring. Hanging calming or amusing posters on exam room walls or hanging a mobile from the ceiling over the exam table lightens up a potentially tense part of the visit. It's this kind of sensitivity that can make your back office people sensitive and comfortable, a good place to get quality medical care.

The environment sets the stage, but it's the personal interaction between physician and patient that gives the visit a rating of 10, or 0. Many physicians who are known for their successful relationships with patients point out that not all patients and physicians can effectively work together. "I'm as picky about my patients as I am about my staff," says Saul Schreiber, MD. "I can't effectively treat everyone, and I'm honest about that up front. If I feel we aren't communicating, I point that out and advise the patient to find another doctor, someone they will work better with." Dr. Cohn employs a similar strategy: "The first visit introduces us to each other; if I can see that the patient is argumentative or combative and we can't work together, I politely tell him that we're not compatible."

CREATING RAPPORT: PLAIN OLD PEOPLE SKILLS

Establishing rapport in a brief office visit isn't magic. It takes plain old "people skills," and they come more naturally to some than to others. Here are a few tips that were gleaned from physicians around the country:

- Familiarize yourself with the patient's history **before** you enter the exam room. One patient commented, "I was pleasantly surprised when my doctor made reference to something personal in my life. He had probably read it in the chart, but at least it showed me he **had** read the chart." Don't read the chart and ask questions at the same time; patients need your attention and eye contact. You may be impressed by your abilities to read, write, and ask questions at the same time, but your patients won't be. A high-tech yet patient-pleasing approach to history taking is used by Ray Hughes, MD, the Phoenix, Arizona physician. For many years he has used a computer in the examination room to take the patient history. Patients love it—he focuses on them as he types on the keyboard, and they get a printed copy of the diagnosis, treatment plan, and summary at the end of the visit. It's a rapport builder, a time saver, and a referral generator, Dr. Hughes reports. "When they see the detail and documentation that goes into the chart, patients get a better understanding of what goes into the diagnostic and treatment process," he says. Other benefits: Patients get tangible, educational information to take home for review with family; staff members can review the chart any time after the visit and know exactly what took place in case patient or referral source calls come in; and risk management experts give him rave reviews (see one of the many letters Dr. Hughes has received in Exhibit 18-1).
- If you've asked patients to fill out a medical history, particularly a lengthy one, take the time to read their answers. Patients say they don't mind filling out questionnaires if they feel that the information is used, but they resent filling them out and then being asked the same questions verbally with no indication that their written responses were reviewed.

Exhibit 18-1 Risk Management Letter

Cigna Private Practice Plan of Arizona
11001 N. Black Canyon Highway
Suite 400
Phoenix, AZ 85029

August 3, 1992

Ray Hughes, MD
717 W. Glendale Avenue
Phoenix, AZ 85021

Congratulations! Your scores for Provider Performance Appraisal/Facility Review were shared with me by our Quality Management Nurse Reviewer, Barbara Jones. It is a rare occasion that we have the pleasure of seeing scores of 100% on both chart and facility audits. Mrs. Jones told me that it was definitely a first for her. This is the type of environment we would like all of our members to experience.

Sincerely,

Robert F. Beauchamp, MD
Vice President and Medical Director

cc: Provider File
Provider Representative

Source: Courtesy of Ray D. Hughes, MD, 717 W. Glendale Avenue, Phoenix, Arizona.

- Ask a personal question first. It shows the concern patients look for. Ask if anything has changed since the patient's last visit (job, relationships, family matters, economics, etc.). An internist saw a 40-year-old woman for aching joints. She hadn't seen the patient in more than a year and learned only through casual conversation that the woman had had a baby in the interim. One way to find out about any changes in a patient's health status is to ask for this information at registration by giving the patient a quick form to fill out. This should include questions about any new medications or reactions to previously prescribed ones as well as about other physicians consulted since the previous visit.

> "Well, I see by your (medical) chart that you have a nice life," says the doctor with easy charm. Then, to my astonishment, he asks my husband about himself. That small gesture establishes instant rapport. "I see you're a journalist," he says, turning to me. . . . (It's not that I want VIP treatment. I just want to be seen as an individual, not just another anonymous jowled "before" face.)[1(p.123)]

- Wash your hands in the exam room, in front of the patient. Patients appreciate your attention to basic hygiene.

A LIGHT TOUCH IS ALL IT TAKES

Make physical contact with the patient; extend your hand for an adult-to-adult handshake. Touch the patient on the shoulder or arm on leaving the room. Don't forget the parent or spouse; acknowledge him or her with a handshake also. Dr. Hales, the New Orleans pediatrician examines babies on his lap, undressing them as he examines them. Older babies sit on Mom's lap; toddlers and older children sit on a chair. "I use the examining table if necessary, but most of the time I don't. You can give a very thorough and competent exam this way without ever freaking the child out," he says.

Sit down when you talk with your patient. Says Dr. Hales, "In medical school, we were taught to stay close to the door, to never allow the patient's mother to get between us and the door. That keeps your visits brief, but it doesn't do much to foster communication."

Look at your patient when you speak to him or her. If an interpreter is needed for someone whose language you don't speak or for someone who is deaf or hearing impaired, make eye contact with the patient, not the interpreter or signer, when you reply.

Pay attention to body language. Folded arms may say, "I'm skeptical." Leaning forward says, "Tell me more." Match your communication style to the patient's. An anesthesiologist said, "Some people want to know every detail while others want simple, old-fashioned reassurance that I'll take good care of them. Period. Sometimes the patient wants reassurance and the family wants details. Sometimes it's the other way around. The patient is my first priority, but I really try to accommodate everybody with what they need from me. Everybody is different."

Make a note in the patient's chart for problems to follow up on. If today's appointment is for an earache but the patient was in for a bruised hip a year ago, ask about the hip. Even for insignificant problems, follow-up makes sense and lets patients know you're tuned in to them. If you won't be seeing a patient for a while and you're concerned about a potentially serious problem, call the patient at home and inquire. A pediatrician was concerned about a newborn's breath-holding spells. She placed the baby on a home apnea monitor and called the parents each morning for a week, inquiring about how the baby did the night before. The worried and exhausted mother said, "I felt better, just knowing she was checking on us."

If you're wrong, admit it. Convey to patients early in your relationship that medicine isn't an exact science. Establish an open, honest, adult-to-adult relationship. Let them know that you're in this together and that an effective doctor-patient relationship will have its share of ups and downs. (Check with your malpractice insurance policy if you're inclined to do this. Some policies don't allow the physician to admit to any kind of problem.)

ASK PATIENTS WHAT THEY WANT

Ask patients, "What is your goal for this visit?" At the end of the visit, ask, "What else do we need to discuss today?" If the patient brings up another major problem that doesn't need immediate attention, let him or her know you're concerned and that you want to take adequate time to address it. Say something like this: "Let's schedule an appointment for next week when we can talk specifically about that. I want to give your problem the time it deserves." Plastic surgeon Gustavo Colon, MD, leans on his assistant, a social worker by training, to spend time with patients who seek standard information about surgery: "Say a patient comes in for a quick follow-up after surgery, and during the visit she says she's considering a face lift. We've only scheduled a brief amount of time for her follow-up appointment, but realistically we now have a new patient. That's when I depend on the skills of my assistant to help answer the patient's questions. I explain that this is something she is very good at, and I want the patient to get the best answers, which my assistant can provide." Of course, he has trained his assistant to give answers that reflect his views.

Ask, "What's the best thing going on in your life right now? The worst thing?" Besides shedding light on the patient's psychological status, the answers may give you a clue as to what's going on medically. A grandmother who was in for low back pain joyfully reported that the best thing in her life was a recent visit from an out-of-town grandson. Her astute internist asked, "What does he weigh?" Only then did it occur to the woman that her back pain might have resulted from an active little guy named Ryan.

Avoid using medical jargon. Think of how you might describe a condition or treatment to your mother—or better yet, your sixth-grade child—and speak so that he or she could understand you. A pediatrician learned this lesson by first-hand experience. He explained to some new parents and their family that their baby was born with respiratory depression. The problem was transient, and the baby was fine after only a few minutes of stimulation and oxygen therapy. The family members, however, heard only one word: depression. At the baby's discharge from the hospital, when the grandmother earnestly asked, "How can we cheer him up so he's not depressed?" the pediatrician realized the miscommunication.

Use physician and staff gatherings to come up with ordinary terms for, and simple ways of explaining, medicalese. Say *gall-bladder surgery* rather than *cholecystectomy, blood in the urine* rather than *hematuria*, and *fluid in the joint* rather than *effusion*. When discussing diet, say *beans* rather than *legumes*.

When treating a patient, emphasize that you are interested in the outcome: "If you aren't better in 7 days, please call me. There are some other things we can consider, but let's try this first."

GET AGREEMENT FOR GREATER COMPLIANCE

When concluding an office visit, say, "Let's be sure we agree on our plan." Getting your patient to participate and believe in your treatment plan by explaining options and alternatives and the merits and negatives of each ultimately is an approach that aids compliance and assures you that the patient understands what to expect.

Consider having a nurse or medical assistant with you when seeing patients. Some physicians use the staffer as a recordkeeper, a scribe who takes notes as the physician and patient talk. This keeps the physician's attention on the interaction with the patient. The staff member can also act as eyes and ears, pointing out body language, facial expressions, and other subtle signs of disagreement or unhappiness you may miss.

Dictate your findings and treatment plan in the exam room in front of the patient. This makes good use of your time; it also allows the patient the opportunity to correct any misinformation as well as to ask questions that he or she may have forgotten. If you, like many physicians, include psychosocial assessment you don't wish your patient to hear, add this after the visit before you go on to the next exam room.

Call patients after surgery or hospitalization, when you've prescribed a new medication with potential side effects, or after consults with referral physicians. Your call shows concern and continuity of care between providers, and it may head off problems before they develop. With today's abbreviated hospital stays, a telephone call is particularly appropriate. A number of practices call every new patient within a day or two of the visit. If you feel that you don't have the time yourself, have a staff member make this call. Record in the medical chart every patient contact, whether it occurs in person, by letter, by telephone, by you or a staff member.

One surgeon reported calling a patient at home the day after a breast biopsy: "Her husband said, 'She's doing fine, except for all that itching.' I asked, 'All what itching?' and he very casually explained that she couldn't sleep because of itching all over. She had developed an allergy to codeine, and her pain pills were the culprit. She and her husband thought the problem was a new kitten her kids had given her. My phone call solved the problem before it got any worse." Besides conveying concern and ferreting out potential problems, these phone calls are practice builders, strengthening customer loyalty and encouraging patient referrals. A number of physicians told us that they use drive time routinely to call patients seen the day before, and they attribute practice growth to this personal touch.

KNOW WHAT YOUR PATIENTS ARE WORRIED ABOUT

Make the patient's priorities your priorities. Most orthopedic patients have endured more than a few jokes about surgeons operating on the wrong leg, but the possibility of such a mix-up is more the fuel for pre-op nightmares than for hilarity. Dr. Schreiber addresses that head-on: He writes "No" on the good knee. The message? "I know you're worried about it. And by addressing the problem, I save you the concern and the embarrassment of telling me you're worried."

Conclude your clinical visit in the exam room or a private office. Don't continue your conversation in the public hallway or at the check-out desk. It's too easy to say things such as, "Now if you have any more of that rectal pain, we'll need to see you again." Patients may seem cordial during such an exchange, but they're probably secretly plotting how to humiliate you in front of your employees.

RAPPORT RESULTS IN SATISFACTION—YOUR PATIENTS' AND YOURS

As we've seen, the connection created between physician and patient is the thread that weaves patient satisfaction and a successful practice. It's what makes patients loyal, makes them follow instructions, pay their bills on time, forgive mistakes, feel confident about your competence, and send friends to your practice. The rapport you create with your patients brings them back. As ophthalmologist Joe Noreika, MD, observes, "We have to come to work day after day. If we do everything we can to make it a positive experience for our patients, we'll enjoy what we do a whole lot more as well." ❧

Action Steps for Creating Rapport

1. Step into your patients' shoes; see through their eyes; hear through their ears.
2. Give each patient your undivided, caring attention during the exam or consultation.
3. Furnish and decorate your exam rooms with special touches that show sensitivity and personality.
4. Read the patient's chart before entering the exam room, and make a note of something personal on which to comment.
5. Touch your patient lightly on the arm or shoulder or with a handshake, and look directly at him or her when you speak.
6. Ask patients what they want or expect from the visit, and at the conclusion ask if their needs were met.
7. Seek compliance by asking for agreement to a treatment plan.

Reference

1. Shopping for a new face, *Allure* (August 1992): 117–131.

19

Follow-Up and Follow-Through for Satisfied Patients

Ask anyone who has had even a slight skirmish with the health care system about the source of irritation, and chances are the answer will concern billing and the paperwork involved. And anybody who has had a **real** battle—lots of office visits, a hospital stay, prescriptions, and follow-up therapy—will tell of stacks and stacks of bills, unintelligible letters from insurance companies, and telephone calls to Medicare offices that result in only more confusion.

And frustration. Plenty of it. Says a retired executive secretary, "Handling my husband's death was hard enough. But the frustration I felt in trying to untangle the mess of his medical bills was almost more than I could bear. I'm fairly good at keeping track of paperwork and telephone follow-up, and I was lost. The worst part was trying to get clarification from the doctor's office, the insurance company, the hospital, and Medicare. Nobody seemed to understand the situation any better than I did. If I asked the same question of two different people, I got different answers."

When you walk in your patients' shoes, you'll see that money and paperwork issues are probably among the most nagging irritants in health care. But there are other issues that can sweeten or sour the relationship with you. Delayed lab results, incomplete follow-up, and problems left unresolved can all lead a patient to less-than-positive conclusions about your practice, even when **you've** done a great job of communicating and partnering with your patient. What to do? Be a leader: Get out there in the practice, and find out what's going on outside your consulting office and beyond the exam room. How's the follow-up after the exam-room door closes? Satisfying? Merely satisfactory? Or do you and your staff consider good patient follow-up to be collecting payment? Let's take a look at some ideas for enhancing customer satisfaction after the patient leaves the exam room:

- Have a private check-out desk or office for patients to settle financial matters. Let them know that any financial concerns can be freely and **privately** discussed with your office manager. Post a sign to that effect in the reception area, and place business cards nearby. Dr. Noreika designates a certain day and time for billing questions to be addressed by phone: "We tell patients that if they have a problem with a bill, they can call Tina each week during this time. Tina knows when these calls come in what the topic is, and patients feel we're prepared to solve their problems."
- Although many physicians post signs in their reception areas saying "Payment is expected at time of service unless other arrangements are made," others are still willing to bill patients. Dr. Hales says, "It feels more professional to me. I don't like the feeling of having a 'cash register' in my office. So we still send bills." Richard Abrams, MD, takes the same approach and says it works. "Health care is not like buying a bag of groceries. We don't ask for payment at the door—but we have a very good collection rate." Do what makes sense for you and your patients as long as it keeps your accounts receivable at a reasonable level.
- Do you file insurance for patients? In some areas of the country, it's still customary for the office staff to file insurance at no charge to the patient. In others, this service has been stopped in an effort to cut costs for the practice. Some practices will file insurance for a processing fee, and if that is the case it should be clearly posted that this service is available to patients who wish to pay for it. (Charging a fee for filing insurance is not, however, a patient-pleasing practice; we don't recommend it.)

QUIETING LAB RESULT JITTERS

How do you report lab results? Are patients expected to call you? Do you call them? Waiting for lab results can be an agonizing experience for patients. Was the mole malignant? Is the pregnancy developing normally? Is the glucose tolerance test normal? Think about how you would react to such unnerving questions if you were the patient, and then think about how you would deal with worrying about them over a long holiday weekend, while your doctor is out of town, or while the lab results make their way across town by wagon train to the office.

Tell your patients what to expect in the way of getting results. If it will be a week before they know the results, tell them it will be 10 days. If it will be 3 days, tell them it will be 5 days. Periodically compare lab turnaround times and accuracy of results. If the lab you use is not providing fast, accurate service, find another one. The lab you use reflects the quality of your service. If you're still using the "no news is good news" system of informing patients, reconsider it. More than one suit has been won by a patient who was told, "We'll call you if there's a problem on your lab test," when in fact the lack of a telephone call meant simply that the lab work was lost or the report was misplaced. There are too many chances for a questionable result to be overlooked and thus for the patient and problem to be lost to follow-up. Some physicians send a letter (not a postcard so that the entire family can read that Dad's sexually transmitted disease has cleared up) explaining lab results.

ADDING WARMTH TO FOLLOW-UP CARE

After surgery, call your patients at home. It's a gesture of goodwill and sometimes results in helpful follow-up care. Even the most jaded healthcare consumers are still pleasantly surprised by the personal call from their physician, no matter what the reason. An RN who works as a health care consultant recalled getting a phone call from a new dermatologist, whom she had seen about 6 weeks earlier for a mild skin problem: "I was so shocked I thought something was wrong, that the lab had mixed something up. But no, the nice part is that he just calls new patients several weeks after he sees them to see if the treatment was effective."

Ophthalmologists and other surgical specialists have captivated many a patient by sending post-op flowers or a green plant in a mug imprinted with the practice name. One obstetrician sends a birthday card on baby's first birthday. Another sends a piggy bank inscribed with baby's name and birth date. Family physician Robert Bright, MD, and his staff often get favorable comments when they telephone patients with acute conditions a day or two later "to see if they're feeling better." He recalled a patient who had celebrated his 74th wedding anniversary and his 96th birthday when he was found to have an obstructing cancer of the stomach: "Everyone thought he was going to die." The elderly man went into the hospital, had surgery, and went home. Four weeks post-op, Dr. Bright stopped by the house to say hello. "He and his family were so pleased, because they didn't expect the visit," he said. It's the little unexpected things that sometimes win the biggest raves.

A TEAM APPROACH REASSURES PATIENTS

When a patient calls with a problem over the weekend and speaks with your associate or a covering physician, call the patient yourself the following Monday. It shows that you and your associates work as a team and that you're concerned about your patients.

If a patient is unhappy about a problem, make sure that it is handled swiftly and followed to resolution. Many practices find it's helpful when an employee who is meeting with little success at efforts to explain or resolve a situation tells the unhappy patient, "Please speak with my supervisor." This makes the patient feel that he or she has been heard, and often that's all the patient wants. Instruct your staff to bring problems to your attention, and don't point fingers or punish when they do, or they will cease doing so for fear of reprisal. Sometimes it helps for the physician to call the patient.

"THANK YOUS" KEEP REFERRALS COMING

Thank anyone who refers patients to you. Keep referring physicians informed of their patients' progress, and not only with the standard "Thank you for referring Mrs. Jones" letter that describes the diagnosis and treatment. Although faxed referral summaries are becoming more common, take all precautions to protect the privacy of your patient. Many offices use a cover sheet stating, "This FAX contains confidential medical information. Please treat it accordingly." If treatment is protracted or involved, send copies of lab and diagnostic test results and interim progress reports, and let your patient know you keep the referring physician informed in this way. This communication not only keeps referrals coming but tells the patient that there is continuity of care between primary and referring physicians. All referrals, whether they come from patients, friends, or other physicians, require a friendly note saying, "Thank you for recommending me. I appreciate your trust." Don't name the referred patient in these thank-you letters; it violates confidentiality. One San Antonio, Texas physician sends a note and a red rose to anyone who sends him a patient.

Speaking of referrals, if you send a patient to a specialist, find out from the patient his or her perception of the physician, the staff, and the visit. Find out whether the subspecialist has a medical care philosophy similar to yours. It's best to determine this before sending him or her patients. A surgeon referred a patient for work-up of a potential prostate problem to a urologist new in town and conveniently across the hall. The urologist did an extensive (and expensive) work-up, which the surgeon felt was definitely overkill. The surgeon said, "I felt that he took advantage of my patient, doing a lot of unnecessary testing that was uncomfortable and expensive. When I learned what he had done, I called him and asked if this was his customary approach. He assured me it was, and I explained that I wouldn't be sending him patients any more unless he could take a less aggressive, more practical approach to routine problems."

PATIENT EDUCATION

It's always a good idea to discuss with patients not only the reason for a referral but what to expect. Sometimes the consultant to whom you send a patient does not reflect your service quality and patient care attitude, but he or she may be the best for your patient's problem. Explain this to your patient; remember, patients judge you according to the quality and service provided by the physicians to whom you send them.

Take time to educate patients. There are plenty of ways to do this (you can read about them in Chapter 29). The physician doesn't have to do it all. Dr. Bright knows that "if I and my staff spend time with a patient, it's all credited to me. Patients don't see the visit as divided: 10 minutes with the doctor, 20 minutes with the nurse." He points out that patients sometimes are concerned about taking too much of the physician's time, so "they don't always hear important things I have to say about lifestyle issues." Many of the physicians we spoke with acknowledged that patients often hesitate to bring up questions for fear of appearing "stupid." These physicians overview with the patient the problem and treatment and then turn him or her over to a nurse or patient educator who is trained to give indepth information and to probe for underlying concerns.

EXTENDING CONDOLENCES

When a patient dies, what should you do? Some physicians send flowers or cards and even attend funerals of patients to whom they were especially close. If you know the family members, and especially if they are patients of yours, a telephone call or letter offering sympathy and support is especially appreciated. Surviving family members are often overwhelmed with paperwork after a death, and much of the paperwork may be from your office or from a recent hospital stay. If you have the resources, offer your office manager's time and talents to help sort through the tangle. Make it clear that this is done gratis, as a courtesy to the family.

PATIENT EXIT INTERVIEWS: THINGS YOU NEED TO KNOW

How do you follow up when a patient leaves the practice? If a request for transfer of records to another local physician comes in, do you simply transfer the records without question? Smart practices contact the patient, conducting telephone exit interviews (either the physician or the office manager should do this) or sending a personal letter with a survey to determine the source of dissatisfaction. This can be an enlightening experience; you may learn things you don't know about your staff, your style, your charges, and other matters. These insights may be unpleasant, but they're things you need to know to improve and provide quality service.

STAYING IN TOUCH BETWEEN VISITS

Do you have any contact with patients between visits? Countless practices send newsletters to patients as a way to keep in touch, to help them stay healthy, to comment on the latest medical news, and to personalize the practice with news of staff and physicians. Is this communication technique worth the time and expense? Ask anyone who has discontinued a practice newsletter whether it's effective. If it was a regularly mailed and well-done publication, people miss it when it's gone. Patients appreciate this subtle reminder of the practice, even if they never comment on it. And you never know when it may yield results. Many physicians report getting calls from people who said they had been receiving their practice newsletter for several years and never needed their specialized services until now.

Your interaction with patients is just a fraction of their entire experience and perception of your practice. There are plenty of details that occur after your office visit that will compel your patients to send you their friends, co-workers, and neighbors or that will propel them to another practice. These "after-the-exam" details may seem minor matters, but they can have a major impact. Pay attention to them, for your patients do, and they tell others, such as the woman who worked in an office of 20 people. She returned ecstatically from her first visit to a new family doctor and promptly sent out a humorous electronic-mail message over the network computer to all 19 of her co-workers. Here's the message she sent:

> I found, after much searching and discarding, a family
> physician who (1) knows what she's doing; (2) has an office
> staff who seems to know the score; and (3) really listens to
> and cares about her patients.

For $500 I'll tell you her name.

Calm down. I'm not that much of a capitalist. The doctor is:

Kim Ottwell, MD
Scottsdale (Arizona)
Tel.: 661-1755

Dr. Ottwell may not have been aware of the impact she and her staff had, but at least 19 people did after her new patient informed them (and now countless others reading this book know as well!).

Pay attention to all of the details that take place among patients, you, and your staff, because your patients surely do. ❧

Action Steps for Effective Follow-Up

1. Know what happens when patients leave the exam room. Follow-up is important to your patients' perception of care.
2. Provide a knowledgeable person and a private place for patients to discuss insurance or financial matters.
3. Make your payment policy flexible and personal. Do what's best for you, your patients, and your bottom line.
4. Call patients at home after surgery or an acute illness.
5. Handle problems swiftly and completely. Patients appreciate this.
6. Thank those who send you referral patients, and when you send a patient to a referral physician, find out his or her perception of the physician.
7. Send a get well or sympathy card when a patient or patient's family member is hospitalized or dies.
8. When a records transfer is requested, do an exit interview to find out why the patient is leaving.

20

"Doctor's Office, Please Hold . . ."

How the phone is answered is a key to a successful practice.
The receptionist needs to be able to stand in for me with my
patients.

Robert Bright, MD, Bremerton, Washington

You can spend many hours communicating to your staff your
philosophy of personalized care and your belief in quality service. You can recognize considerate acts, reward extraordinary
actions, and feel justifiable pride in the patient sensitivity of your
practice.

But all this significant progress toward putting the customer first
can be chipped away by the following all-too-common scenario:

> *Ring-ring-ring.*
> *Ring-ring-ring.*
> *Ring-ring-ring.*
> *"Doctor's office. Please hold."*

The telephone is the first connection, a vital connection between your practice and a potential or actual patient. Faceless,
untouchable, and remote, the voice that comes through to the
caller carries emotion and attitude. The voice says very clearly
what the practice is like, what *you* and your physician colleagues

220

are like. The way your telephone is answered helps set up patient expectations.

What does it say when the caller hears the telephone ring . . . and ring . . . and ring again and again before a voice responds?

What does it say when the person on the other end sounds bored, uncaring, or rushed?

What does it say when the voice on the other end of the line is an answering service employee who mispronounces the physician's name and knows nothing about the practice?

What does it say when the voice on the other end is not a person at all but an automated electronic maze requiring endless, confusing button pushing before the caller finally reaches a person?

And what kind of service and medical care expectations might someone have after getting connected to your practice in any of these ways?

THE TELEPHONE: A DIRECT CONNECTION

The telephone is the first and most direct connection to your practice for most of your patients. Is that first "moment of truth" a positive, pleasant one? Does the voice of your practice speak well of you?

A *Medical Economics* survey found that 15% of patients are dissatisfied with the way physicians and their assistants handle telephone calls[1] (see Figure 20-1.) That's one out of seven patients. What are they unhappy about? Being put on hold too long, lack of courtesy by staff members or the answering service, and delays in return calls by the physician. Some of those unhappy customers may become irritated or frustrated enough to quit calling. They'll look for a practice where the telephone is a priority. Some will complain, as this patient did:

> *I called my doctor's office the other day, and when the receptionist answered the phone with her standard greeting, "Dr. M.'s office," I waited, because usually, that phrase is followed by "Please hold." It doesn't matter what time or what day I call, I'm usually put on hold. I was stunned when I wasn't—in fact, I laughed and told her I had ex-*

Figure 20-1 Problems When Patients Telephone

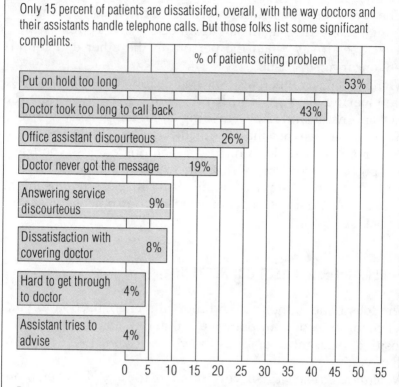

Only 15 percent of patients are dissatisifed, overall, with the way doctors and their assistants handle telephone calls. But those folks list some significant complaints.

% of patients citing problem

Problem	%
Put on hold too long	53%
Doctor took too long to call back	43%
Office assistant discourteous	26%
Doctor never got the message	19%
Answering service discourteous	9%
Dissatisfaction with covering doctor	8%
Hard to get through to doctor	4%
Assistant tries to advise	4%

Percentages add to more than 100 because of multiple responses.

Source: Reprinted from M. Crane, Making Things Easier for Patients Pays Off. *Medical Economics,* April 23, 1990, p. 73.

pected to be put on hold, and she said, "Well you'd better hurry and talk or you will be." I've told my doctor about his telephones, I've told his staff about it, and they tell me it's always like that, the phones are always busy. End of discussion. If I hadn't been going to him for 10 years, I wouldn't put up with it. I'd hang up and find a doctor whose office doesn't treat telephone callers like a bothersome interruption.

We empathize with the people who answer the telephone in a medical practice. It's a tough job. The lines ring continually; each caller expects personal, immediate attention. Some want to describe their problem, from hemorrhoids to hernias, in infinite, intimate detail. Meanwhile there's a patient standing at the front desk trying to get the receptionist's attention, and the nurse is standing at her shoulder with a question about the caller on line three. And Dr. Burston is on line five waiting to speak to Dr. King. And we're saying the person answering the telephone should smile and be friendly?

We are. **Especially** because the telephone connection is faceless and impersonal, the voice at the other end—the voice of the practice—needs to respond with a smile and a name and a helpful tone. To ensure that this occurs, the practice leadership and management must understand and respect the significant role and responsibility of the person answering the phone. This means hiring sharp, compassionate individuals who understand the impact they have and then training those who answer the phone not only to handle calls appropriately but to convey the values of the practice as well as the services available.

The office manager in a four-physician group found when she joined the fast-paced practice that "the people answering the phone were trying to keep up with the physicians' pace. They were answering the phones hurriedly, not identifying themselves or the practice, putting calls on hold immediately so they could get to the next ringing line. They were doing what they thought they were supposed to do—keeping up with the calls and the doctors, but in the process, no one was paying attention to patients and their needs."

TELEPHONES NEED SPECIAL TECHNIQUE AND SKILLS

If your phones are ringing constantly and callers are frequently put on hold, your practice may need additional phone lines, additional personnel to answer them, or better training for staff. Most phone companies offer a service to identify peak busy periods for incoming calls; they can also determine how often callers are turned away with a busy signal. Either problem can be adjusted with more staff handling calls during busy periods or by adding a phone line if necessary. A mature well-trained telephone receptionist also can handle calls efficiently, taking care of callers quickly while maintaining a congenial, helpful tone. In many practices, unfortunately, the person who answers the phone is a minimally educated, minimally trained, minimum-wage individual whose previous telephone experience is limited to lengthy conversations about what happened to Tiffany and Ted last Saturday night. The technical skills are there; the employee knows all about picking up the handpiece and pushing the right buttons, but the important concepts of service, responsiveness, and attitude are missing. It's not the employee's fault. If no one conveys to him or her that he or she is the focal point for connecting patients to the practice, the employee may short-circuit patients and the practice because of lack of training and awareness.

A TELEPHONE SURVEY

We called 15 practices at random. The good news: All but one answered the phone within three rings. One-third of the practices we called responded with a friendly "Good morning" followed by the name of the practice and the receptionist's name. Five voices were borne across the line on a smile. The bad news: Eight voices were rushed or routine. One was recorded: An answering machine picked up the call after 9 a.m. One was an answering service—friendly, but why a service during calling hours? Five of our calls were put on hold. Two-thirds of the practices did not identify the person responding to our call.

How would your telephone be answered?

The practice telephone is a service with significant impact on patients' impressions of the quality they'll encounter; it deserves priority attention. The benefit is not only in patient satisfaction but in improved efficiency and productivity. When you take the time to train staff in telephone etiquette and to implement telephone triage policies, you reduce unnecessary telephone transfers, reduce the number of unnecessary calls, and free up phone lines for important calls. In the rest of this chapter, we'll give you guidelines for making quality come across the telephone line, so that every moment of truth "on the line" is a happy one for your customers.

PERSONALIZE THE PHONE VOICE

Telephone conversations are more difficult than face-to-face interactions. The telephone poses a barrier that can impede communication. What to do?

First, recognize the importance of the telephone contact. Hire and train the appropriate number of individuals—people with the personality, maturity, and wisdom needed to handle incoming calls. Standardize telephone interactions without depersonalizing them. These are minimum customer service requirements:

- Phones should be answered within three rings.
- The name of the practice or the physician(s) should be given. "Doctor's office" should be banned as a greeting.
- The person answering the phone should give his or her first name.
- No caller should be put on hold without first being asked for permission. Here's an example of acceptable handling:

  Receptionist: The Jones and White Medical Group. This is Anna. Can you hold for a moment, please?
  Caller: Yes, I can.
  Anna: Thank you.

  Unacceptable: "The Jones and White Medical Group. Hold please."
- The telephone receptionist should be taught (and believe) that he or she is the voice of the practice.
- A triage system should be established to ensure that patient calls are handled efficiently and professionally.

The telephone creates a connection, but it also poses a barrier to communication. The "voice without a face" at the end of the line has the potential to seem impersonal and uncaring. To overcome this, your staff need to know how to use personal action to knock down the communication barriers created by this technology (see Exhibit 20-1).

Several physicians we spoke to said they occasionally test their telephone lines by calling their own practice or by having a friend

Exhibit 20-1 Knock Down Telephone Barriers: Get Personal

Barrier	Action
Misunderstandings that occur when facial expressions, attitudes, and enunciation aren't clear	◆ Speak clearly and at a moderate rate. Remember that people recall what they see better than what they hear. Complicated problems may require more time as well as visual follow-up (mailing of a brochure or article, etc.). ◆ Smile as you speak. Even if you don't *feel* like smiling, a more positive attitude and tone will come through. Keeping a small mirror at the reception desk can serve as a reminder to the receptionist that facial expressions speak loudly.
Distractions that deter listening and understanding	◆ Focus exclusively on the caller. The person answering the phone should not attempt to tend to other matters at the same time he or she is handling a caller's question or problem. If the telephone scheduler is also responsible for greeting and checking in patients, he or she should excuse himself or herself **briefly** from the phone call to acknowledge the person standing before him or her, saying, "Good morning, I'll be with you as soon as I complete this call." ◆ Show respect to co-workers who are on the phone. Keep background conversations and noise to a minimum; don't interrupt or try to get the attention of the person on the phone.
Lack of rapport	◆ Give your voice **personality.** Identify yourself as you answer. *Example:* "Women's Center for Health. This is Brenda. How can I help you?" *or* "How may I direct your call?" Smile before answering. That smile comes through loud and clear! ◆ Use a friendly conversational tone of voice. Callers to a medical practice are often anxious; try to ease anxiety by being calm and helpful. ◆ Use the patient's name in conversation. ◆ If a call must be put on hold, ask the caller's permission, and wait for a response before doing so.

do so. (For more about this technique, see Exhibit 20-2). One physician who had a medical condition requiring surgery told us this story:

In the course of getting treatment I had to call several doctors' offices. I was struck by the telephone manners when I called. Often I was put on hold, sometimes disconnected, or I would be on hold forever, then a voice would come back on the line: "Doctor's office, may I help you?" One time I had called an office for the second time trying to make an appointment, and while I was talking to the scheduling person, another line began ringing. She took that call and completed it before coming back to me, which I found

---

Exhibit 20-2 Mystery Shopper Survey

Date: _____ Time: _____

Reason for call: _____

Phone number called: _____ Number of rings: _____

How answered: _____

Put on hold? ❑ yes ❑ no How long? _____

Transferred? ❑ yes ❑ no If so, to whom? _____

Rate the friendliness of the receptionist:
❑ excellent ❑ good ❑ fair ❑ poor

Rate the helpfulness of the receptionist:
❑ excellent ❑ good ❑ fair ❑ poor

First available date of scheduled appointment: _____

Were you asked what type of insurance you have? ❑ yes ❑ no

Were you asked if transportation was needed? ❑ yes ❑ no

Did receptionist offer to send practice brochure or other information? ❑ yes ❑ no

Comments: _____

_____

_____

*annoying. I found my initial contact with doctors' offices
not very favorable. I formed an impression of the practices
by the way the phone was handled. What it told me was that
these doctors may be great physicians, but no one is paying
attention to what the employees are doing.*

What do patients experience when they call your practice?
Find out with a mystery shopper survey. Have family members
or friends call the office at different times of the day and days of
the week. These potential patients can call with questions about
the practice or to schedule an appointment. Have them complete
the form shown in Exhibit 20-2 to document the responses and
attitude. The use of the mystery shopper survey should be explained to staff in a positive manner. It can stimulate a discussion
about patient expectations, first impressions, and techniques for
managing multiple calls in a positive manner. To further evaluate
your practice, take the telephone test in Exhibit 20-3.

Exhibit 20-3 A Telephone Test

*Is the telephone voice in your practice a friendly one? Use the following list of
questions to evaluate telephone responsiveness in your practice and to
determine barriers to service, gaps, and potential problem areas.*

1. How much specific training in telephone etiquette is given the person who
   answers the phones?
2. How much and what kind of information about the practice, the physician(s),
   and the services provided is given the person who answers the phones?
3. How is the telephone receptionist instructed to answer the phone?
4. How many telephone calls does your office receive each day?
5. What are the reasons for these calls? (e.g., appointment, information, speak
   to the physician, emergency, etc.)
6. How are telephone calls documented?
7. How often do patients complain about the telephone, and what do they
   complain about?
8. What form of telephone triage instructions and training does the telephone
   receptionist receive?

You can find out how patients feel about your telephone service with a postvisit survey (Chapter 14). Structure five or six survey questions on a 3- by 5-inch card to focus specifically on telephone etiquette by asking about courtesy, whether the patient was put on hold, whether the time on hold was excessive, and the like. Use the responses for staff meeting discussion and to determine whether changes need to be made.

PATIENTS WANT CALLBACKS PROMPTLY

Patients who are displeased with telephone courtesy in their physicians' offices are often unhappy with the amount of time the physician takes to return their phone calls. Dr. Abrams commented, "I want my patients to feel comfortable to call me. I encourage it. It creates extra work for me, but I try to keep people from interrupting their lives because they're waiting to talk to me. I know that when people finally make the decision to call the doctor, they're afraid to leave the house or office for fear they'll miss a return call. They can handle a wait of 15 minutes, but not 2 or 3 hours. And they certainly don't want to wait until the end of the day to get an answer."

Dr. Abrams takes patient calls throughout the day, but his approach may not work for you. A practice telephone policy can solve the problem. First of all, every practice and every physician should have a triage protocol posted by each phone. The triage protocol lists symptoms or problems that are emergencies requiring immediate attention, questions that can only be answered by a physician, and questions that can be answered by a nurse, physician's assistant, or other clinical staff member. The triage protocol should also list policies for prescription refills and for documentation of telephone calls. To establish a protocol, gather staffers who handle patient calls, and have them name the questions most commonly or frequently asked. (You may wish to have those who regularly take patient calls keep a log of the questions for a week or two.) Make a list of the 10 or 20 most common questions, and specify appropriate answers and/or to whom the call should be referred. This is both time saving and patient pleasing, because answers can often be given immediately. See Exhibit 20-4 for a sample matrix.

Exhibit 20-4 Telephone Triage Protocol

1. List symptoms or conditions commonly seen in practice that require an immediate appointment or response by doctor or nurse.
2. Develop a written protocol for prescription refills; e.g.:
   • Who can approve refills
   • List of medications okay to refill without appointment and number of refills allowed
   • Conditions or circumstances that require an appointment before a refill
   • Medications requiring a lab test before refill
   • Who takes questions about medications and medication reactions
3. Develop a list of commonly asked questions and appropriate responses. Emphasize that additional questions not on the protocol list should be referred to the appropriate staffer.

EXAMPLE

Question	Answer
What does the physician charge for an office visit?	An initial visit exclusive of any laboratory tests is $46.
How long does it take to remove a suspicious mole, and when are the results back?	The minor surgery procedure is performed here in the office. It takes 30 to 45 minutes and the pathology report is usually available in 2 to 3 days.

Staff should know each physician's schedule or time for making return phone calls to patients. Many physicians return calls at midday and at the end of the day. If a patient calls at 8:30 a.m. with a nonemergency question and is politely informed that the doctor will return the call between noon and 2 p.m., the patient knows that he or she doesn't have to sit by the phone waiting for the call. If you prefer to return calls throughout the day between patient appointments, your staff should be instructed to tell patients, "Dr. Avery makes patient calls in between appointments. He will call you back sometime between now and noon. Is that convenient?" Managing return phone calls is similar to managing waiting time: Patients simply want to be informed and know what to expect.

WHEN YOU'RE ON OVERLOAD

Bell Road Medical Group, a four-physician family and internal medicine practice in Phoenix, Arizona, discovered several years ago that all eight of their incoming lines were often lit up at once. Callers frequently got a busy signal. Monthly patient surveys were returned regularly with negative comments about difficulties getting through. Office manager Tina Dombrowski tackled the problem by expanding incoming lines from eight to twelve, adding an "on-hold" tape service that provides personalized messages about the practice, and implementing a stringent policy about putting people on hold: Ask first, wait for an answer, and **listen** to the answer because some callers don't want to be put on hold. Patients and referring physicians give the "on-hold" service rave reviews. Patients comment that they often get the information they need—office address, directions, and so forth—from the taped message and that it makes time on hold seem shorter. Three front office staff answer phones among other duties; if too many lines are ringing, they call the office "floater" to assist with telephone duties. A dedicated line for pharmacies is linked to a voice mail system. Pharmacies leave information about the patient name and requested prescription refill, and office nurses check the line periodically throughout the day. For continuous improvement of skills, office staff attend a telephone seminar once or twice a year, and improvement of telephone service is a regular agenda topic at monthly staff meetings. Does this practice take its telephone connection with patients seriously? You bet.

The telephone is a technological device, but in many ways it's the heart of the practice, linking patients to you and saying far more about the practice, staff, and physicians than the words that come through the line. When the connection exceeds patient expectations, patients gain a professional, personal image of the practice. The telephone is often the first opportunity to tell a patient, "We're knowledgeable. We care about you. You can count on us." But telephone excellence—attentive, responsive, friendly, and personal service—doesn't happen by accident. It's a team effort, the result of education, motivation, and good management. ᵛ

Action Steps for a Great Connection

1. Hire and train telephone receptionists who are mature and intelligent. The person who answers the telephone is the voice of the practice.
2. Establish standards for telephone response, and make sure they are followed.
3. Periodically, have someone conduct a telephone "mystery shopper survey" to monitor how callers are treated.
4. Don't overburden the telephone receptionist with responsibilities. In a busy practice, handling the phones is a demanding job. The telephone receptionist should be able to focus on the caller.
5. Have the office manager review the telephone test shown in Exhibit 20-3 to determine the friendliness and responsiveness of your telephone connection.
6. Make sure patients know when a return call from the physician can be expected. Develop a phone triage schedule so that staffers know what calls to route and to whom to route them.
7. Consider a telephone company evaluation of your system if patients frequently encounter a busy signal or are put on hold.

Reference

1. M. Crane, Making things easier for patients pays off, *Medical Economics* (April 23, 1990): 60–80.

—— 🐌 ——

21

Dealing with the Waiting Room Dilemma

Q: How do you make an elephant stew?

A: Keep him waiting in the doctor s office.

Whew! If you want to get an earful, just ask someone what bugs him or her more than anything else about going to the doctor. Here are a few sample reactions:

> Our **former** doctor always kept us waiting. On one occasion we were "lost" in the waiting room after signing in, then put in a crowded storage room after I complained about the excessive wait, and were "lost" again in that room. It was 1 hour and 40 minutes after our arrival that we finally saw the doctor. When I complained to him, he said he was sorry, he didn't have enough information to explain what happened, and he'd look into it. I never received any follow-up explanation or apology.
>
> We have a new family doctor now.
>
> *   *   *
>
> It's most important not to be kept waiting for more than 15 minutes beyond my appointment time. My time is valuable too. In most doctors' offices we all play the waiting game. This is a real peeve of mine!
>
> *   *   *

I get annoyed with doctors who are in such a rush because of their late schedule that they don't have time to talk to you, and leave you with unanswered questions.

* * *

No single subject brings forth such wrath, righteous indignation, and downright anger on the part of patients as waiting time. Perhaps Plato was sitting in his physician's office watching the minutes tick by when he wrote, "Since the doctor cuts us up, and orders us to bring him money . . . as if he were exacting tribute, he should be put under rigid control." Plato also suggested that physicians be elected by the public and severely penalized "if they fail to carry out the letter of the law." It's a good bet that today's public would want a provision in the law specifying a maximum waiting time.

Somewhere along the path of medicine's progress, disregard for patient appointment times became institutionalized in the structure of many practices. (Just take a look at the size of the waiting rooms in some medical practices!) People have become accustomed to calling the office before an appointment to learn "how late the doctor is running" so that they can plan accordingly. Some have learned to bring along projects: knitting, homework, or massive novels. Everyone jokes about it, but there is an increasingly bitter edge to the laughter.

WAITING MAKES PEOPLE INCREASINGLY IRRITABLE

You may have noticed that your own patients are more irritable about spending too much time in your reception area. Consumers across the United States are less willing to wait and more vocal about it. In 1976, 4 of 10 patients said that after 15 minutes beyond their appointment time their resentment grew with each additional minute. In 1990, 7 of 10 felt that way.[1] With the choices available in the health care marketplace today, few people are likely to willingly choose someone who blatantly disregards their time. "My time is valuable too," commented the CEO of a New York stock exchange company. "I can't afford to spend **my** productive time reading old magazines in my doctor's office, and doctors need to understand this.

"When I go to a doctor's office, I tell the receptionist, 'I'm starting the clock now,'" he said. "'You have 25 minutes, and if you haven't called me by then, I'm gone.'" He has never had to wait the full 25 minutes, he said; but who knows, his threat to leave may wield some clout, getting him in ahead of other patients.

But isn't it unfortunate that people feel they have to resort to threats and demands to gain the service due them (which is what honoring an appointment is all about)? In talking to patients and physicians for this book, the subject of waiting time came up again and again, often unbidden. Our interviews and our research have led us to this conclusion: Waiting time is a far more serious service lapse in medical practices than **anyone** (except patients) gives it credit for. Furthermore, too many practices—very **good** practices with excellent clinicians and very fine service and care—are losing patients because they minimize the impact of this problem.

Fortunately, it is a manageable problem. We know it is, because we have encountered a number of very busy, very successful practices where patients don't wait. These physicians and their staffs realize that their patients expect them to honor the schedule, barring emergencies and similar problems. These physicians are as vehement about **not** keeping people waiting as their patients are. These physicians have made a commitment to being on time and have found ways to stay on schedule without short-changing their patients in the exam room or consultation room.

Too many physicians, however—the same ones who speak with sincerity and enthusiasm of the importance of service—confessed that their patients wait—sometimes an inordinate amount of time. One of these physicians (who will remain nameless just in case he mends his ways) said that a physician's responsibility is **not** to keep patients waiting, but "I'm vulnerable on the waiting issue," he said. Later he added that the patient's responsibility is "to be on time on the miraculous chance I might be on time too."

NOT A SUBJECT TO BE TAKEN LIGHTLY

This physician (and some others) make light of waiting time, but patients, for all their joking, do not treat it lightly. A practice that regularly keeps patients waiting without justification not only incurs patient wrath—it also penalizes itself. A reception area chock full of patients glancing at their watches is symptomatic of a problem. The problem is inefficiency, and the symptom is poor service. This inefficiency has these harmful effects:

- People and processes are not as productive as they could be. This means lost income and higher overhead.
- Patients are displeased. Displeased patients often express their unhappiness to staff members, creating stress and dissatisfaction in these employees. These displeased patients may not return. They definitely won't give you or your practice rave reviews. This translates directly to lost income because most practices depend on patient referrals for continued growth.
- A lengthy wait affects patient perception of quality. The longer patients have to wait to see their physician, the less satisfied they are with their medical care.[2]

When we asked good physicians who said they believe in quality service about waiting time, we heard excuses such as this: "Well, we're doing everything else right. Our patients like us and appreciate what we do for them. We have the latest equipment and techniques. So patients really don't mind waiting."

Really? Ask them sometime. Patients who have been with your practice for some time may tolerate the long wait (changing physicians is a major hassle, after all); nevertheless, it taints their perception of your quality. New patients unfamiliar with the practice and the physicians don't get a favorable impression when the visit starts out with an extended introduction to the reception area wallpaper pattern.

Moreover, think of the endorsement a long-time patient may offer to a friend: "My doctor is great. She listens to you, she's always on target with her suggestions, gives you plenty of information. Really a good doctor. Of course, you usually have to wait an hour to see her. But you just plan ahead for that, and bring plenty of stuff to do." Few of today's time-deprived health care consumers would select such a doctor, given other alternatives.

WAITING TIME CAN BE MANAGED

Fortunately, many physicians are aware that patients seethe as the minutes stack up, and they're paying closer attention to their schedules. Perhaps, like some of the physicians we spoke with, they've received one too many blistering comments from patients tired of restructuring their daily schedule after an unplanned chunk of time in their waiting room. There has even been significant improvement in waiting time. In 1990, the median wait was 15.5 minutes, compared with 24.0 minutes in 1976. Patients say they'll tolerate a wait of 13.5 minutes past their appointment, so the gap is closing.[3]

Take waiting time as seriously as your patients do. Pediatrician Stephen Hales is fanatic about waiting time. "We don't waste people's time, we don't make people wait, even if I see 40 or 50 or even 60 patients on a hectic day." It's rare for someone to wait more than 5 or 10 minutes in Dr. Hales' office. He accomplishes this smooth-flowing schedule by:

- Not taking walk-in appointments
- Leaving room in the schedule throughout the day for emergency call-ins
- Allotting visit time according to the complaint
- Communicating to patients the expectation that **they** must be on time
- Communicating clearly to his staff his commitment to an on-time schedule, and gaining their cooperation and commitment
- Cross-training all his staff to ensure maximum efficiency

What Dr. Hales gains from his no-wait policy: a booming practice that thrives in the midst of group and multispecialty competition, and the professional satisfaction that comes from knowing that patients are pleased.

Denver, Colorado internist Carol Gilmore, MD, runs a tight schedule, so tight that one of the biggest complaints from patients is that they can't be late. "I've had patients who arrived late for their first appointment and their excuse is that doctors are always late. They can't believe we run on time," Dr. Gilmore says.

SCHEDULE EFFICIENTLY BUT NOT RIGIDLY

There are as many approaches to efficient scheduling as there are styles of practice. And that's the key: A rigid schedule is meaningless and ineffective if it does not take into account the individual style of the physician. We know of a dermatologist whose appointment book is set up in 10-minute slots, yet he's a chatty fellow who generally spends no less than 25 minutes per patient. Fortunately for his patients (but unfortunately for him), his practice has fallen off (perhaps because patients stacked up in the reception area grew tired of hour-long waits), so the 10-minute slots have plenty of gaps in between to accommodate his chit-chat.

Take a look at your schedule and personal style, as Dr. Schreiber, the orthopedic surgeon, has. On the charge slip, the patient's arrival time is noted along with what time the patient was brought back to the exam room. To speed the flow, Dr. Schreiber doesn't always see patients in order; he'll see a quick patient ahead of one he knows will require more time. "I could see more patients if they were booked more closely and if I spent less time with them. But I like what I'm doing and the way I'm doing it," he says. It's likely that his patients do, too.

Pat Medeiros, human resources manager for Wilmington Health Associates in Wilmington, North Carolina, lists waiting time as one of the four common patient expectations. "Patients don't want to wait," he says. The practice uses patient surveys to learn if patients believe they're waiting too long and then follows up with the physician to resolve the problem.

A time audit can be helpful in analyzing bottlenecks within the practice. The audit can be done by staff members on every patient for a week or two. Exhibit 21-1 shows a sample audit form. It documents not only patient arrival and departure time but the amount of time spent in each phase of the encounter. Analysis of these audit forms can show if blockages are caused by too many walk-ins, not enough time allotted for certain conditions, and so forth.

THERE WILL BE THOSE DAYS . . .

Even the most efficient practice occasionally (and sometimes frequently) has days when the calendar is crammed, emergencies

Exhibit 21-1 Time Audit Form

Reason for visit/procedure _____

Patient _____

Date _____ Appointment time _____

Arrival time_____ Time shown to exam room_____ Time seen by doctor_____

Time finished _____ Total time in office _____

Walk in?_____ Emergency?_____ Referral?_____

(Check All That Apply)

overrun the normally smooth schedule, patients arrive late with stories of traffic back-ups, and every patient seems to have several complaints in addition to the presenting problem. When the inevitable delays occur and the waiting room is indeed a "waiting room," it helps to have alternative strategies to ease the frustration for patients and to help them while away the time.

> *John Lambis glances up at the clock suspended on the waiting room wall, then returns to the rumpled pages of a magazine.*
>
> *The clock ticks. The air smells of rubbing alcohol. Someone coughs. Fifty minutes have passed since Lambis entered the doctor's office—on time for his appointment.*
>
> *"Have you ever noticed how we all sit quietly, seemingly engrossed in a magazine, but in fact are listening intently for our names to be called?" says Lambis, 40, of Marietta, [Georgia], describing his most recent experience at the doctor's office. "Physicians consistently double-book, stacking us up in the waiting room like planes on a runway. At least with the airlines you get a free drink."*
>
> *But has Lambis ever expressed his irritation to his doctor or asked why there are delays? No. "I can't bring it up because it would put me in a funny position."*[4(p.1)]

The predominant service strategy for unexpected delays is to tell the patient. Patients appreciate being informed: An explanation or apology from a staff member makes them feel better, even though it doesn't change the fact that they must wait. Acknowledgment from the physician helps too. Several physicians told us, "I make it a point of apologizing if I've kept my patients waiting too long." They also said that many patients are amazed to hear a physician say, "I'm sorry you had to wait."

Like many of the service-minded physicians we encountered, Denver ophthalmologist Jerry Meltzer, MD, tries to avoid keeping patients twiddling their thumbs in his reception area. For the occasional days when patient problems and work flow flood the schedule, he has interesting books and publications (the *Reader's Digest Encyclopedia of Drugs,* the *Wilson Quarterly,* and the *Utne Reader*) and televisions in the reception area and exam rooms with laser disk and cable "so patients can tune in to their favorite soap opera." A nutrition center is stocked with coffee and donuts or cookies to stave off the munchies. And when patients must wait, not only do they get an apology but their fee may be reduced by 20% to 50%. The goal of the practice is to acknowledge the patient's arrival within 1 minute, to have the patient conversing with a technician in 10 to 15 minutes, and to have him or her out of the office within an hour for most visits. When an emergency throws the schedule off, patients are called ahead of time.

A PERSONAL APOLOGY HELPS

Adds radiologist Lawrence Cohen, MD, "When patients wait, it's helpful if I go out and talk to them and say 'I'm sorry, we had an emergency' and offer to pay for their parking or try to do something to make them comfortable. A demonstration of sincerity and an explanation that this is not a routine situation get a positive response."

Waiting time may seem to be an insignificant component of the health care experience—and that's how some physicians view it. They believe that the ultimate goal—diagnosis and treatment of an individual's problem—should outweigh the inconvenience of the outer office waiting game. But today's consumers don't agree.

They're greedy. They want it all: a readily available appointment, minimal waiting, instant diagnosis and cure, and low cost.

It may be difficult to meet the rest of their expectations, but addressing waiting time is a good start. Because waiting time is such a significant element of patient satisfaction, we've devoted a whole chapter to the subject of creating a schedule that minimizes excessive waiting time. If you have a waiting time problem in your practice (and you know if you do), pay special attention to the next chapter.

Your patients will thank you for it. ❧

Action Steps To Minimize Waiting Time

1. Do a time audit to monitor patient waiting time in the reception area and in the exam room.
2. Regularly measure patient expectations to determine what is acceptable to your patients. Target a waiting time *under* this minimum time.
3. Analyze physician practice style. Accommodate the schedule to physician style. It won't work any other way.
4. Analyze the types of patients you see and the time they take. Adapt appointments accordingly.
5. Delegate tasks to use physician time efficiently and effectively.
6. Convene staff to identify problems and discuss realistic solutions. Use the analysis techniques in the next chapter to develop a schedule that minimizes waiting time.
7. Listen with an open mind if you are pinpointed as part of the waiting time bottleneck.
8. If consistently excessive waiting time is a serious problem, outside assistance may be a solution. Don't hesitate to get professional help. Patient satisfaction and practice growth may depend on it.

References

1. M. Crane, Making things easier for patients pays off, *Medical Economics* (April 23, 1990): 61.
2. L. Herkert, Communication affects patient satisfaction, *Internist* (May/June 1988): 38.
3. M. Crane, Making things easier, 61.
4. T. Friend, Both sides need a shot of empathy, *USA Today* (August 15, 1991): 1. Copyright 1991, *USA Today*. Reprinted with permission.

ò

22

"My Time Is Important Too!" Scheduling for Patient Satisfaction

---

Q: What is the one thing physicians should do to ensure a more positive and satisfying experience for patients?

A: Maintain a good schedule. Don't bring us in and have us wait. I used to see one doctor who would schedule 10 or 15 patients for the same time, and this was before he ever got to the office. This was routine, so if you were not very early, you could wait 2 hours.
                                                              —A patient

---

As we saw in the previous chapter, excessive waiting time is a prime irritant for patients. It causes patients to leave for good, and those who stay may not recommend your practice to others. Excessive waiting time is inefficient and reduces productivity for physicians and staff. On the other hand, a smoothly flowing schedule that minimizes waiting time is a significant ingredient in your recipe for patient satisfaction and practice success.

How do you accomplish this? Create a practice schedule that's personalized to your style, your staff, and your patients. That's what we'll help you do in this chapter, because you can't afford to irritate your patients and cut down on your productivity and your staff's efficiency with a schedule that's not doing the job it should.

Let's look first at the most widely used scheduling methods. Each has advantages as well as drawbacks. Then we'll go step by

Scheduling Options

Type of Schedule	Advantages	Drawbacks
Stream	• Easy • Standard books available	• Not flexible • Excessive patient waiting time • Idle time for physician and staff
Wave	• Reduces idle time of physician and staff	• Excessive patient waiting time • Crowded waiting room
Modified Wave	• Reduces idle time of physician and staff	• Possible patient backlogs

step through a process to choose options to create a customized scheduling method that will work for your practice.

THE STREAM METHOD

With stream scheduling, one appointment is scheduled after another in a sequence of uniform blocks throughout the day. For example, one patient is scheduled at 9 a.m., the next at 9:15, and the third at 9:30. The advantage: It's easy. Most appointment books are organized for this method. But stream scheduling doesn't work unless all patients require exactly the same amount of time. Patients who are late or don't show up can cause wasted time. On the other hand, a patient who needs a longer procedure and extra time for conversation can throw the whole day off schedule.

THE WAVE OR BLOCK SCHEDULE

With the wave or block system, a specified number of patients are scheduled at one time, and then none is scheduled in the subsequent time slots. Six patients may be scheduled at 9 a.m. and the next six at 10 a.m. Wave scheduling eliminates down time for the physician and staff; even if some patients are late or don't show up, there's always someone waiting for the doctor. But patients aren't very pleased with this system. When several people arrive together, those who wait longer are likely to become upset. And once established patients figure out this scheduling system, they are likely to do what one staff member reported occurs in the medical practice in which he works. Knowing that several appointments are made for the same time and that the person who arrives earliest is seen first, patients now arrive an hour or more ahead of their scheduled appointment, just to be sure they're seen first. What an inefficient scheduling system! Just imagine what patients must say about this practice while they're whiling away their valuable time in the waiting room.

THE MODIFIED WAVE SCHEDULE

With the modified wave schedule, a cluster of patients is scheduled at the beginning of each hour, and then individual appointments are scheduled every 10, 15, or 20 minutes for the rest of the hour. For example, three patients are scheduled at 9 a.m., one at 9:30, and one at 9:45. An alternative modified wave method books two patients at the same time, at the beginning of a time slot long enough to see two patients—for example, two patients at 11 a.m. and two at 11:30.

This method increases the likelihood that a patient will always be available when the physician is ready, and it can work if auxiliary personnel use the waiting time for the second and third patient to complete paperwork and to do preliminary procedures. If the time required doesn't match up with the time available, however, patients can get backlogged. Also, some patients might wind up waiting 20 or 30 minutes, which is longer than they're likely to tolerate without becoming irritated.

USING THE COMPUTER FOR SCHEDULING

More than half of all physician practices use computers as a practice and financial management tool, but only 25% use an automated scheduling system. A computerized scheduling system may cost upwards of several thousand dollars or more, but it can pay for itself in reducing lost charges, improving efficiency, and providing risk management documentation.

Scheduling software is usually tied to billing and automatic recall systems. A good program can search for available time slots and coordinate appointments with the physician and ancillary services. Computerized scheduling is especially helpful for large group practices and practices with multiple locations. The computerized "appointment book" can be used simultaneously by several users in different places.

In investigating computerized systems, be sure to work with a company that specializes in medical practice management systems. Ask questions such as these:

- How will the system integrate with current hardware and software?
- Does it schedule by time slot or appointment type, or can it accommodate both methods?
- Can it note other information, such as reason for visit or referral source?
- Can it list appointments by patient as well as physician or time?
- Can it block out times automatically for standing commitments?
- Can it generate automatic mailings?

WHAT WILL WORK BEST FOR YOUR PRACTICE?

The success of your customized schedule depends on gathering key information about the characteristics and style of your practice. The first step is to be sure that you understand your preferences, your practice style, and your staff and patient needs. Enlist the help and ideas of the entire staff in your evaluation process. Answer the following questions, and think about other preferences that need to be reflected in your scheduling procedures:

- What types of patients do you see? Patients in various age groups and with certain demographic characteristics have different demands on their time that affect when they are able to schedule appointments.
- Are you comfortable grouping similar procedures, or is mixing different types of appointments more effective? Grouping similar appointments can increase efficiency.

- What tasks can be delegated to staff members so that your time can be used more efficiently: patient education? initial work-up? phone calls? recording patient information?
- What time should each office session (morning and afternoon) start and end? You need to make a commitment to be at the office and ready to see patients at the agreed-upon starting time. Patients should not be scheduled significantly before your arrival.

An office manager for a practice with a physician who was consistently 45 minutes to an hour late each day told us how the staff cured the problem: After pleading and pointing out how angry waiting patients became, the office manager left the first hour unscheduled for several days. When the physician arrived, late as usual, and learned that there were no patients for her to see, she was at first irritated (livid!), but the next day and thereafter she arrived on time. (We don't necessarily endorse this procedure; not all employers are likely to be as understanding or to change their behaviors as easily.)

DO A TIME AUDIT, THEN ORGANIZE YOUR INFORMATION

The second step in tackling your schedule is to find out what's really going on in your practice. For 2 weeks, attach a time audit form similar to the one shown in the previous chapter to each patient's chart. List the patient's name and the reason for the visit, and fill in times as the patient moves through the visit.

The third step is to organize your information. Group the time audit forms for similar procedures and examinations into stacks. For each stack, add the "total time in office" numbers. Then divide this sum by the number of forms in the stack. This is the average time required for each category. Look back through your appointment book to see if any procedures were missed in your audit. List them with the approximate time required.

Classify each day as busy, average, or quiet. Analyze daily and weekly patterns of visits. Are Mondays busy? Are Thursday afternoons quiet? What is your pattern of urgent appointments, walk-ins, and physician referrals?

The time audit will help you see each physician's personal style of practice. If patients are typically allotted a 15-minute interval and you're spending an average of 25 minutes per patient, adjustments need to be made. Either more time needs to be given to each appointment, or you need to change your style (not realistic if you've been practicing medicine for any length of time). Another option is to use staff members to perform routine tasks that hinder your productivity—but leave yourself enough time during the appointment for rapport building with patients.

YOU'RE READY FOR SCHEDULING PROTOCOLS!

Now you're ready to develop written scheduling protocols that reflect the preferences and patterns of your practice. A staff member should take the information gathered during the time audit and make a list of the 15 or 20 most common examinations and procedures performed in your practice. Next, use a scheduling key form similar to the one in Exhibit 22-1 to create an easy-to-use chart listing the time needed for each kind of visit. In your scheduling book, each time or procedure category should be color coded to indicate scheduling preferences or groupings. Use the same color code in the circles on the scheduling key. In deciding on appointment lengths, remember that allowing adequate time

---

Exhibit 22-1 Scheduling Key

Color Code	Procedure/Reason for Visit	Time Slot Required
◯		
◯		
◯		
◯		

Instructions: Color code different slots in the appointment book to indicate scheduling preferences or groupings. Use the same color code in the circles on this key.

for tasks increases efficiency and decreases wasted time. Then hold a staff meeting with front and back office personnel and the physicians to discuss the issues listed below as well as any other concerns unique to your situation. The most important thing is to identify your needs, set reasonable protocols, and then stick to them!

Make sure patients know that you value their calls. Staff should offer alternative times and days in a friendly, accommodating way, balancing patient convenience with your need to fill appointment slots efficiently. The scheduler should be well trained to screen patients effectively. To ensure that the proper amount of time is allocated, patients should be asked these questions:

- What is the reason for your visit?
- What symptoms have you been experiencing? For how long?
- Have we seen you in this office before?
- If yes, have we seen you for this problem before?

Some patients are reluctant to state the reason for the visit. The scheduler should explain that knowing the problem allows the correct amount of time to be allotted. The scheduler should be trained in asking tactful questions about sensitive conditions.

Look at your busy/average/quiet pattern. Schedule longer visits and routine follow-up appointments during less-busy times. Maintain a few open slots for urgent visits and referrals, even on busy days. Flexibility is especially important when booking referrals: If you're unable to respond quickly to referring physicians, they'll refer elsewhere. The Neurology Center in Chevy Chase, Maryland has built its large and growing practice on an adamant policy of always fitting in referral patients without sacrificing the schedule.

Keep slots available for new patients. New patients don't want to wait a long time for an appointment. They'll find another doctor if the wait is too long; they have no bond yet with your practice. If you have a heavy managed care load, be sure to assign some open slots for non–managed care patients. Allow time for telephone calls, hospital consults, meetings, lunch commitments, and so forth. Consider grouping appointments on slower days for similar procedures and diagnoses. You might call certain blocks of appointments a "specialty clinic" for a certain condition or disease. Your patients will appreciate your special concern for their problem, and they may like the opportunity to interact with others with similar problems.

Maintain a waiting list of patients who would prefer an earlier appointment or who are available for cancellation slots or unused slots held open for referrals. Consider offering early morning and/or evening office hours once or twice a week. The total number of office hours could remain the same. You can come and leave earlier or later. What about Saturday morning appointments, or using a weekday noon hour for appointments? In Chapter 17, Dr. McHargue, the Virginia dermatologist, reported great success and patient satisfaction with offering evening appointments. Survey your patients to learn if there's interest in nontraditional hours, or simply try it for a month or two. If you do this, be sure that patients know that these appointment times are available. They aren't likely to ask for evenings or noontime appointments if you've never had them available previously.

Patients who don't show up for appointments are a major drain on practice efficiency. The most common reasons people become no-shows:

- They are afraid of the procedure or diagnosis, or they don't understand the reason for or importance of the appointment.
- The appointment time is not convenient, or they are annoyed at long waiting times at previous visits.
- They've neglected to record the appointment date and time and simply forgot it.
- Your policy is to ask for payment at the time of the visit, and they don't have the money.

Keep these issues in mind when dealing with patients, and try to communicate your concern and willingness to discuss and solve problems. You'll find a guide to reducing no-shows in Exhibit 22-2.

YOUR CUSTOMIZED BOOK

You now have the facts to create an appointment book that is tailor made for your practice. Here's how to design a book that works for *you:*

Exhibit 22-2 How To Reduce No-Shows

Patients who don't show up for appointments reduce practice productivity and efficiency. (This may also reflect dissatisfaction and can pose a liability risk, so it's a good idea to keep track of no-shows and to follow up with them.) Here are tactics to reduce no-shows:

- Send a welcome letter and information about the practice in advance of a new patient's appointment. This creates an affiliation with the practice that reduces the chance of cancellation or no-show. The Manchester Heart Center in New Hampshire accomplishes this with a personalized membership card that's sent to every new patient.
- Call patients 1 day before the appointment to confirm.
- Office managers should keep a "no-show notebook" with patient name, day and evening phone numbers, time and date of broken appointment, reason for visit, and response. Call patients to ask the reason they didn't show up; note the reason, and make a new appointment if the patient is willing to do so. If a patient does not reschedule, inform the physician; he or she may need to follow up with the patient.
- For medical-legal reasons it is important to document all no-shows and the practice's attempts to contact them. If a no-show is a referral, send a written notice to the referring physician. Periodically review the reasons given by no-shows; this information may be useful as you make practice decisions.
- Give follow-up patients a reminder card to take home. There are cards available with a peel-off sticker for patients to put on their personal calendars. The card should indicate your cancellation policy: "Please call 555-0000, 24 hours in advance if you must cancel so we may give your time to another patient and make another appointment for you."
- Give return patients a "treatment plan." Note the date and time of the next appointment, why the patient is coming back, what is planned, and how the patient can participate in his or her care. Informed patients will be more likely to understand the importance of the next appointment.
- New to the market are automated appointment reminder systems, which call patients, state a personalized reminder and then request and log the patient's confirmation. They also allow patients to change appointments if necessary by pushing specified buttons on touch-tone phones. Automated systems offer the benefits of confirmation calls without making demands on busy staff members; they are, however, impersonal. Weigh the convenience benefit against this significant disadvantage.

- Look back at your scheduling key. What is your mix of visit lengths? It's likely that you have visits that range from 5 minutes to an hour. Next, review your written scheduling protocols. Keeping in mind the appointment lengths needed and the agreed-upon protocols, sketch out an ideal book.
- Establish slots of various lengths depending on the specific needs of your practice. Combining the modified wave schedule with appointment lengths customized to your needs is the best solution for many practices. Alternating long and short blocks can help keep you on schedule.
- Include sufficient space in each block to record name, address (to ensure that the correct chart is pulled), day and evening phone numbers, and the reason for the appointment (this is essential to allot enough time, to assign the appropriate exam room, and to assemble equipment). Include any other information that would help in your office.
- Use the information in your protocols to color code different slots to indicate scheduling rules and preferred patterns or groupings. For example, shade short appointments for post-operative patients green and longer appointments for initial visits blue. Use the same color code on your scheduling key. Post the key near the appointment book, and use it to assign an appropriate time slot on the basis of the reason for the visit. If you know that a particular patient will take more time than average, assign a longer slot. In a group practice, develop a customized page style for each physician to reflect individual lunch hours, standing meetings, and preferred patterns.

A loose-leaf format is best for your appointment book. The book can be either horizontal or vertical, but it must open flat. Be sure that the pages are Mylar-reinforced at the binding edge. Many physicians like to have a copy of the daily schedule for reference. Order customized pages through an appointment book supply company or a local quick printer. Print time slots in the units that you have decided will be most useful. You may want to preprint lunch, telephone, and referral/emergency/new patient slots.

STAYING ON SCHEDULE

Now that you have a schedule that works for **your** practice, stay on schedule with these tips:

- Have staff make a welcoming call to new patients to gather basic information and to provide directions (thus reducing the risk of late arrivals). Or, mail patient history question-naires before the appointment if there's time. If paperwork isn't sent in advance, ask new patients to arrive 15 minutes early to complete forms. Dr. Lana Holstein's office simply tells new patients that their appointment is 15 minutes before the time written on the schedule to **guarantee** that they arrive in time to fill out paperwork.
- Designated phone time should be booked into the schedule. It's generally not wise to squeeze in calls or interrupt exami-nations. Many practices find that 15-minute blocks in the morning and afternoon streamline callbacks.
- Authorize staff members to let physicians know when they are running behind schedule.
- If patients arrive at the same time, see the ones who require less time first.
- Many practices hold a 5-minute stand-up meeting for physi-cians and staff at the beginning of the day to identify poten-tial problems and bottlenecks and to ensure proper room use planning.
- Some patients need extra time and attention. It's important to take time to talk, but at times a patient's needs extend well beyond the stated reason for the visit. If a patient makes an appointment for one problem and then brings up several others during the examination or brings other family mem-bers to be seen, it's wise to schedule a separate appointment, explaining that the problems deserve appropriate time and attention.

When you follow the steps described above to create a sched-ule that satisfies everyone in the practice—physicians, patients, and staff—you put patient satisfaction on schedule. ❧

Action Steps for a Satisfying Schedule

1. Enlist the help and ideas of the entire staff in developing protocols.
2. Be sure that everyone participates in and understands the rationale for and objectives of changes. When people make an investment in new ideas, they are more motivated to make the system work.
3. Monitor and nurture your new system, and make adjustments as necessary.

23

Can We Talk?

---

*I always felt like my rheumatologist wasn't listening to me. Before
I could finish answering one question, he would ask me another.
I think I'm pretty concise; I don't ramble or bring up things that
don't pertain. This doctor wasn't really interested in my responses
at all. I don't know why he bothered to ask.*

If you think communication is all talk, just listen.

Communication is the glue that cements the physician-patient
relationship. Too little, the wrong kind, or communication without empathy has been pinpointed as the impetus for malpractice
suits that otherwise may have been avoided.

Communication is the heart and soul of quality service in health
care. Without it, not only do doctor-patient relationships not last,
they don't exist. Communication is the ruler patients use to gauge
the overall quality of the encounter. In fact, patients who are
satisfied with their physician's communication style tend to be
more satisfied with the medical care as well.[1]

As the previous chapter pointed out, there's a great deal that
goes into building a strong and positive relationship between
patient and physician. Communication, however, is the basis of
the relationship. But what is good communication? Research has
found that patients are most satisfied with communication that
encompasses the following characteristics:

- information
- technical and interpersonal competence
- partnership building
- social conversation
- positive rather than negative talk
- longer duration (Duration is a matter of perception. Communication that takes place as part of a satisfying interaction will be perceived favorably no matter how long or short the actual time span.)[2]

This kind of effective, interactive communication is healthy for patients because it gives them a sense of control in what can be an otherwise intimidating experience. A researcher at Fox Chase Cancer Center in Philadelphia, Pennsylvania found that active, involved patients who were not afraid to ask questions and get answers had less physical discomfort and more positive attitudes and felt more in control. Moreover, when their physicians showed understanding for these patients' concerns, the patients experienced less stress and greater ability to deal with their problems.[3] According to COMSORT, a continuing medical education consortium specializing in communication and compliance issues, physician-patient communication has been associated with improved recovery from surgery, greater tolerance of pain, and physiological changes such as decreases in blood pressure and blood glucose levels.

MORE THAN JUST WORDS

Although communication usually results in some sort of verbal interchange, there's much more to it than words. In fact, patients often judge the quality of communication not only by words but by a handshake, eye contact, and the "white spaces" when no words are spoken but an emotional or personal connection is made. This connection must be sincere and honest; a caring attitude can't be simulated.

When this connection occurs between physician and patient, it's like plugging an electric cord into a wall socket. The room lights up. "I get a real satisfaction when I take the time to explain something to a patient. They're so appreciative, it's a real bonus to my day," says radiologist Lawrence Cohen in describing how he reacts to communication that connects. If the physician reacts so favorably to this type of interchange, imagine how the patient must feel!

Effective communication in the physician-patient encounter is two way and free flowing. This can be difficult for physicians who were taught the traditional medical approach that calls for control, power, and authority. The traditional approach is physician-focused. It says to the patient, "Listen to my questions, give me the answers I want, and wait for my authorization to speak."

For some physicians, communication means **talk.** In the belief that patients consult them for their wisdom and that wisdom is evidenced by sage advice and extensive use of medical terminology, these physicians talk. A lot. Perhaps they believe that the amount of talk is directly proportional to perceived value. The more words (and the more jargonesque they are), the greater the value.

All this talk gets results, but not necessarily the desired results. The ratio of physician chatter to patient satisfaction is inversely proportional: The more the physician talks compared with the patient, the less satisfied the patient is. In one study this was found to be true no matter how long the visit or how much each spoke.[4] Another study found that half the time physicians did not elicit patient complaints or patient concerns during the interview.[5]

Similarly, psychosocial and psychiatric problems, which are all too common in medical practice, were missed in up to 50% of the cases in another study.[6] Again, researchers found that in half of all health care encounters physicians and patients did not agree on the nature of the main presenting problem.[7]

It appears that there's a pattern unfolding here. Lots of talk but little communication. Sociolinguist Richard Frankel, MD, of the University of Rochester Medical School reviewed medical interviews between internists and their patients and found that 51 of 74 physicians interrupted their patients within 18 seconds of the patient's explanation.[8] Another study found that physicians spend less than 2 minutes of a 20-minute visit actually providing information.

Patient reactions back up the poor communication performance these studies documented. A 1989 *Time* cover story focusing on the doctor-patient relationship cited a poll of 1,000 adults who were asked about their satisfaction with physicians. Although 72% said that doctors do a good job of keeping up with medical knowledge, nearly half criticized them for their listening skills, and one third felt that they do a poor job of being "caring" with patients.[9]

WHEN PATIENTS START TALKING

Enough negative talk! The question is, what can you do to improve communication and patient satisfaction? After all, patients do need to hear your diagnosis, your instructions, and your advice. It is for your wisdom and medical expertise that your patients come to you. But first, they must have **their** chance to talk. If given the opportunity to talk freely, patients will actually take less time to summarize their complaint. They are more likely to divulge (or at least hint at) everything that's on their minds, including the hidden agenda that brings them to you.

Many physicians, however, believe that the message is the medium. They focus solely on what they are saying without paying attention to the receiver or the results (e.g., did the patient not only hear the message but understand it correctly?). Concerned about time, physicians hesitate to use open-ended questions or statements (e.g., "Tell me what you're concerned about, Mr. Phelps") for fear that they will open the verbal floodgates.

In truth, an uninterrupted narrative usually takes about 1 or 2 minutes on average, or about 2.5 minutes at most. During this narrative, the physician's role should be to engage in *active listening*. As a surgeon explained, "You're trying in a very few minutes to judge a patient's personality and his problem and integrate it. You need to pay attention to your patient and use every communication technique available."

An active listener responds in this fashion: "And what did that pain feel like?" or "What I hear you saying is. . . . " Active listening lets your patient know that you have **heard** what he or she has said. It is also listening between the lines, listening to voice tone, watching body language, and hearing references that may offer significant clues. Active listening is empathic listening. It shows concern and interest. It positions the physician as both medical expert and interpersonal communicator, roles to which patients give equal value. As one patient complained, "Some doctors seem not to be too concerned about me as an individual— I feel like I'm just one of the numbers in the rows of medical charts on the wall. Doctors need to be genuinely concerned about the patient's needs. This means **listening!**" Asked if her own physician does this, she nodded affirmatively, adding, "He makes me comfortable. He talks with me, eases my nervousness and answers my questions, usually to my satisfaction."

Yet many physicians believe that nonempathic listening is faster, more efficient, and more productive. It gets the job done without wasting time, they believe. Using "yes–no" questions, and focusing tightly on the apparent medical problem may generate information, but chances are it's not the best information, or all the information needed to make an accurate, comprehensive diagnosis.

PROVEN TECHNIQUES FOR GOOD COMMUNICATION

Try the following techniques for patient consultations that take minimal time and yet satisfy your patients. The satisfying interaction is one in which the patient gets the chance to tell you the facts about his or her symptoms **and** his or her opinion of where the problem lies.

Begin with social conversation. It can quickly establish empathy and personal interest. Some physicians make notes in the patient's medical record to remind them of nonmedical subjects— a daughter graduating from college, a new job started last month, an award. These notes jog the memory when you haven't seen the patient in 4 months. Edward Buchbinder, DPM, an Arizona podiatrist, starts out by asking his patient, "How are you doing from the feet up?" This technique takes new patients aback; it also tells them, "You're a person to me, not merely a foot or ankle problem to be fixed."

Dr. Buchbinder would be classified as an "affiliative" physician, one whose communication style establishes a positive relationship with patients through friendliness, interest, empathy, a nonjudgmental attitude, and a social orientation.[10] That's the style of family physician Lana Holstein, MD. "I like to know about my patients' lives," she said. "I enjoy discussing the good things in people's lives. I think it's good for them. It shows I value them as a person. It fosters a conversation rather than a 'medical interview.'" It doesn't take much time, either. Witness the following interchange between Dr. Holstein and her 68-year-old female patient who had just returned from a European vacation:

> *Dr. Holstein:* Hi, how are you doing? How was your trip? (*She holds the medical chart in her hands but puts it aside as she sits in a chair next to the examining table where her patient is sitting*)
>
> *Patient:* Wonderful. It was cold in England, but then it always is. We had a marvelous time in Germany—the changes since the Berlin Wall came down are remarkable.
>
> *Dr. Holstein:* I'd love to go . . . maybe next year if my schedule allows it.
>
> *Patient:* You'll enjoy it, especially if you've been before, because you will notice such a difference.
>
> *Dr. Holstein:* When I do, I'll consult with you about it! . . . Now, how are you feeling? Any new problems?

This nonmedical conversation took 25 seconds.

In addition to the typical "yes-no" questions, use open-ended questions. For example, before asking, "Do you experience faintness during the day?" say this: "Tell me how things are going these days, Mrs. Crane." She may describe her frustration over the fact that she doesn't have the stamina to put in a full day at the office and that she sometimes feels lightheaded for no reason. Open-ended questions elicit information and revelations that don't come out of "yes-no" questions. They also are interactive, nurturing the doctor-patient relationship.

Listen. Bite your tongue, put your hand over your mouth, do whatever it takes to stay silent until Mrs. Crane is through speaking. Most patients will synopsize the problem and complete their explanation within a few minutes. Dr. Schreiber, the orthopedic surgeon, says that you have to give patients a chance to "tell their story," even if it's unrelated to their medical complaint. Until they do, he says, they're not ready to hear what you have to say, no matter how important it may be. If someone does begin to ramble, you can gently bring him or her back by saying, "I'd like to focus on the chest pains you just mentioned. Next time you come we'll talk about your problems with your daughter-in-law."

Don't give in to the urge to dive into a break in the conversational flow. Not only is silence golden, it can be productive. When your patient is fumbling for words, he or she may be overcoming nervousness or formulating a difficult statement. Give him or her the space and time to verbalize it.

Don't be afraid of "emotional hand-holding." Use nonverbal techniques to show that you're listening and to show compassion. Put down the chart and **look** at your patient while he or she describes the problem. Dr. Schreiber doesn't write a word in the chart. He uses a staff member to document everything said during the interview, which leaves him free to focus on the patient. A risk assessment firm that reviewed his practice gave him the highest marks possible for this and other communication techniques he uses.

A gentle touch on the shoulder, nonjudgmental comments ("I'm worried about your weight loss"), and appropriate "uh-huhs" and "hm-ms" are simple ways to visibly demonstrate that you're listening and to convey the concern and interest you feel.

Probe for the hidden agenda. Many patients have one; it's the *underlying* reason for visiting you, not what they list on the patient information form. Watch for nonverbal cues or agitation after you've supposedly discussed the presenting condition. The patient with a hidden agenda expects, or hopes, that you will dig it out through insightful or open-ended questions. Many physicians conclude their discussion and examination by asking, "Is there anything else you want to talk about today?" This gives the patient the opportunity to bring up the hidden agenda.

Paraphrase the patient's complaint, restating it as you heard it. You might say, "Mrs. Crane, what I hear you say is that you're concerned about your lack of energy and especially the occasional faintness you're feeling. And since your mother had a stroke a few years ago, you are afraid these symptoms might be indicative of something more serious. Is that right?" Paraphrasing shows active listening on your part while allowing you to probe for the meaning in your patient's statements. It also allows your patient to confirm, correct, or add to what you heard.

ACTIVE LISTENING YIELDS CLINICAL BENEFITS, TOO

Most patients want their physicians to ask for their opinion. They want a say in treatment options, or at least a chance to express their hesitation or fear about a recommended procedure and to offer their point of view. Active listening gives patients the opportunity to state their views, and it gives you a chance to assess your patients' knowledge about their condition. As Sir William Osler counseled in 1889, "Listen to the patient, he is telling you the diagnosis." Active listening yields clues you aren't likely to gain through a series of limiting questions.

When you conduct the medical interview in the traditional physician-centered way, you may believe that you've collected what you need to know in the most efficient way possible. You may even gather the information and complete the visit more quickly. Your belief may be that quality medical care has taken place. You've made a diagnosis, prescribed a treatment, shaken Mrs. Crane's hand and wished her a good day, and maybe even smiled at her as you walked from the exam room. You've fulfilled your technical role, but was the physician-patient relationship enhanced? It's doubtful. You may be satisfied—you've efficiently accomplished your objective of dispensing medical care—but your patient is not. The building blocks of the relationship are stacked in place, but the glue—effective two-way communication—is missing. Without it, so are the results you seek: patient compliance, a better outcome, and, most of all, patient satisfaction. 🙢

Action Steps for Communicating Effectively

1. Practice active listening with your patients. Here's how:
   - Paraphrase your patients' statements to demonstrate that you *hear* what they say.
   - Ask probing follow-up questions.
   - Don't interrupt. Allow your patients to state their case or express their views.
2. Ask open-ended questions; they are interactive and elicit information that "yes–no" questions can't.
3. Use nonverbal techniques to show interest:
   - Establish eye contact.
   - Touch the patient lightly on the shoulder or arm.
   - Don't write in the chart every moment you're with the patient.

References

1. L. Herket, Communication affects patient satisfaction, *Internist* (May/June 1988): 38.
2. J. A. Hall, D. L. Roter, and N. R. Katz, Meta-analysis of correlates of provider behavior in medical encounters, *Medical Care* 26 (1988): 657–675.
3. D. Cole, Listen Doctor . . . , *Self* (July 1991): 114–134.
4. K.D. Bertakis, D. Roter, and S.M. Putnam, The relationship of physician medical interview style to patient satisfaction, *Journal of Family Practice* 32, no. 2 (1991): 175–181.
5. M.A. Stewart, I.R. McWhinney, and C.W. Buck, The doctor-patient relationship and its effect on outcome, *Junior College General Practice* 29 (1979): 77–82.
6. P. Freeling, B.M. Rao, E.S. Paykel, L.L. Sireling, and R.H. Burton, Unrecognized depression in general practice, *British Medical Journal* 290 (1985): 1880–1883.
7. B. Starfield, C. Wray, K. Hess, R. Gross, P.S. Birk, and B.C. D'Lugoff, The influences of patient-practitioner agreement on outcome of care, *American Journal of Public Health,* 71 (1981): 127–132.
8. D. Goleman, All too often, the doctor isn't listening, studies show, *New York Times* (November 13, 1992): 1.
9. N. Gibbs, Sick and tired, *Time* (July 31, 1989): 47–51.
10. K.K. Bertakis et al., The relationship, 175–181.

—❧—

24

The Patient Is Your Partner

"I always try to do my homework before I go to the doctor. If I have a specific problem or complaint, I read up on it or check with other professionals who may have some knowledge about it. I do this so that I can ask intelligent, specific questions and so that I can be certain all my fears and concerns are addressed.

"Some doctors don't seem to like this. Sometimes I think they resent my knowledge. I think it makes me a better patient if I understand the problem. It certainly has the potential to make it easier on the doctor, because he or she can focus on my questions more easily."

—A patient

"I don't think patients want to knock doctors off their pedestal. They've gone to medical school; they've earned the right to be there. We just want to climb on the pedestal and talk to doctors side by side, instead of yelling up at them."

—A patient

"Who knows what patients want. . . . You give them information, then they want to make the decision, too. What do they need the doctor for? Why don't we just hand them a medical encyclopedia and a PDR. . . ."

—A frustrated physician

Partner: *A person associated with another in some activity of common interest.* Partner *implies a relationship in which each has equal status and a certain independence but also implicit or formal obligations to the other or others.*

The paternalistic "Doctor knows best" model in medicine has a rich and lengthy history. Hippocrates counseled physicians to conceal "most things from the patient while you are attending to him . . . turning his attention away from what is being done to him; sometimes reprove sharply and emphatically, and sometimes comfort with solicitude and attention, revealing nothing of the patient's future or present condition."[1(p.124)]

Small wonder, then, that some physicians have a hard time with patients who question their decisions or demand to see X-rays, lab reports, and test results. It's not their style, and it's certainly not medical tradition to share information fully with patients or to seek their opinions. In a 1989 speech to the 36th National Health Forum sponsored by the National Health Council, Diana Dutton, PhD, said, "The idea of doctors and patients as equal partners is still controversial today; it must have seemed downright heretical when it was first proposed in the mid-1950s" by two psychiatrists who proposed a previously unknown level of equality between physician and patient. Now, in the 1990s, Dutton added, "We've come full circle. No longer is the goal merely an equal partnership with doctors; now it is the **patient's** turn to take control!"[2]

Researcher Jack Ende, MD, of Boston University found that what people seek from their doctors is not control but collaboration, with a healthy dose of information. Patients yield to the physician for the final decision, but they want to know how and why he or she arrived at the decision, as Dr. Ende and his colleague, Mark Moskowitz, MD, found in 1989 when they asked 312 people about their preferences.[3] This relationship is described by Mary, a patient who said that her physician exhibits the qualities she expects: "My doctor is very explicit in describing what the problem is and allowing patients to see lab results and X-rays. As a patient, this makes me feel more like a part of having whatever needs to be done carried out. Being a part means helping to make the decision, though not making the decision myself."

Mary is pretty typical of today's health-educated consumer. Nevertheless, the partnership concept is difficult for some physicians to accept. It's not enough that managed care firms, hospitals, employers, the government, and every other agency is telling you what kind of care to provide, how often, and when. Now it seems that patients want to dictate to you as well, prescribing treatment, medication, and follow-up. After they've consulted a lay health care network of family and friends and the latest Oprah, Donahue, or Dr. Dean Edell show and self-diagnosed their illness, that is. The print media plays its part, too. Pick up any popular magazine or best-seller list, and you'll come across article titles such as "Learn To Become a Participating Patient" and books such as *Taking Charge of Your Medical Fate* as well as a host of tips for putting doctors in their place, wherever that may be.

WHAT SHOULD THE DOCTOR-PATIENT RELATIONSHIP LOOK LIKE?

Are patients taking control, or are they simply asserting their rights? What should the doctor-patient relationship look, sound, and feel like? How should it work?

The evidence, as well as consumers and physicians we interviewed, says that most patients prefer to defer to the physician or surgeon when it comes to the ultimate recommendation. What they want is information and discussion before the decision is made. Most people don't want to make the final choice between pro or con, but they want to know what the pros and cons are, and they want the chance to weigh them, even if they ultimately let you tip the scales.

What does the patient-as-partner concept have to do with quality service? If you view the physician-patient relationship as a service relationship, it's easier to understand. Let's say you go to a department store to buy a business suit. You probably have some idea in mind as to the style, cut, color, and price of your intended purchase. You want some assistance in making the decision, however, and you look to the salesperson to act as an informed partner in the decision. Depending on the price range in which you're shopping, your previous experience in suit buying, and the information and knowledge the salesperson demonstrates, you may defer to a greater or lesser degree to the store employee's recommendation. In some cases, you may even let the salesperson's opinion override your own.

The amount and apparent depth of information that the salesclerk offers ("Pewter is the newest color for fall; it's also a classic that will never go out of style. The vertical stripes make you appear taller and leaner") and his or her honesty ("The $400 suit is actually made better than the one for $500") are likely to influence your perception of the quality of the service you receive. The salesperson acts as a partner in helping you reach a decision, making recommendations based on his or her knowledge of tailoring, fabric, and your needs. The help provided makes your decision easier, because it's based on information. If he or she takes over the decision process without offering information or data to support it, you are likely to feel resentful and patronized. You're also not likely to buy a suit from the salesperson.

WHAT PATIENTS WANT: AN INFORMED PARTNERSHIP

Although buying a suit is not the same as visiting the physician, many people have similar expectations regarding the relationship they have with their physician. They seek an informed partnership that's grounded in trust and built on facts and judgment, a partnership in which significant decisions or recommendations reside with the most knowledgeable party. In the medical encounter, that's you. You can help patients understand how you view the relationship by describing it verbally or in writing. A sample "Partners in Care" letter can be found in Exhibit 24-1.

A physician told us the following story that seems to affirm the patient's perspective regarding the physician's role in the partnership. The physician learned that he had an elevated PSA (prostatic specific antigen) and consulted a urologist, an old friend and well-respected physician in the community: "He examined me and said that everything seemed normal. Then he told me, 'You can have an ultrasound if it will make you feel better.' I'm not faulting him, but I think he could have reworded his advice. As a patient, I wanted to

Exhibit 24-1 "Partners In Care" Letter

A Message to My Patients

As patient and physician, ours is more than a relationship; it's a partnership. A partnership is based on mutual trust and confidence. I want to ensure that you get an accurate diagnosis and the treatment that's best and most satisfactory for you.

To give you the best, most thorough care possible, I need some things from you:

1. Communication: If you don't understand what I'm telling you, if you don't understand a treatment, prescription instructions, or my diagnosis, tell me. If I explain again and it's still not clear, say so. With a complex topic, sometimes it takes two or three explanations to clarify all the details. I'm willing to explain as many times as needed; I simply need you to remind me.

2. Clarification: Tell me what you need to know about your condition. If I've told you to take it easy until your condition improves, and you want to know if you can go to work, watch television, or go shopping, ask.

3. Satisfaction: Be sure you're comfortable with what I've recommended, and if you're not, tell me. We can discuss alternatives, or, if there are no options, I'll try to do a better job of making you feel more at ease and explaining the choices you face.

4. Understanding: Understand that medicine is a science, but it's also an art. Doctors don't always have the perfect, no-questions-asked diagnosis, treatment, or cure. I'll use my knowledge to evaluate your condition. I can do a better job of treating you if you will keep me informed, ask me questions, and give me honest, complete information about your medical history and current symptoms or problems.

5. Information: Tell me or one of my staff when something is troubling you, whether it's that my front door is difficult to open, that one of us was short-tempered with you, or that the prescription I gave you doesn't seem to be working. If I know when you're unhappy or not fully satisfied, I can do something about it. If you keep it to yourself, I'll never know—and sometimes the information you keep to yourself may affect the course of your treatment or recovery.

In return for your involvement and communication, I promise I'll communicate with you. I believe the result will be better medicine and a stronger relationship.

Physician's Signature

know from the 'authority' what my options were, and what his recommendation was, so that I could make an informed decision."

Others tell similar stories of wanting recommendations backed up by detailed information. Recalls Peter, a runner:

> *I had to see an orthopedic surgeon about a back problem. My back hurt, and I wanted to be able to continue to run. The doctor took an X-ray, then explained that the problem was a congenital defect. He prescribed a limited course of an anti-inflammatory drug and recommended a series of exercises.*
>
> *What I remember most was how much time he spent listening to me. He didn't make assumptions about my needs or what I wanted him to do. He took the time to listen to what I had to say and what I wanted to do, then helped me figure out how to do it.*
>
> *I didn't expect to tell him how to treat my condition, but I did expect that he would inform me about treatment options. I didn't want to make the decision, I just wanted to know the data that went into making the decision. And that's what he gave me.*

Involved patients are happier patients. They're also healthier patients, studies suggest. A group of patients with chronic ulcers was trained to read their medical records, to ask questions, and to negotiate medical decisions. Compared with a control group, these patients reported less disability and fewer physical limitations from their condition; they were twice as effective in obtaining information from their physicians and just as happy with the care they received.[4]

To create this partnership with your patient, you need to understand **who** he or she is as well as what symptoms and complaints he or she may have. The more you understand of your patient's education, economic and social status, personality, medical and family history, and previous health care experience, the more clearly you can determine how the partnership should be weighted.

Even so, avoid making assumptions about your patient's level of knowledge. A friend who works in health care recalls consulting her internist about a fairly uncommon condition from which she suffered: "My doctor was aware of my profession and assumed, albeit innocently, that I had a broad understanding of clinical issues. He rarely offered any explanations relative to my condition. I finally had to remind him that I was a **marketer** who knew virtually nothing about the problem we were discussing other than how to spell it."

Physicians who advocate patient satisfaction and quality service seem to understand the benefits of partnership. Lawrence Cohen, MD, believes that the physician should inform and guide the patient toward a decision: "It's important for us not to make decisions for patients, but to educate and inform them about the choices, alternatives and consequences of their decisions, then offer advice to help them reach the best decision. If you give them information, most patients are very capable of making their own decisions, and they appreciate the respect it shows you have for them."

YOUR PATIENTS LIVE WITH THEIR CONDITION, SO GIVE THEM INFORMATION

"Let's face it," pointed out cardiologist Alan Kaplan, MD. "A patient may have 20 minutes together with me in the exam room. That's only a fraction of the time he will spend living with his condition. My role as a doctor is to help the patient understand how to make decisions so he can have some independence in his care."

Encouraging questions helps patients make informed decisions. Dr. Kaplan's practice provides "cues" to prompt questions, such as a clipboard with a notepad in the reception area and exam rooms. "I want patients to know everything they should about their condition, medications, and treatments," he said. To encourage patients to recognize and report problems, he gives them information sheets describing side effects of drugs prescribed. "If they know what to expect, they won't just stop taking the drug, they'll call me and tell me what's happening." The result: healthier, more compliant, more satisfied patients.

WHAT STYLE OF PARTNER ARE YOU?

Partnership doesn't mean that only one provider style is acceptable. In an article in the *Journal of the American Medical Asso-*

ciation, Emanuel and Emanuel described four models of the physician-patient relationship: informative, interpretive, deliberative, and paternalistic.[5] Each relationship depends on the physician's understanding of the patient's values. In the informative model, the patient is given all relevant facts to make a decision; the physician's role is that of "technical expert." The interpretive model is more collaborative; the physician helps the patient by providing facts, risks, and benefits and then also aids in determining an appropriate course of action. The deliberative model requires the physician to act as friend or teacher, providing information and then, through dialog with the patient, recommending a course of action. In the paternalistic model, also referred to as the parental model, the physician acts as guardian to the patient, sharing selected information and encouraging a course of action for the patient's well-being.

The authors point out that there may be an appropriate time and place for each model. An emergency may demand quick action without patient consent, for example, making the paternalistic model acceptable. But overall, they believe that the deliberative model is the ideal physician-patient relationship.

PARTNERSHIP, YES, BUT PATIENTS WANT YOUR EXPERT OPINION

Physicians whose perspectives and approaches range from semiauthoritarian to collegial acknowledge that collaboration that occurs through education is the most effective and productive decision-making process. Dr. Cohn, the author-internist, said, "I tend to be authoritative. I don't pretend to be the best doctor for every patient. I try to inform them, and I encourage them to be informed, but I definitely get my two cents worth in. I think the outcome is best if the physician determines the course of treatment. When I take my car to the garage, I'm seeking the opinion of an expert. I don't expect him to draw me into a diagnostic discussion: 'Dr. Cohn, do you think it's the carburetor or the emissions system?' I want to hear my patient's point of view, but I also want to give patients a sense they're seeing someone with experience and expertise."

No matter what your partnership style and how much decision-making responsibility you turn over to patients, the personal concern must be there. Patients give higher satisfaction ratings to physicians who demonstrate a warm, open, and sympathetic style.[6] James McNamara, MD, of the Sansum Clinic in Santa Barbara, California believes that what physicians want from patients is "a feeling we're in this together." Dogmatic, dictatorial physicians are out of touch, he believes, although "older patients want me to direct them, and I will, if necessary. But I much prefer to develop a friendship relationship, so that I can do what's best for the individual by knowing his background."

Health care consumer guardian Charles Inlander, president of the People's Medical Society, believes "respect is the ultimate goal of the physician-patient relationship." He expects the physician to explain things, "to allow me to ask questions, to make decisions in the partnership. It should not be a parent-child relationship, which may be more expedient and easier. Instead, there should be equality in decision making." The physician partners with the patient through candid disclosure of skills, expertise, knowledge, and information, he said.

Even in a partnership, however, the person with greater knowledge and expertise must sometimes take over. Thomas Zink, MD, a St. Louis, Missouri physician, believes "when a crisis occurs, people turn to someone who is credible, someone in authority. When there's a tornado warning from the weather bureau, people turn on the radio because they want to hear someone who knows where the shelter is, when to go there, what to take. It's the same with medicine. The doctor needs to have the backbone to say, 'I don't recommend this' to patients who are demanding something that may not be appropriate." What if the patient isn't convinced? "The problem may be that the doctor hasn't established a strong relationship with the patient to begin with," Dr. Zink says. We couldn't agree more.

PARTNERSHIP IS PATIENT CENTERED

Partnership in health care is a patient-centered approach. It is the kind of relationship most often sought by knowledgeable, informed consumers. And studies are beginning to show that partnership may improve outcome and quality of life. A new questionnaire developed in part by Interstudy, an Excelsior, Minnesota health care "think tank," recognizes the significance of the patient's perspective. The quality of life survey form, called SF-36, is being used to help physicians determine appropriate treatment and to help pharmaceutical firms determine the effectiveness of certain therapies. The questionnaire asks thirty-six questions about a person's ability to perform physical activities such as carrying groceries or taking a walk around the block. The questionnaire also asks about mental or emotional attitude. SF-36 proponents believe that use of the survey can help physicians determine appropriate treatment by getting them to focus on the patient's own quality-of-life assessment, not just on lab test results and quantitative data.

WHAT PHYSICIANS SAY ABOUT PARTNERSHIP: "IF MY PATIENTS WOULD ONLY. . ."

Partnership implies shared responsibility. If the physician has certain responsibilities, what are the responsibilities of the other partner—the patient? According to Timothy Cavanaugh, MD, "Patients shouldn't come to me with the attitude, 'I've got a problem and the doctor is going to fix it.' They need to understand their part and their responsibility."

As Washington, D.C. neurologist Herbert Baraf, MD, says,

Doctors aren't omniscient. I can't put my hand on a patient's forehead and read his thoughts. Patients need to tell me what's wrong. They need to understand that the process of diagnosis and treatment requires good communication. And if I don't ask the right questions, the patient has the responsibility to point it out to me.

The consensus of physicians about the patient's responsibility was this: "Patients need to ask questions and give us information. We can give better care when we have all the facts." They said that patients receive better, more effective care if they are:

• actively involved
• honest

- informed
- questioning
- compliant

In fact, most physicians, we found, would like their patients to be more assertive and proactive in the health care relationship. "Patients are often concerned about taking too much of the doctor's time," explained Robert Bright, MD. "They have concerns but they won't express them, or they don't always hear what I have to say about lifestyle issues" out of concern that they are usurping more than their fair share of the appointment schedule.

How Physicians Say Patients Could Be Better Partners

Here s what physicians had to say when asked to complete the following sentence: **"I could give better care and my patients would be more satisfied if they would only . . ."**

. . . become more educated about their health and their type of insurance and coverage. (Lawrence Cohen, MD, Silver Spring, Maryland)

. . . follow advice on preventive care. (Gerald Angoff, MD, Manchester, New Hampshire)

. . . help us learn where we can improve. Don t be so in awe of us as doctors that they fail to express concerns or talk about aspects of service care they don t like. (Timothy Cavanaugh, MD, Kansas City, Missouri)

. . . accept personal responsibility for their lifestyle choices. (Donald Parsons, MD, Denver, Colorado)

. . . be patient, and never leave without asking the questions they have. (Dan Burrus, MD, Nashville, Tennessee)

. . . be as open as possible about expressing their needs from the visit. (Bruce Dixon, MD, Nashville, Tennessee)

. . . this sentence shouldn t be finished. It should be changed to If I would only. . . . (Marvin Korengold, MD, Chevy Chase, Maryland)

PATIENTS SHOULD BE ACTIVELY INVOLVED

Dr. Baraf says, "Quality care involves patients fronting for themselves. Sometimes they fail to realize that if they're having problems at night or even during the week, we should be informed." But he put the burden back on physicians: "It's incumbent on physicians to break down the barriers with patients who are not forthcoming." His point is well taken. Doctors need to help patients become actively involved in the partnership. You need to make them feel **comfortable** in doing so. Create proactive patients by:

- giving them information and emphasizing the importance of reviewing and understanding it so that they become knowledgeable about their health, their illness, symptoms, medications, and treatment
- asking for feedback and responding to it ("Are we meeting your needs? Do you have any questions?")
- encouraging them to bring along a family member to support them and to speak up if necessary
- posing questions yourself to let them know you want to hear their questions (e.g., "You may wonder why I chose this particular implant. Let me explain . . . .")
- developing a handout of commonly asked questions relating to a specific condition and going over it with patients
- **telling** your patients that you expect them to ask questions

Passive patients who don't question their physicians tend to receive lower-quality care, many physicians believe. Charles Mittman, MD, president of the Central California Faculty Medical Group in Fresno, California believes that "all too often patients don't ask questions or insist upon clearly understanding the care being provided." Dr. Thomas Zink, former medical director of the Sanus Health Plan in St. Louis, Missouri agrees with Dr. Mittman. He says that patients often let themselves be intimidated. They have difficulty asking even routine questions.

So how do you get these patients to participate? While he was employed by Sanus, Dr. Zink developed a pamphlet entitled "How To Communicate with Your Doctor." It's an excellent primer for encouraging enlightened, active patients. Part of the text is reproduced in Exhibit 24-2.

Helping patients assume their role in the health care partnership sometimes takes prompting. Uninformed surgery patients are a particular liability risk. "I hate to see a patient leave when they haven't asked any questions or participated in their care, then the next day they'll call because they didn't understand what or why they were told something," Dr. Cavanaugh said. At the Hunkeler Clinic, surgical counselors are instructed to inform Dr. Cavanaugh if a patient doesn't seem to understand the scheduled procedure. He will then explain it in more detail. This special attention increases efficiency while enhancing satisfaction because it reduces the chance of the next-day phone call that takes staff members or physicians away from other tasks.

Patients don't always know or think of the right questions when they are in the physician's office. Anxiety, stress, and "white coat syndrome" fog some people's thinking. Carol Gilmore, MD, sends her patients home with explanatory material "to give them time to digest what they learned. Then they can call with questions. I do a lot of telephone follow-up."

HONESTY IS THE BEST POLICY

The truth, the whole truth, and nothing but. That's what physicians want from patients. The hidden agenda remains hidden unless the physician excavates it. Posing an open-ended question during the conversation such as, "Anything else you want to talk about?" helps patients feel free to say what's on their minds. Concern and compassion on the part of the physician also accomplish this. Allowing the patient to put it in writing can also encourage openness.

It's clear that most physicians recognize that a patient who participates actively in the medical encounter is likely to get better care. It's also clear that physicians and staff members must encourage this partnership by giving patients the **knowledge** they need to make informed decisions and the **comfort** that allows them to speak up and ask questions. ֍

Exhibit 24-2 Sanus: Self-Care and Your Health

Through its member newsletter *Healthy Update,* Sanus Health Plan in St. Louis, Missouri provides information to help people know when self-care is appropriate and when to call the physician. This sort of educational information is a patient-satisfying strategy for any practice. It shows concern for patients "in sickness and in health." A typical *Healthy Update* article points out, "Because 80% of all health care problems can be managed at home, there is much we can do for ourselves."

The article lists symptoms that call for a telephone call to the physician. They include:

- Fever of more than 102°F along with any symptom related to the throat, ear, or sinuses or a cough
- Fever accompanied by a skin wound or rash, marked irritability, confusion, severe headache, stiff neck, severe back pain or abdominal pain, vomiting, diarrhea, or painful urination
- Fever of 101°F lasting more than 5 days
- Headache described as the worst headache ever
- Headache associated with severe stiff neck and fever
- Headache accompanied by slurred speech, vision disturbance, weakness in extremities, or fainting
- Sore throat associated with a skin rash; great difficulty swallowing, talking, or breathing; hoarseness; or enlarged lymph nodes for more than 2 weeks
- Cough accompanied by wheezing, difficulty breathing, shortness of breath, chest pains, and bloody, brown, or green mucus
- Nasal congestion lasting longer than 3 weeks or associated with bloody, green, or brown discharge or serious pain in the forehead, cheeks, or upper teeth
- Earache with hearing loss, dizziness, ringing noise, pus, or bloody discharge
- Vomiting or diarrhea associated with signs of dehydration, the inability to hold down clear liquids, abdominal tenderness, and yellow skin color
- Vomit or diarrhea that appears bloody, black, or like coffee grounds
- Indigestion not relieved by antacids and lasting longer than 3 days
- Back pain after an injury
- Back pain associated with severe abdominal pain or frequent, painful, bloody urination
- Back pain accompanied by loss of bowel or bladder control, numbness, or weakness in the lower extremities
- Injury that causes large bruising, deep laceration, and uncontrollable bleeding
- Injury with marked swelling, extreme tenderness, coldness, discoloration, and numbness of an extremity
- Injuries that result from strong forces, such as tackles, falls, and traffic accidents

This list of symptoms is not meant to be a substitute for appropriate medical care. It may, however, help you determine when it is best to call your physician for advice.

Source: Courtesy of Sanus Health Plan, St. Louis, Missouri.

Action Steps for Creating Partners out of Patients

1. Be aware that each patient has different partnership expectations depending on his or her age, education, medical condition, and urgency.
2. Encourage informed patient partners by giving them information for decision making.
3. Don't make assumptions about a patient's level of knowledge. Ask.
4. Learn as much as you can about your patient. It fosters the relationship as well as the partnership.
5. People consult a physician for expertise and knowledge. Don't strive so hard for an equal partnership that you turn over your decision-making responsibilities. Most patients want information and guidance from the medical expert.
6. Let your patients know what you need and expect from them in the partnership.

References

1. J. Katz, Disclosure and consent: In search of their roots, *Genetics and the Law II*, eds. A. Milunsky and G. Annas (New York, N.Y.: Plenum Press, 1980): 124.
2. D. Dutton, Healing encounters: Patient-provider collaboration reconsidered (Paper presented at panel on The Psychology of Collaboration, March 28, 1989, Baltimore, Maryland): 3, 5.
3. T. Friend and D. Sperling, Learn to become a participating patient, *USA Today* (April 6, 1989): 7D.
4. S. Greenfield, S. Kaplan, and J. Ware, Expanding patient involvement in care: Effect on patient outcomes, *Annals of Internal Medicine* 102 (1985): 520–528.
5. E. J. Emanuel and L.L. Emanuel, Four models of the physician-patient relationship, *JAMA* 267, no. 16 (1992): 2221–2226.
6. L. Herkert, Communication affects patient satisfaction, *Internist* (May/June 1988): 38.

Part 4

Continuity: Get It, Keep It, Grow It

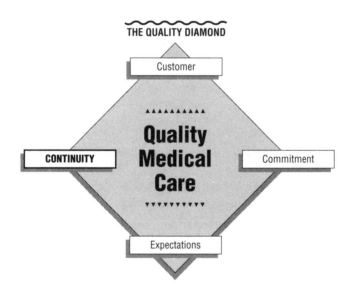

THE QUALITY DIAMOND

Customer

Quality Medical Care

CONTINUITY

Commitment

Expectations

Quality doesn't stand still. But you know that. It's why you attend medical meetings and conferences regularly—because medicine is changing, improving, continually finding new therapies and procedures that will keep people healthy. Techniques that seemed perfectly reasonable 10 years ago—or even yesterday— may seem prehistoric tomorrow. Service quality is just the same. It demands continually "upping the bar," looking for ways to satisfy patient needs a little more thoroughly, a little more personally, a little more efficiently.

Continuity calls for setting standards, monitoring what's working (and what's not), fixing things that go wrong and preventing them from ever happening again, paying attention to patients, paying attention to other practices, other businesses, other industries. Continuity is the CME of service—continuous improvement for practice success. 🕩

25

Quality Is a Moving Target

"There's no standing still in the world anymore," Peterman says. "You are either going up or down. I've decided to go up. We deliver wonderful things, so people keep buying. We do this among lots of challenges. I know that when the quality challenges stop, when we think we've solved all the quality problems, we're through."[1(p.4)]

It's an ironic fact of the quality journey: The better you are, the better you must be. As the level of quality and service soars, the customer's expectations for the service escalate. At the same time, a service error or omission, however slight, becomes more noticeable.

Quality, in other words, is a moving target. To maintain quality service, you must keep moving, continually improving. Because where quality, service, and patient satisfaction are concerned, staying where you are is a slow slide backward. And that's a direction a practice can ill afford to take in today's competitive and demanding health care environment. As one patient told us:

> *I always brag about my doctor to my friends. I've never had to wait an excessive amount of time; her staff is always friendly and professional; and she always asks about my personal life and about how I'm doing, even though I only see her once a year for a routine check-up. To me, she's the*

epitome of what a doctor should be—concerned, knowledge-
able, efficient.

But I went to my annual appointment last week, and I was
disappointed. Not because she was unfriendly or uncaring,
but because the visit was routine. I think I had bragged
about her so much, I expected something extraordinary. I'm
not sure what—just more than a routine visit.

An innovative, patient-oriented team—the team you and your staff now are, or are on your way to becoming—must constantly look for ways to provide better service and soar above patient expectations. This service attitude is akin to cardiovascular conditioning. Newly quality-conscious organizations are like novice runners. At first, the daily run of 1 or 2 miles leaves them gasping and fatigued, but eventually they build endurance so that 3 or 5 miles becomes routine. Then they begin looking for challenges—hills, a faster pace, more miles to cover, a 10K race, even a marathon in which to test themselves. Seasoned runners continually seek improvement. When they break 3 hours in a marathon, they strive for 2:50. They become conditioned to achieve. If you are intent on achieving patient satisfaction, no one—physicians or staff—can ever be satisfied with the most recent accomplishment or accolade. Enjoy it, then move on, striving for service excellence through improved processes. Here's how.

ADOPT A "GOOD ENOUGH ISN'T" ATTITUDE

Like runners seeking constantly to improve their cardiovascular condition, pace, and running style, you and your staff must build on each success in the practice. Look for continual small steps you can take toward better care and better service. Continuous improvement should be a regular topic for discussion at staff meetings and during departmental, committee, and physician meetings. Make it a specific responsibility of every member of the practice; write it into job descriptions to reinforce the expectation that quality is everyone's job. Don't leave "well enough" alone. Improve it. Then work on making it better still. Set standards for waiting time, patient education, communication, billing, return calls, and all other areas of your practice. Monitor patient and staff expectations and reactions (see

Chapters 14 and 27). When you find that you're consistently reaching the standards you've set, move the bar a little higher.

One practice started by deciding to make the time more productive and pleasant for patients waiting in the exam room for the physician. First, magazine racks with current issues of popular magazines were installed so that patients had something to read. Patient comments were favorable. Then a staff member said one day, "Why don't we hand patients a brochure or information about the condition for which they've made the appointment and recommend that they read it while they're waiting so if they come up with questions, they can ask the doctor?" Patients were impressed with this evidence of concern, but the staff didn't stop there. They placed notepads and pencils for patients to write down their questions, which was another patient pleaser. There were so many compliments about the patient education effort that the practice set up a patient education library in a little-used office, stocking it with magazines, pamphlets, videos, and audio cassettes. Staff members created a scrapbook of articles from current popular magazines and even some medical journals, and the physicians wrote comments or "perspective" articles in response to those they felt required additional insight or clarification. Patients interested in more information about a disease, a condition, or personal fitness were referred by the physician or nurse to specific items in the library.

But one day a medical assistant commented, "You know, we've got the right idea, but shouldn't we be looking at the real issue— the amount of time patients are waiting in the exam room? I wonder if we've become so eager to fill the time, we've forgotten that patients shouldn't have a whole lot of time to occupy." Thus came about the next service improvement: monitoring the time the patient waited before the physician came in to the exam room and setting a maximum of 10 minutes as a target. The staff are now evaluating the scheduling system to find better ways of moving patients through the practice without affecting their favorable perception of the overall visit.

CONTINUOUS IMPROVEMENT WORKS

Continuous improvement as a formal business growth strategy is a relatively new concept in the United States. Significantly, the

English language does not have a single word to express the concept of continuous improvement, whereas the Japanese understand its value and processes culturally and linguistically, using the word *kaizan* to express it. Although there may not be a succinct way to say it, patient-centered practices understand the importance of continuous improvement. The physicians and staff in these practices talk and share ideas among themselves, formally and informally; they look for other practices and other firms against which to benchmark, and they look for problems before patients call their attention to them. You'll find a short history of the concept of Total Quality Management in Appendix 25-A at the end of this chapter.

Practices in which patient satisfaction is a targeted objective spend an incredible amount of time communicating with each other. Seldom did we encounter a practice whose office manager or physicians said, "We don't have time for staff meetings." These practices meet in groups of 2 or 10 or 50 and more—daily, weekly, monthly, or annually depending on the purpose of the meeting and the members of the group. They meet to **communicate,** to share ideas and take action. For example, the Hunkeler Eye Clinic in Kansas City, Missouri uses "huddles" to activate incremental improvements. Each huddle consists of five or six employees and a physician. The huddle members meet daily to discuss a problem and work on solving it or to learn about issues that affect the practice.

In late 1991 and early 1992, Medicare's new reimbursement system was a topic for each of the huddle teams. The practice believed that it was important for employees as well as physicians to understand the impact of this new form of resource-based reimbursement, especially for more common surgical procedures in the practice. The huddles are a formal means of effecting incremental improvements and ensuring constant attention to quality. The huddles are only one of a number of organized communication efforts within the practice.

BECOME FANATIC ABOUT IMPROVING SERVICE

Service excellence does not occur accidentally, nor does it occur through occasional or casual attention. In talking with physicians whose practices displayed a strong customer orientation, we were struck by a common characteristic. These practices, and the physicians who lead them, take an almost rigid stance where patient satisfaction is concerned. They believe, and act on the belief, that patients are paramount in the practice. They ensure a patient orientation by hiring, training, continually educating, and constantly motivating and rewarding staff members. In these practices, improving patient satisfaction and finding ways to bring it to an even higher level are frequent discussion, and action, topics.

The Neurology Center in Chevy Chase, Maryland is a good example. The practice culture, according to marketing director Terri Goren, is "quality all the way. State-of-the-art equipment, state-of-the-art service. We don't cut corners." Although technology, ambience, and furnishings get plenty of scrutiny, employees are held to high standards, and front-line people are recognized as important service providers who make a lasting impression. Headed by Marvin Korengold, MD, founding partner of the 21-year-old practice, the physicians and staff pride themselves on being "user-friendly." Dr. Korengold says, "The whole name of the game is to serve the people. No matter how good your diagnosis, how expert you are, if you haven't done that, you haven't done anything."

As a referral-based practice, the Neurology Center is fanatic about accommodating patients no matter what the circumstances. Dr. Korengold says, "We believe in 'flexible convenience'—the doctor and the staff will stay later if necessary to get the patient in." (And they often do.) Referral sources expect and appreciate this bend-over-backwards approach, he says. In addition to satisfying patients through timely appointments, the practice is attentive to the special needs of individual patients.

This may mean ordering lunch for a diabetic who is undergoing a lengthy test or scheduling a series of diagnostic examinations for an elderly person over several days rather than 1 day, as is normally done. "Older people become exhausted more easily. It's difficult for them to see the doctor, have their lab tests and the consultation all in one day," Dr. Korengold says.

Like the ultra-fit athlete who runs compulsively every day, rain or shine, this continual striving for improvement has measurable benefits. "We believe there's a direct relationship between patient satisfaction and the growth of our practice," according to Dr. Korengold. Patient satisfaction is important in a referral-based practice such as the Neurology Center: "You can have the best doctor with the best diagnosis, but if the patient is dissatisfied because of the way the secretary talked to them, or if the doctor's rapport with the patient is poor, or the patient is not handled very politely on the phone, the patient will go back and report to the referral doctor, 'I don't care for that doctor you sent me to.' That could be the end of that relationship." He adds a reminder that every customer-centered practice seems to keep in mind: "A satisfied patient is a practice builder."

ACT ON EVERY LITTLE THING

Practices that take service seriously regard minor matters as major concerns. "We answer every patient letter we get," Dr. Korengold says. He recalls once receiving a two-page, single-spaced, typed letter from a patient who was angry because the magazines in the waiting room were too old. "I wrote a letter in response to the patient and thanked him for calling it to my attention," Dr. Korengold says. "The problem was important to him, so it was worth a response."

Like Dr. Korengold, Richard Abrams, MD, believes in paying attention to everything patients say, even "off-the-wall" criticisms: "There's always some truth in them." Saul Schreiber, MD, insists that his staff pass along to him patient complaints or criticisms that they hear. He follows up with the patient, determines the source of the problem, and ensures that corrective action occurs.

Does this "small is big" attitude seem excessive? Perhaps even fanatic? Fanatic, yes. Excessive, no. Service that stands out is a result of fanaticism. Service fanatics are people who say, "Good enough isn't," who believe that tiny complaints, ignored because they're believed to be insignificant, pile up to create an immoveable mountain. They believe it's wiser to pick up a few rocks in the road than to let them accumulate to the point that you need a backhoe.

BE SYSTEMATIC ABOUT IMPROVING

The patient-oriented practices and physicians we encountered don't wait for problems that impede progress. Nothing is left to chance. These practices plan for continuous improvement. They have systems. The Hunkeler Clinic has its huddles, among a host of other strategies. The Heart Center holds two board retreats a year for long-term planning, but physicians and staff are besieged with (and believe in) a continual emphasis on patient satisfaction: lunchtime in-services, round-table meetings with department heads, profit sharing to encourage improvement, instant bonuses to reward good ideas, scenario discussions that focus on problem identification and resolution, and, most of all, an attitude that "everyone here is a patient advocate." Robert Bright's family practice in Bremerton, Washington has end-of-the-day review meetings. The Palo Alto Medical Foundation and the San Jose Clinic haven't left continuous improvement to chance. Both practices have implemented formal continuous improvement, hiring a quality consultant, Jim Shaw of Shaw Resources in Cupertino, California, to facilitate the effort. Under Shaw's direction, the practices have created teams charged with streamlining processes such as registration, scheduling, collections, and other "administrative" functions that often exasperate staff as well as patients, clog productivity, and gnaw away at profits.

These practices look for barriers early on, querying patients, referral sources, staff, and each other. They analyze and evaluate every aspect of their practice and their service, from the accessibility of the bathrooms to the clarity of their instructions. They offer countless opportunities for patients and staff to speak up and speak out by using suggestion boxes, follow-up phone calls, question cards, and visit-concluding "Anything else?" questions. They don't stop there. They fix the glitches and goof-ups by using the knowledge they gain from the repair process; they regard mistakes as the classroom for learning and improvement.

The purpose of this continuous attention? Prevention. Look for problems to prevent, and you'll find opportunities to improve.

THIS OBSESSION PAYS OFF

The physicians, practice managers, and staff members we spoke with take a stringently radical approach to service. Like a house cleaned by an army of white-glove housekeepers, these practices sparkle physically **and** emotionally. The physicians and staff may appear obsessive, but they also seem happier than the typical practice, and their patients radiate enthusiastic satisfaction. A patient commented about practices such as this:

> There is one thing I hate about well-managed physician practices. From the moment you check in, there is absolutely no time to read the magazines in the reception area. Have you ever noticed these are the only practices with current, interesting magazines?
>
> No one drives this point home better than my doctor. Each and every visit to his office is a good experience. I always leave feeling like a valued customer whose time is important. This practice is made up of a team of people who do things right the first time.

When patients are regarded as customers in a practice, and when customers are moved to the top of the organization chart, physicians and staff take on a whole new attitude. It's an attitude we noticed in our interviews and visits. It's what you notice when you stay at a Ritz-Carlton hotel, which claims a "born at birth" approach to quality. In practices and organizations such as these, there's an aura that says "You're special." Not "We're special." The focus is **you,** the customer.

FROM CUSTOMER FOCUS TO TOTAL QUALITY MANAGEMENT

Eventually, this customer focus may lead you, as it has other physicians in other practices, to decide to adopt a comprehensive quality improvement or total quality management (TQM) approach to every area of the practice. TQM, you may recall from Chapter 2, is a comprehensive, systematic, and process-focused method of analyzing, implementing, and continually monitoring and upgrading the quality of *every activity* in an organization. For some organizations (including several of the practices interviewed for this book), it is a natural progression of the effort to keep getting better. For others, it's an economic decision, even a matter of survival.

That was the case for the San Jose Medical Group, a 70-physician clinic that was having severe financial problems several years ago. TQM was a meaningless acronym to the physicians. "Before we started TQM, I'd never heard of it," confessed Harley Negin, MD, associate medical director. The clinic was in economic disarray. It had people problems. Patients weren't just dissatisfied, they were disgusted and disgruntled. Staff morale was minimal, with frustrated employees taking sick days to avoid work. Recognizing the depth of the problem, that's when the practice administrator brought in Jim Shaw, a consultant, to salvage the situation. Shaw believes that quality improvement in a medical practice calls for the same approach that would be used in any organization. You improve the processes. But where to start? San Jose had chronic, multisystem problems in medical records, patient registration, accounts receivable. . . .

Where to start is a common point of contention in organizations trying to improve quality. Without a logical approach, many organizations try to "fix" activities or people rather than processes. They spend huge wads of money and chunks of productive time killing ants with a blowtorch, while termites destroy the foundation. To select key processes for improvement, Shaw recommended looking at the organization as patients see it. With this perspective, the San Jose quality improvement team targeted medical records retrieval, which affected scheduling, clinical care, and follow-up. By using a formal assessment and documentation process, San Jose's medical records quality improvement team flowcharted the medical records retrieval process; measured volume, defects, and other "countable" pieces of the process; listed the customer suppliers for each step; designated a process "owner" (an individual responsible for ensuring cooperation and task completion); and identified performance measures and failure factors. The continuous improvement cycle then began: Establish requirements (standards), implement changes (improvement), measure results, and achieve target.

The result? You read about it in Chapter 2: more than $200,000 in savings in improved efficiency and productivity. Is the San Jose Medical Group done? Not if you believe in **continuous** quality improvement as they do. The organization now has a quality council charged with creating the environment in which continuous quality improvement is an inherent cultural attitude in the organization. San Jose continues to target other practice processes with similar success and continues to monitor and upgrade its efforts in medical records and other areas.

"WE'RE MOVING FORWARD"

According to Dr. Negin, "We have a sense of moving forward rather than floundering. We have a structure and a process in place; it gives us confidence." Like many physicians, Dr. Negin once interpreted quality to mean quality assurance. It was hardly a favorable interpretation. Today he's a TQM enthusiast. But he's realistic. "You have to unlearn old things, and that's hard for doctors," he says. They're learning that the expectations of health care consumers are the same as customer expectations of Disneyland, the Ritz-Carlton, or the neighborhood grocery store: "You need processes to work well. It reassures you. It gives you value for your dollar." And it makes for quality care: "You have to look at your organization's processes as all hanging together. It's no good to talk about quality of care if you can't get the patient registered, if you can't get their chart to the doctor who's caring for them, if you can't get a bill to them."

Improving service quality isn't easy. It means change, and people don't easily accept change. The human brain becomes patterned to sameness, adapted to predictability. Change means work: "You want me to think new thoughts, move in new directions, create new paradigms? No thanks, I'll do it the old way." Expect resistance, and prepare for it by incorporating individual values and goals with organizational values and goals. When quality is bred into the organization, people understand their role as individuals and team members, whom they serve, and what they are striving to accomplish. Quality service breeds pride, satisfaction, and success. Eventually, everyone in the practice will view what they do, and the effort to improve it, in the same way that Leon Gorman of L.L. Bean does. He says, "Service is just a day-in, day-out, ongoing, never-ending, persevering, compassionate type of activity."

QUALITY IS WORKPLACE WELLNESS

Is TQM a fad that will soon fade? No more than technological improvements, new surgical procedures, and new drugs are fads in medicine. Quality improvement is a fundamental way to do business as well as a fundamental way to give medical care because it provides a system for **preventing** errors by nurturing people who believe best is better, and by designing processes that give good outcomes rather than continually **fixing** things that are flawed. Think of continuous quality improvement as workplace wellness. As a physician, you prefer to see your patients stay healthy. You promote wellness by encouraging good dietary habits, exercise, and safety at home, in the car, and on the job; you educate them with information about these subjects. It's far less costly, as you know, to keep a person well than it is to treat them when they become ill or injured.

Think of quality in your medical practice as a way to keep your practice healthy by encouraging good work habits through continuous improvement. It's a healthy attitude for you and your staff. ❧

Action Steps for Keeping the Quality

1. Build on each success by looking for incremental, continual ways to improve.
2. Monitor expectations and set standards, and when you consistently reach the highest level, move the bar a little higher.
3. Communicate internally with everyone, often. It's the best way to keep up the quality.
4. Put patients at the top of your organization chart both on paper and in your actions.
5. Act as if minor errors are major concerns. Fix them fast.
6. Be fanatical about service, and institute systems for improving it.
7. Consider a TQM process for a serious, long-term quality improvement effort in the practice.

Reference

1. To deliver genuine quality, create a customer experience, *On Achieving Excellence* (December, 1992): 2–4.

Appendix 25-A

A Short History of Quality Improvement in Business

The concept of quality as a corporate strategy began in the 1930s with Walter Shewart at Bell Laboratories, who formulated the concept of statistical process control. Quite simply, this was the theory that minimizing variation in processes would reduce errors. Fewer errors, lower cost, better financial return.

Later, W. Edwards Deming promoted the idea of management responsibility for quality by changing systems that created problems and giving workers the methods and tools for good work. Japan embraced his ideas in 1950; it took another 30 years before the United States accepted the benefits of quality as a management tool.

Joseph M. Juran also achieved success in Japan with his quality ideas. He promoted fitness for use, that is, the ability of the consumer to depend on the product or service for its intended purpose. He also advocated that management understand and tally the cost of quality, pointing out that defects, failures, and redos all cost money. He proposed the original "continuous quality improvement concept" (although his theory had an end point). Keep improving quality, he said, until there is no longer a positive economic return. In truth, quality must be continually improved because customer expectations escalate as the level of quality rises.

Phillip Crosby, a former quality executive at ITT, founded the Crosby Quality College in 1979. By this time, corporate America was enthusiastic about the benefits of quality and sought to understand better how to achieve it. Some 35,000 executives attended his "college." His view was that management needed to see quality as a tangible product; he defined "conformance to requirements," a variation on the no-process-variations theme, and suggested that zero defects as a corporate standard and not simply a motivational slogan would help American business compete in the world marketplace. Ultimately, Crosby said, quality is free because improvement in processes lowers costs and hikes profitability.

All the "quality gurus" proposed essentially the same concept: Continuous quality improvement is good management. It's how to run a business. Does it work? Ask any practice that has begun the quality journey. Says the administrator of one practice that has set as its goal winning the Baldridge Quality Award, "Our referrals are up, our revenues are up, our profits are up since we began total quality management. It pays." ❧

26

Standards: Minimum Requirements for Maximum Service

"I didn't know that's how I was supposed to do it!"

"Chris only calls patients if there's a positive lab test, so I figured that sounded good enough to me."

Do statements such as these have a familiar ring? Do employees in your practice follow precedent or habit, right or wrong, because there are no guidelines, no standards that prescribe minimum requirements or objectives to aim for? Does everyone have his or her own acceptable limits for everything, from how long a patient should wait for a return phone call to how medical records are completed?

Would you accept such imprecise language or variability in treating your patients? Hardly. Precise, quantitative measures and accepted normal values are important means of ensuring quality medical care. There are standards for everything, from positive blood glucose levels for diagnosing diabetes to hemoglobin counts in pregnant women. In medical practice, you're familiar with clinical parameters—generally accepted principles or ranges for management of patient problems or medical conditions. These parameters serve as a gauge for measuring the validity of the diagnostic and treatment process and the outcome.

In the nonclinical activities of a medical practice, standards eliminate variation in activities and results, reduce confusion, clarify expectations, and simplify routine decision making. Standards help ensure **reliable methods**—precise, consistent, explicit, and tested ways of achieving a sought-after outcome. They also serve as a base for measuring performance and service quality. These are just a few of the areas in which standards may be applied in a practice:

- Telephone response
- Patient greeting
- Office appearance
- Medical chart organization
- Waiting time
- Patient education
- Complaint follow-up
- New patient follow-up

STANDARDS SIMPLIFY DECISION MAKING AND REDUCE ERRORS

"We've developed protocols for every procedure—even down to how a report should look. It makes decisions easier and prevents errors," says Tony Demetracopoulos, the Heart Center's administrator. Setting standards frees you and your staff to concentrate on significant activities, because each standard removes uncertainty ("Mrs. Brooks has been waiting for 30 minutes in the exam room. I wonder if I should tell Dr. Egan he's running behind?") and makes the appropriate action clear ("Mrs. Brooks has been waiting for almost 10 minutes. I'd better let Dr. Egan know, and I'll tell Mrs. Brooks that the doctor is running a little behind and see if she would like a magazine to read.").

Standards provide the physician(s) and staff with personal and collective goals; unlike goals, however, standards should be immediately and consistently achievable. Goals may be a target to aim for, with the expectation that they may not immediately be realized.

SETTING STANDARDS: A PHYSICIAN, STAFF, AND PATIENT TRIAD

But don't make the mistake of setting standards only according to your wishes or needs or those of your staff. Physicians and staff should jointly determine appropriate standards, with patient wishes or expectations used as a gauge. A story is told of a U.S. carpet manufacturer several years ago who sold a large order of foam-backed carpeting to a European customer. The customer provided his own testing specifications and was politely brushed aside with, "Don't worry; we have the highest-quality standards. You'll get the best there is." The manufacturer tested the carpet according to its stringent standards for foam stability, molecular weight distribution, particle size conformity, percentage of unreacted monomer, adhesion strength, and other technical measures. Upon passing these tests, the carpet was then shipped to the customer. Three times the customer sent the order back. Finally the manufacturer's representative called the client to learn what the problem was. "It's simple," the customer said. "Your carpet doesn't pass my roll-stool test." "Roll stool test?" the manufacturer's representative asked, mystified. The customer explained that an office chair on casters was weighted and then spun on a sample of the carpet continuously for several days. If the carpet didn't delaminate from the foam, it passed the customer's test. In this case, the carpet didn't pass.[1]

Set standards in your practice, but make certain that they are designed to meet your patients' "roll stool test." The techniques described in Chapter 14 for measuring patient expectations and ideas in other chapters will help you determine where to set standards and what they should be.

HOW TO DEVELOP STANDARDS AND PROTOCOLS FOR SERVICE

1. Developing service standards is a group effort, so bring together the practice staff or department staff. Focus on only one service process at a time—for example, patient check-in.
2. You'll need to know not only what each step in the process is but also what your patients' expectations are. Use surveys, focus groups, and direct patient responses. The person providing the service for each step should **ask** patients how they would like the interaction to occur and what behaviors, words, and attitudes would represent a maximum service level.
3. Create a flowchart that depicts each step in the patient check-in process. Verbally "walk" a patient through the process,

noting the action that occurs on the part of the patient as well as the actions of staff members for each step or "moment of truth." Also list the patient's expectation for each step.

4. Using the expectation as the criterion, establish a protocol for behavior or a numerical standard that at minimum meets the expectation. It's important that expected behaviors be described as clearly and specifically as possible. For example, rather than "Patient will be greeted in a friendly manner," the standard should specify "Patient will be greeted by name, using Mr., Mrs., Ms., or Miss and the last name, with a smile and hand-shake, within 10 seconds." This clearly indicates that the behavior is to be professional, friendly, and courteous. These "soft" standards are important determinants of patient satisfaction: Evidence shows that patient satisfaction is significantly higher when friendliness accompanies competence.

5. List "value-added" behaviors that will surprise patients and exceed their expectations. For example, the patient's expectation upon signing in may simply be that he or she will be acknowledged within a reasonable period of time. If the receptionist looks up within 30 seconds of the patient's arrival, smiles, and says, "Hi, please have a seat," the patient's expectation is met. But if the receptionist smiles warmly and says, "Hello, Ms. Chang, it's nice to see you! You're here to see Dr. Milos today, aren't you? May I get you some coffee or juice?" the patient is pleasantly surprised and pleased.

6. Repeat this process for every service encounter your patients have. You may wish to do this activity over a period of many weeks or months, depending on your practice size and current level of patient satisfaction.

7. Develop a follow-up action to determine how you're doing. This also provides an opportunity to reassess patient expectations and practice protocols.

WALK THROUGH THE PRACTICE LIKE A PATIENT

One technique for determining standards is used by a pharmaceutical company sales representative, who figuratively walks the staff members through a typical patient appointment. In playing the role of "Joe Patient," he helps practice staff identify bottle-necks and less-than-excellent service encounters at each point or moment of truth in the practice. From the initial telephone call for an appointment through diagnostic testing, exam room interactions, check-out, and billing, "Joe Patient" prods for problems: "Okay, I've checked in at the front desk and you've told me to have a seat. What happens now to me? And what's happening in the front office and back office to get ready for me?" This step-by-step process forces staff and physicians to see and hear actions and responses through the patient's eyes and ears and thus helps them determine where improvements should occur and standards need to exist. This is a detailed variation on the "mystery shopper survey" technique discussed in Chapter 20. The advantage of this approach is that the practice team can observe the patient's experience and reaction, even if only through role play.

Most employees are acutely aware of the glitches and goof-ups that are likely to occur as a patient makes his or her way through the maze of people and processes in the practice. Often, however, it's an eye-opening exercise for physicians. You become aware of barriers, hoops, and hurdles that patients confront in your office—barriers that are often shielded from your view.

This systematic process of setting standards complies with the "manage by facts and data" dictum of quality improvement. The act of evaluating activities, behaviors, and expectations and then setting appropriate standards incorporates reliability and predictability into practice activities and processes. This allows greater flexibility and productivity; staff energies are focused on patient care and patient satisfaction issues rather than on repairing mistakes and apologizing for problems that could have been prevented (see Figure 26-1).

TAKE PROCESSES APART TO ESTABLISH STANDARDS

In setting standards, processes are dissected as a series of activities, with each step of the activity or encounter broken down to determine the individual events that create the final outcome. This analytical research should reveal where flaws, faults, extraneous steps, and missing information within each step of the

Figure 26-1 Typical Patient Encounter in an Ophthalmic Office

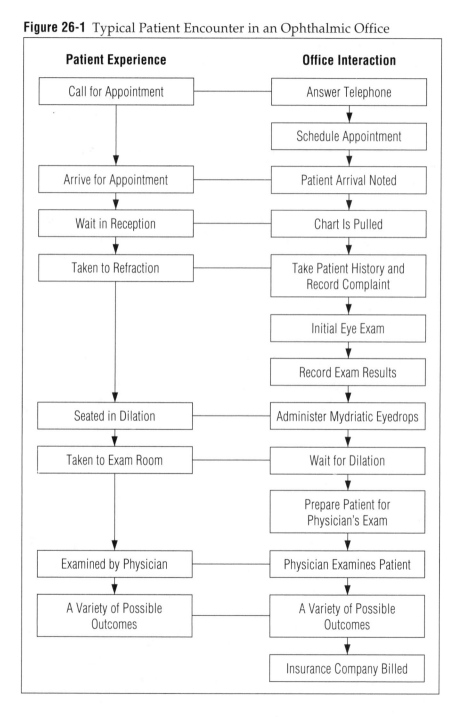

process are likely to be creating unreliable, nonstandard processes. When this occurs, services and outcomes are often unpredictable or of poor quality.

In addition to documenting the steps of the process, the *customer* and the *owner* of each activity must be acknowledged. (By *owner*, we're referring to a physician or staff member ultimately responsible for the activity.) In specifying the customer and the owner, understanding dawns that the customer at certain points in the process may be a fellow employee rather than the patient. In other words, practices and physicians have internal as well as external customers.

Just as the highest-quality clinical care occurs when standards are adhered to, developing and following service standards in your practice will help you achieve or surpass patient expecta-

Exhibit 26-1 Charting Standards for Patient Experiences

Patient		Office	
Expectation	**Experience**	**Interaction**	**Standard**
Phone answered promptly	Call for appointment	Answer telephone	Telephone will be answered within three rings, with a smile, using practice name and first name of receptionist
Friendly acknowledgment of arrival	Arrive for appointment	Acknowledge patient	Greet patient by name with a smile within 30 seconds of arrival
Wait no more than 15 minutes	Wait in reception area	Ask patient to have a seat until called	Inform patient approximately when he or she will be called to examination room; inform patient of unavoidable schedule delay and length of delay
Staff will be pleasant and courteous	Called to exam room	Call patient to exam room	Acknowledge patient by name and personally escort to exam room

tions (see Exhibit 26-1). Staff members should be encouraged to come up with ways to exceed expectations either via the standard or through an unexpected "value-added" process or product.

In setting standards in a practice that has not previously followed them, it's vital that all staff believe in and comply with the standards. Otherwise, you may have the situation described by Kathy Peart of Thomas-Davis Medical Clinic in Tucson, Arizona: "You get a new employee all fired up after going through orientation, and they go to their workstation and there they find the long-term, old-fashioned employee who says, 'What do you mean pick up the phone on the second ring? Let it ring for a while; we're too busy!' They can undo all the good you've done in employee orientation. So you've got to go back to the people who have been with the system and get them to believe in it and help develop the standards."

She goes on to make an important point: "New employees are probably the least empowered because they don't have any longevity or power base or support group or credibility. You must build belief and gain commitment throughout the organization, particularly with the long-term staffers who may be resistant to change." (How to do this? Review the suggestions in Chapters 8 through 11.)

STANDARDS ARE COMFORTING TO STAFF AND PATIENTS

Standards provide continuity and consistency, evidence of quality, and a level of comfort to physicians, staff, and patients alike. Standards also bring risk, however. When practice standards are rigidly monitored and adhered to, any deviation is glaring. Patients become acclimated to service excellence; eventually it becomes their expectation. If your schedule runs smoothly and efficiently 99% of the time and patients are escorted to the exam room within 10 minutes, this becomes the expected standard. Patients will overlook an occasional knot in the schedule that causes them to wait (although they're more likely to be forgiving if an explanation and apology accompany the error). But when waiting time lengthens to 20 minutes on several occasions, patients are likely to become suspicious and skeptical. They have learned not to expect this. Setting standards escalates expectations. Failure to achieve the standards increases customer disappointment.

The benefits to the practice that establishes, follows, and continually improves standards are many. For physicians, it's the reduction in recurring problems and questions and the improved productivity that efficiency brings. For staff, it's the continuity, freedom, and diminished uncertainty that documented requirements provide. For patients, it's the pleasure of a predictable and positive experience. For all members of the practice team—physicians, patients, and staff—there's an atmosphere of pride, pleasure, and accomplishment. And, of course, satisfaction, all the way around. ❧

Action Steps for Setting Standards

1. Bring staff members together to analyze areas and activities in the practice for which standards should be applied.
2. Set standards according to patient expectations and needs, not merely for the convenience of physicians or staff.
3. Review standards with all employees, new and old, to ensure consistency of attitude and actions.
4. Review practice standards regularly to determine whether they need to be moved higher. As service quality improves, patient expectations will increase.
5. Set standards not only for areas and activities that patients see but for internal processes: paperwork, staff-to-staff behavior, and the like. Remind employees that internal customers are as important as external customers.

Reference

1. S. Smith, How to quantify quality, *Management Today* (October 1987): 86–88.

27

Monitoring Techniques: How To Know What's Working

Remember Childress Buick, the Phoenix, Arizona auto dealership? A computer disaster forced the company to focus on customer satisfaction. Today Childress has 42 different ways to monitor the results of the company's customer service efforts. Just one example: A new car buyer gets a customized booklet on preventive maintenance with a schedule indicating when service is needed. The customer receives a "recall" postcard before the recommended service due date. No response? A Childress service representative calls the customer. The customer retention file is reviewed every week.

Customer retention is a bottom-line focus for everyone at Childress. Each customer is viewed as the equivalent of $142,000 in revenues (or loss). Childress Buick would not have achieved the gains it has over the past few years without continually monitoring quality and customer service efforts. Like any business, large or small, a medical practice can't expect to achieve consistent, continued improvement and customer satisfaction without consistent, continued monitoring. "What are we doing right? What needs to be fixed? What do our patients need, want, and think of us?" Every practice should ask these questions in a number of formal, reliable, trackable ways. As you learned earlier in this book, patient satisfaction measurement is a tool used increasingly by payers, including employers and managed care firms. Rather than wait for payers to evaluate their service and tell them whether their patients are pleased (or why they are not), proactive

303

practices will monitor patient satisfaction regularly. This consistent and comprehensive approach allows problems to be corrected before they become imbedded. Then, of course, the smart practice reports patient satisfaction survey results to third party payers as tangible evidence of service quality.

MONITORING QUALITY FOR PROOF TO PAYERS

Joseph Noreika, MD, has taken this one step further. Several years ago he began collecting clinical and demographic data on all his cataract surgery patients. Information about the patient age, diagnosis, related medical conditions, surgical procedure performed, type of intraocular lens implant, outcome, and other details go into a computerized database. Currently Dr. Noreika compiles reports from this database and provides it to optometrists in the form of patient report cards to inform them about the patients they referred to him, but he says he also intends to use information in the database as evidence to managed care firms of his clinical quality. The approach he has taken could be adapted by every practice. Rather than waiting for health plans to survey your patients about their satisfaction, why not provide copies of your annual patient survey results to the health plans for which you're a provider? In fact, it's smart to be proactive in providing documentation of positive feedback you receive from risk management evaluators and other sources as well.

SERVICE COMMITMENT CALLS FOR ONGOING MONITORING

In Chapter 14, a number of tactics and techniques were listed for determining what patients want and need. Most of these methods were simple, on-the-spot actions that could be taken without a great deal of effort or cost. In addition to letting you know expectations, these techniques also provide feedback regarding satisfaction in some cases. But if it is truly committed to service and to patient satisfaction, a practice must also monitor in a comprehensive and thorough manner the success of ongoing efforts to determine the level of satisfaction and where improvement needs to occur.

Think of monitoring quality service efforts as "service recall." You do it with your patients routinely. If you diagnose a 6-month-old baby with acute purulent otitis media, you'll probably prescribe a course of antibiotics and ask the parents to bring the baby in for a follow-up visit in a week. You want to make sure the treatment is working. Formal patient satisfaction monitoring is how you make sure the "treatment" is working in your practice. It's service follow-up. You evaluate satisfaction to be certain that the service offered is accomplishing your objectives and meeting or surpassing patient expectations. When you evaluate results and measure them against standards or goals, you know if you're successful.

BE FANATIC ABOUT SOLICITING AND ACTING ON OPINIONS

Successful practices—patient-centered practices—are fanatic about monitoring and measuring what they do. Like Childress Buick, they use a variety of techniques. They're not satisfied with one or two. The Noran Clinic in Minneapolis, Minnesota, a 15-physician, 185-employee neurology practice with 4 locations, mails 3-page patient questionnaires to a random sampling of its 30,000 annual patients 4 times a year. Countering the oft-heard argument that "people don't have time to fill out surveys," the Noran Clinic gets a 41% average rate of return. This lengthy evaluation is done in addition to the short postvisit survey cards used for immediate feedback (see Chapter 14 for an example). According to associate administrator Phil Riveness, the practice also does random telephone surveys.

When patient surveys are returned and tallied, the results are shared with physicians and staff. But it doesn't stop there. Riveness compares each physician's individual scores with the group mean **and** with his or her previous scores. Areas of weakness are discussed, and the physician is then required to put in writing a specific action plan for improvement. Riveness then follows up in 6 months to determine progress. Rather than complaining about this intense survey process, the neurologists are "impressed at how meaningful the process is," Riveness says.

Patient questionnaires are probably the most relied-upon way to measure and monitor the results of, and satisfaction with, the service and care offered in a practice. Once implemented, a patient survey provides a baseline against which future surveys (and the success of new service measures) can be evaluated. Because information about this technique is available from a great many sources and organizations and has been covered extensively in two previous books written by the authors, we won't go into detail here. Nevertheless, we urge physicians to consider implementing a patient survey if one has never been done in the practice. This survey gives you a starting point for service improvement activities. We emphasize the action step: Don't implement any form of survey unless you intend to act on the findings, because a survey of any type implies that you plan to fix what's wrong and to improve whatever patients rate as "acceptable."

You'll find a detailed discussion of patient satisfaction surveys in *Promoting Your Medical Practice: Marketing Communications for Physicians*[1] and in *Marketing Strategies for Physicians: A Guide to Practice Growth.*[2] A sample patient survey can be found in Appendix 27-A at the end of this chapter.

TELEPHONE SURVEYS YIELD QUALITY INFORMATION

Telephone surveys are an effective alternative means of determining where improvement needs to occur in the practice, according to Penny McLaughlin, a marketing consultant for Clinical Radiologists of Silver Spring, Maryland: "I've always believed that written surveys only reflect the views of people who are extremely angry or extremely happy. You don't get those who are in the middle or on the fence—and they tend to be the majority," she says.

One day a month she makes telephone calls to 50 to 60 patients seen that day in Clinical Radiologists' main location. The best time to call, McLaughlin says, is from 5 p.m. to 8 p.m. The surveyor must be very familiar with the practice and its policies, services, staff, facilities, and billing; in fact, a tactful staffer with the ability to probe may be best qualified to elicit details from patients. "You can't have a market research firm make these calls and get the kind of information you need," McLaughlin believes. A former radiology technician, McLaughlin spends a great deal of time in the Clinical Radiologists practice offices, talking to physicians and staff; as an "insider," she is able to probe for detail with the patients she calls.

She's been doing the telephone surveys for nearly 3 years, long enough that her calls now are conversational rather than rote, although she still follows a general format for discussion. A sample questionnaire used by clinical radiologists for telephone surveys is shown in Exhibit 27-1.

How do patients respond to being called during the dinner hours? Very favorably, McLaughlin says. "Some people are skeptical at first. I introduce myself as the patient care representative for the practice and explain that I'm calling to find out how satisfied they were." She recalls reaching one patient who commented skeptically, "Right, lady, and I'm a neurosurgeon. What are you trying to sell?" After McLaughlin explained that the purpose of her call was legitimately to find out his opinion of the service at the practice, the patient apologized for being rude and answered her questions.

Most people appreciate the call, she says. "They find it unusual that physicians are seeking their opinion." Upon completing the telephone calls (she usually reaches about a third of the 60 patients), McLaughlin prepares a written report summarizing favorable and negative comments, problem areas, and specific concerns. The report is distributed to supervisors in the practice, who are required to address problems and share positive comments with staff. The supervisors' action plans and/or specific responses to individual patients are distributed along with the comprehensive survey report to the 23 physicians in the practice.

McLaughlin notes that physicians and staff will often tell her on a particularly hectic day, "Please don't do your telephone calls today. This was a terrible day!" That's the day she'll target, she says. Interestingly, those "bad" days often get glowing reviews from patients, who say things such as, "Oh yes, they called me at home and said there was a delay. I knew there were problems, but everyone was wonderful!" (Service recovery tactics can have remarkably favorable results, as you'll discover in the next chapter.)

PAY ATTENTION TO PROBLEMS: PLAN IMPROVEMENT

As with any monitoring technique, telephone surveys require continual attention to identified problems. It's not enough to realize that a problem exists and to target a plan for improvement. The

Exhibit 27-1 Telephone Survey Questionnaire

Patient Questionnaire

Area Sampled_____   Time Frame_____   Total Sampled_____

_____ % Perfect Score (#) Remaining_____ (#) Rated Our Services in the Following Percentages

Aspects of our Services	"4" High	"3" Mid-Neutral	"2" Low	"1" Very Low
Calling our office to make an appointment				
Time between making appointment and being seen				
Length of total visit time				
Length of time waiting in dressing room				
Length of time waiting in examination room				
Amount of time spent in reception area				
Receptionist was friendly and courteous				
Procedure performed was explained by the caregiver				
Quality of written patient information				
Sensitivity of caregiver to your illness				
Questions were answered adequately by staff				
How satisfied are you with the overall care you received in our practice?				

Source: Courtesy of Penny McLaughlin, Annapolis, Maryland.

problem and the plan must be monitored to be certain that change occurs and sticks. It's easy to slip back into bad habits and traditional ways of handling a process. Be sure to implement routine "check-ups" into action plans and service recovery processes.

McLaughlin's experience surveying patients by telephone seems to be validated by a study developed by the Family Practice Clinic of the University of California. Researchers did telephone interviews with clinic patients, asking the same questions used on a written patient satisfaction questionnaire. The telephone surveyors probed for clarification of patient responses and often found that a person's initial response did not match the open-ended discussion that followed. For example, a patient responded "extremely well" to the question, "How well does your doctor answer your questions?" Probing revealed the complaint that the physician often ignored the patient's questions or answered with "big words" she couldn't understand. Although praising the "excellent care" they received, most patients had at least one complaint about service, communication, convenience, or other surrogate indicators of care.[3]

Does this mean that written questionnaires are useless? No. Telephone interviews, however, can provide clarification and detail regarding specific issues, new services, and potential trends identified through other monitoring techniques. Telephone surveys serve the same function as focus groups and other qualitative market research techniques: They add depth and substance to the statistics and data of written surveys.

INCIDENT REPORTS PUT PATIENT-FIRST PHILOSOPHY INTO ACTION

The Marshfield Clinic, a 380-physician group practice in Marshfield, Wisconsin monitors patient satisfaction with an "incident reporting system." According to administrator Frederick Wenzel, "We have a tendency to overreact. We encourage reports from anyone on anything . . . from a patient slipping in the hall to rude treatment by an employee." The report must be signed by the person completing it, but anonymity is protected. Each report goes to the nursing staff in the department as well as to the clinic's general counsel, Wenzel, and the assistant medical director, and follow-up action is required for each report. Encouraging the 2,600 clinic employees to complete incident reports when they see something amiss is tied to the practice's overall belief in "operationalizing" the philosophy that the patient is number one, Wenzel says.

"Everything that happens here is based on the attitude that the patient comes first," he explains. An arriving patient parks in front of the clinic's main building and is assisted by a doorman. The reception desk staffer is trained to answer questions; a patient walking down a hallway with a quizzical look gets an immediate "Can I help you?" from any employee passing by. "We try to view quality from the perspective of the patient," Wenzel says. For example, the clinic's professional practice committee, which is charged with dealing with issues of quality, determined that an excessive number of appointments were being cancelled—not by patients but by the scheduling desk. A policy was instituted to eliminate the problem.

Although patient satisfaction surveys are a standard technique for monitoring the results of quality service efforts in a practice, don't ignore the other important customer of most practices: referral physicians. Referral source surveys are a valuable information-gathering technique. Practices such as the Heart Center in Manchester, New Hampshire; the Sansum Clinic in Santa Barbara, California; the Neurology Center in Chevy Chase, Maryland; and many others use this method for learning not only what other physicians think of the practice but what their patients report back about their experience.

Thomas-Davis Clinic, a 13-site group practice in Arizona, conducts patient satisfaction surveys with a market research firm. Five patients per physician per month are randomly interviewed. Survey results are compiled every 6 months and given to the appropriate department head, who reviews the results with each clinic site and individual physicians. A significant problem encountered by Thomas-Davis (and one that is common with other practices where physicians haven't accepted a customer-first philosophy) was physician resistance to the results. Some argued that the data were invalid, although the medical director of Thomas-Davis noted that "the patient satisfaction data [are] consistent with what we sense about these same doctors."

MONITORING SATISFACTION MEANS ACTION AND CHANGE

Thomas-Davis' experience is not unique. Monitoring patient satisfaction requires action and change. Patients expect it. It's implied in the process of seeking opinions, as you learned in Chapter 14 in measuring patient expectations (why else would you do it?). But if physicians or staff are not committed to quality service and do not strongly believe in and act out quality service attitudes, they will not believe the results of any monitoring or evaluation efforts. If you encounter this problem in your practice, go back to Chapter 1. You must achieve buy-in, participation, and involvement. Everyone must believe that quality counts and that patients come first. You must commit to your belief and then measure expectations, monitor the results, and act on what you learn. ❧

Actions Steps for Monitoring Patient Satisfaction

1. Implement at least one formal, comprehensive process for determining patient satisfaction, and repeat it regularly so that improvements or problems are tracked.
2. Once a process is in place, incorporate follow-up—the action that will take place and the individual responsible for it—when problems are identified.
3. Include referral sources in patient satisfaction monitoring. They often receive reports from patients who were referred to your practice.

References

1. S.W. Brown, A.P. Morley, Jr., S.J. Bronkesh, and S.D. Wood, *Promoting Your Medical Practice: Marketing Communications for Physicians* (Oradel, N.J.: Medical Economics Books, 1989).
2. S.W. Brown and A.P. Morley, Jr., *Marketing Strategies for Physicians: A Guide to Practice Growth* (Oradel, N.J.: Medical Economics Books, 1986).
3. G.A. Goldsmith, Patient satisfaction with a family practice clinic: Comparison of a questionnaire and an interview survey, *Journal of Ambulatory Care Management* (May 1983): 24–31.

Appendix 27-A

Patient Survey

QUESTIONNAIRE COVER LETTER

This is an example of the kind of covering message that should accompany your patient questionnaire. You should, of course, tailor it to your own situation.

Dear Patient:

We here at Center Street Family Practice Clinic want to provide you and your family with the highest-quality health care possible in a comprehensive, compassionate, and cost-effective manner. To help us evaluate our effectiveness, we would like your opinions about us. Your answers and suggestions on the following questionnaire will help us continue to improve the health care we provide you and your family. So won't you please take a few moments to give us this important information?

Thank you,
Dr. _____ and Staff

QUESTIONNAIRE

This is a patient questionnaire designed for a family practice. You can easily adapt it to your own practice.

I.   About yourself
Age:_____   Name (optional): _____
Sex:_____
Address: _____
Marital Status: Single _____   Married _____   Widow(er) _____
Name and Age of Spouse: _____
Names and Ages of Children: _____
Occupation: Yours _____ Spouse _____
Education: Yours _____ Spouse _____
Household Income: _____
Best Times for Appointments: _____
   1. Are we the main source of health care for your family?   Yes ____ No ____
   2. If members of your family are seeing other physicians, please tell us who and
      why.
      Spouse _____
      Children _____
      Other _____

II.   Our specialty and services
   3. Do you feel you understand the specialty of our practice?   Yes____ No____
   4. Do you believe you are aware of all the services we offer?   Yes____ No____

III.   Physical plant
   5. Is the location of our office convenient?   Yes____ No____
   6. Do you find our waiting room comfortable?   Yes____ No____
   7. Do you feel relaxed in the waiting room?   Yes____ No____
   8. Are the parking facilities adequate?   Yes____ No____
   9. Do you have to pay to park when you come to see us?   Yes____ No____
  10. If yes, is this a hindrance to receiving your care here?   Yes____ No____
  11. What changes would you make in the physical aspects of our office? _____
       _____
       _____

IV.   Front office personnel
  12. Do you find our office personnel (secretary, receptionist):
                                Friendly? Yes____ No____
                              Courteous? Yes____ No____
  13. Do you find our business personnel (office manager, bookkeeper):
                              Friendly? Yes____ No____
                              Courteous? Yes____ No____
  14. Are your phone calls handled in a prompt, courteous manner?
                                      Yes____ No____

15. Are you receiving adequate help with your insurance?   Yes_____ No_____
16. If you need help with your insurance, can we help?   Yes_____ No_____

_____

17. Have you received a copy of our business policies?   Yes_____ No_____
18. Have our payment and billing policies been explained to your satisfaction?   Yes_____ No_____
19. Do our payment and billing policies create difficulties for you?   Yes_____ No_____

V. Nurses

20. Do you find our nurses: Friendly? Yes_____ No_____
    Courteous? Yes_____ No_____
21. Do you feel our nurses are sympathetic to your illness?   Yes_____ No_____
22. Do our nurses give you enough information about their part in your care, such as telling you what your weight and blood pressure are?   Yes_____ No_____

VI. Doctors

23. Do you find our doctor(s):   Friendly? Yes_____ No_____
    Courteous? Yes_____ No_____
24. Does the doctor tell you enough about your illness?   Yes_____ No_____
25. Do you feel the doctor is interested in you as a person?   Yes_____ No_____
26. Does the doctor spend enough time with you?   Yes_____ No_____
27. Does the doctor give you enough health care information, such as booklets on diet, exercise, and smoking?   Yes_____ No_____
28. Do you feel the doctor is interested in your health?   Yes_____ No_____

VII. Waiting time

29. Is your wait too long in the reception area before you are called to see the doctor?   Yes_____ No_____
30. Do you have to wait too long in the examination room before the doctor sees you?   Yes_____ No_____

VIII. After-hours and weekend care

31. Do you have difficulty reaching us after hours?   Yes_____ No_____
32. Do you know the number for our answering service?   Yes_____ No_____
33. Is our answering service prompt and courteous?   Yes_____ No_____
34. Do our doctors promptly return your calls?   Yes_____ No_____
35. If you see a doctor in this practice other than your regular doctor, are you as satisfied with the care you receive?   Yes_____ No_____
36. If doctors other than those in this practice share after-hours calls with us, are you satisfied with the care they provide?   Yes_____ No_____

IX.   Phone calls
37. Are your phone calls to the doctors during the day returned promptly?
Yes_____ No_____
38. Do you mind if the nurses handle some of your calls?   Yes_____ No_____

X.   Ancillary services
39. Do you find it inconvenient to go someplace else for certain
X-rays or lab tests?   Yes_____ No_____
40. Do you find the staff at these other facilities: Friendly? Yes_____ No_____
Courteous? Yes_____ No_____
If not, at which facilities? _____
41. Is the emergency department we use convenient?   Yes_____ No_____
If no, which one would be more convenient? _____
42. Do you find separate billing by these other facilities inconvenient?
Yes_____ No_____
43. Are you satisfied with the hospital we use?   Yes_____ No_____
44. Is this hospital convenient for you and your family? Yes_____ No_____

XI.   Cost of services
45. Do you feel that our fees are: High? Yes_____ No_____
Average? Yes_____ No_____
Low? Yes_____ No_____
46. Do you belong to a health plan?   Yes_____ No_____
If yes, name of plan_____
47. Are you familiar with our credit and billing policies? Yes_____ No_____
48. Have you used other health services (such as an emergency clinic) because you
felt it would be less expensive?   Yes_____ No_____
If yes, which one(s)? _____

XII.   Scheduling
49. Do you have trouble getting an appointment as soon as you would like?
Yes_____ No_____
50. Are our secretaries helpful in finding appointments that meet your needs?
Yes_____ No_____
51. Are our office hours convenient for you? If no, how could we arrange our hours
to best serve you?   Yes_____ No_____
_____
_____

XIII. Educational information

52. Does your doctor give you enough information about your:

Illness?	Yes____	No____
Medicine?	Yes____	No____
Health?	Yes____	No____

53. Would you like more educational information from us?   Yes____ No____
54. Would you accept this information from the nurses?   Yes____ No____
55. If we had audiovisual tapes available about your problem, would you use them?
                                                                    Yes____ No____
56. Would you want to get a health newsletter from us periodically?
                                                                    Yes____ No____

XIV. Services offered

57. Are you satisfied with the range of services provided by this practice?
                                                                    Yes____ No____
58. Do you believe you know all the services we offer?   Yes____ No____
59. Are there any specific services that you would like to see us provide?
                                                                    Yes____ No____

Pediatric care?	Yes____	No____
Care for elderly?	Yes____	No____
Minor surgery?	Yes____	No____
Diet counseling?	Yes____	No____
Stress reduction?	Yes____	No____

Others? _____

XV. Referral

60. How were you referred to this practice?
     Other patients_____ Friends_____ Yellow Pages_____
     Medical society_____ Another doctor_____ Our reputation_____
     Health plan provider list _____
     Other: _____
61. Are you satisfied with the care we provide to refer other people to us?
                                                                    Yes____ No____

XVI. Comments

Please use the space below for any additional comments you may have.

_____
_____
_____
_____

XVII. Signature (optional) _____

28

Service Recovery:
When Things Go Wrong,
Make Them Right

An error gracefully acknowledged is a victory won.
                        Caroline L. Gascoigne

How are we doing? Can we do better? Have a complaint, idea, suggestion or compliment? Please call me personally. My home phone number is 602-277-1914. I accept collect calls. We really want to know!

                        Listen Update, *customer catalog for*
                        Reddings Books on Tape

No matter how well organized a practice, how understanding and knowledgeable the staff, or how quality oriented the attitude, mistakes **will** happen. Make no mistake about it.

The error is not necessarily in the mistake but in not acknowledging it, making amends, and trying to prevent future mistakes. Most people are incredibly forgiving if they're informed about a situation that may have resulted in poor service or given them a bad impression of the practice. They are even more forgiving if they get a personal apology. It doesn't have to be an acceptance of guilt, just an "I'm sorry this happened to you." And they may become lifetime converts and proponents of your practice if a tangible expression of contrition takes place.

318

This process of acknowledging and correcting errors is called service recovery. We call the steps in service recovery the Triple-A Action Plan (see Figure 28-1):

1. **Acknowledge**
2. **Apologize**
3. **Amend**

Patients tell us (and consumer research confirms) that service errors are forgivable if they are not predictable (that is, if the same or similar mistakes don't happen routinely) and if the organization or individual that made the mistake acknowledges it, apologizes for it, and makes amends.

WHEN THINGS GO WRONG

Recovery is a vital component of service because, as we emphasized earlier, things **will** go wrong. Mistakes will occur. As a result of a mix-up, memory gap, miscommunication, or misunderstanding, someone will misplace a chart, record an appointment at the wrong time, forget to make a phone call, or keep someone waiting too long. These things will occasionally occur even in the best of organizations. In a practice that is moving toward empowerment and innovation, mistakes may even occur more frequently at first as employees become accustomed to making decisions independently. Mistakes can be evidence that someone has tried to accomplish something.

When a mistake occurs, it's important not to criticize the error or chastise the person(s) who made it. This may inhibit future decision making and innovation. Critique the process that caused the problem, and institute a process for recovery and prevention. Encourage everyone within the practice to participate in ferreting out errors, determining the root cause, and responding immediately when a service error occurs. It should be understood by every member of the practice that mistakes can be anticipated in an environment of change and innovation. Service recovery doesn't deny the error, but it allows the practice to learn from it while reinstating patient satisfaction.

Figure 28-1

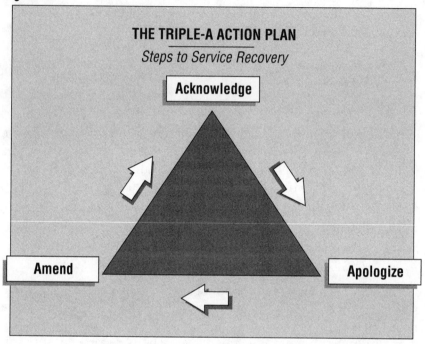

THE TRIPLE-A ACTION PLAN

Steps to Service Recovery

Acknowledge

Amend

Apologize

Recovery is a way of saying to your patients, referral physicians, staff, or anyone who may have encountered less-than-optimal service, "We value you as a member of our practice." It also tells those who may make an error in judgment or fact that occasional rocks on the road to service quality should be considered stumbling blocks, not permanent barriers. Service recovery attacks the process, not the person.

A recovery strategy, even one as simple as an apology, can actually make patients strong advocates for the practice. Cardiologist Alan Kaplan, MD, says, "It never hurts to admit you're wrong. If a mistake is made and you admit it, your patients will become more loyal."

Recovery does not mean that patients and family members should be told about each and every clinical error that occurs. Revealing medical misdiagnosis, incorrect procedures, inaccurate test interpretation, or other clinical mistakes should be approached judiciously and sometimes only after consulting your attorney or insurer (some insurers will not permit policy holders to admit any error). If you have developed a good rapport with your patient, if you make it a habit of communicating thoroughly and personally, and if the error is not the result of sloppiness, laziness, or attempting something you are not fully trained to do, your chances of incurring a malpractice liability suit are minimized.

WHY COMPLAINTS OCCUR

Often, a patient complaint will be unfounded or a result of a misunderstanding about billing, Medicare, or third-party payer requirements or restrictions. Sometimes the complaint is due to miscommunication, lack of clarification, or overuse of jargon on the part of physician or staff. A complaint may be directed at the provider even though the problem lies with clinical problems that are beyond anyone's control, such as slow recovery or medication side effects.

No matter why the complaint occurs, who is at fault, or how minor the problem, it needs attention. Quickly, efficiently, and personally. Because untended complaints can be a source of malpractice liability at worst. At best, they can disrupt practice productivity by demanding unreasonable attention from staff members. And they can result in the "trickle-away" effect: patients and potential referrals trickling away because of the perception that the practice has little concern for patient satisfaction. Develop and adhere to a policy for everyone to follow in addressing and reporting patient complaints.

In the book *In Search of Excellence,* Peters and Waterman point out that top managers treat service problems as "real-time" issues that deserve immediate, personal attention.[1] There's something to be said for that philosophy, and satisfied patients will say it.

THE TRIPLE-A ACTION PLAN

A service recovery strategy ideally addresses prevention as well as recovery. By reading and implementing the recommendations in this book, you're on the path to prevention because attention to service quality and continuous improvement can prevent process errors that lead to service disappointments.

> *Hector Alphonso called his urologist's office at 8:47 A.M. He had had a biopsy 3 days earlier and had been told by Dr. Lane that he would be contacted with the results within 2 days. So far he had heard nothing. The nurse with whom he spoke, hearing the concern in his voice, promised that she or Dr. Lane would check on the test results and call him within the hour. After she hung up, however, Dr. Lane was called to the emergency department about a patient, and the nurse was grabbed by another staff member to correct a scheduling problem with a surgical procedure planned for the next day at the outpatient surgery center. By the time the nurse remembered her promise to Hector, 2½ hours had gone by. When she called him back, his line was busy. After trying a few more times and still getting a busy signal, she decided to try again after lunch. Before she could call Hector, he had called Dr. Lane, furious that he had heard from no one despite the nurse's promise to respond promptly.*

We've agreed that errors, misunderstandings, and misjudgments will occur even under the best of circumstances. So let's get started on the Triple-A Action Plan for remedying service mistakes—Acknowledge, Apologize, and Amend.

Step 1: Acknowledge the Mistake

When a mistake or misunderstanding occurs, no matter who is at fault, the first step is to acknowledge the error and the wronged party's right to be concerned or angry. For example: "Mr. Alphonso, I am very sorry I did not call you back promptly as I promised. Dr. Lane was called to the emergency department and was unable to call you, but I should have made arrangements for someone to contact you. I know you are angry, and I apologize for inconveniencing you." Or: "I'm sorry your Medicare bill was late arriving. I can understand how upset you must be." Acknowledging the problem (without necessarily accepting blame, unless you are clearly at fault) defuses the situation without diminishing the individual's right to be upset.

In acknowledging the situation, thank the patient for bringing an unsatisfactory, disruptive, or disappointing situation to your attention. Encourage people to complain by giving them a formal method such as a suggestion box with a sign requesting "compliments, complaints, and problems you can't or won't talk about." Here's how Stew Leonard, owner of Stew Leonard's Dairy in Norwalk, Connecticut, feels about complaining customers: "Customers who complain are your friends because they are giving you the opportunity to improve, instead of just walking out." He worries more about customers who don't complain when they're dissatisfied—because they leave and don't come back. And you never know they're unhappy, so you don't get the chance to correct the problem. Let patients know you want to hear their complaints. Tell them verbally, encourage staff to elicit and document details when patients seem unhappy, and provide a suggestion box for patients who are reticent. Then let them know you plan to correct them. A complaining customer whose problem is acknowledged and tended to can become a loyal customer for life, even more loyal than he or she was before the error took place.

Step 2: Apologize

Saying "I'm sorry" is a critical step in service recovery. As in acknowledgment, apologizing does not require that you accept blame unless the practice is at fault for the problem. Even if the fault lies with the patient or outside sources, it's easy to apologize: "I'm sorry this situation occurred," "I'm sorry you had to wait," or "I'm sorry you're still in pain." An apology conveys concern, which is one of the key characteristics patients seek from physicians and staff members. If there's even the slightest question as to whether something went wrong, apologize anyway. You can't go wrong, and your patient will be impressed.

A father took his 15-year-old son to a primary care physician for a basketball physical. The physician had been recommended by his employer, who was also a physician. He told us this tale:

I waited for 2 hours to get in to see this doctor. I wasn't a walk-in; we had an appointment. I would have left except that my son had the afternoon off from school, and rescheduling with someone else would have meant taking him out of school. After an hour and a half, I asked the receptionist how much longer it would be, and she told me, 'Oh, any minute now they'll be calling you.' It was 30 'any-minutes' later before we were called back to the exam room. When the doctor came in, he asked me who had referred us. I told him Dr. T. had recommended him, but then I said, "But you're not worth a 2-hour wait." He didn't even apologize—he said something about all those health plan patients who pay a $5 co-pay and want an hour of your time. It just so happens I was one of those health plan patients, so he didn't earn any points with that comment.

Step 3: Amend

No matter how seemingly minor the error may be, a demonstration of contrition shows grace and sincerity. Making amends can be a simple but heartfelt act such as hand writing a note of apology. If the error is more severe—the patient arrived for an appointment only to discover that it hadn't been recorded in the schedule (yet he has a card that was given to him when he made the appointment on his previous visit)—making amends may require working the patient into the schedule, discounting the bill, sending a green plant to his home or office, or a similar display of apology. To captivate the patient, do something unexpected or beyond what's called for. Send flowers to the patient's office; think of the impact when the patient tells 15 curious co-workers, "The flowers are from my doctor. Her office had promised to call in the morning with some important test results, and they didn't call until the next day."

Making amends should mean giving the offended party options. A common action in medical practice is to offer a patient whose appointment time has been delayed the option of waiting or rescheduling for another day. People like being given choices because it gives them a feeling of control. (Conversely, it's because they feel they have no control over a situation that people may get angry when an error is made.) Fred, the allergy patient who routinely shows up unannounced for his shots, should be given the option of calling an hour or a day ahead so that the nurse can prepare the injection and anticipate his arrival, thus minimizing the waiting time; or he can be told, "You can continue to come without calling ahead, but we can't always promise to take you back right away; you may have to wait several hours, depending on our schedule." This approach gives the individual a no-choice option, yet still gives him some control. He knows that if he chooses to show up without calling, he will wait. It's a choice he knowingly makes.

There are two basic requirements that accompany the "amendment" step of the Triple-A Action Plan for service recovery: Employees must convey sincere concern and interest upon learning of a problem, and they **must** be empowered to solve problems and make amends. There's nothing more irritating to a patient than to be told, "I'm so sorry, Mr. Wiu, but I'm not authorized to change a billing statement. I'll have to talk to the office manager, and she'll have to check with Dr. Zimmerman. We'll call you next week."

Stew Leonard's Dairy is renowned for its customer-first and "do whatever it takes" attitude toward service recovery. One example from *The Service Edge: 101 Companies That Profit from Customer Care:*[2]

> *On a Friday afternoon, disaster strikes: A computer failure shuts down the cash registers. Most customers wait (munching a free shrimp, courtesy of the management), but one woman leaves, drives 30 minutes to get home, then calls the store and complains to the manager that because of the computer crash, she now has no groceries for her husband's sixtieth birthday party, which happens to be that night. Within an hour, a car pulls up at her house and out pops a Stew Leonard's employee who delivers her groceries—along with a birthday cake that says, "Happy 60th, George. Sincerely, Stew." Guess what people talked about at that party.*

PREVENT THE PROBLEM

The Triple-A Action Plan for service recovery is meaningful and effective if it's only occasionally required to deal with one-of-a-kind errors. If you or someone in the practice deals consistently with the same problems (same situation, different faces), it may be a sign of a bigger problem—unclear communication, processes without ownership, or unempowered employees, for instance. When a service error occurs more than once, it's wise to look behind the symptom to find the situation's source.

IDENTIFY THE MISTAKE

If you don't have standards and processes in place that encourage patients, staff, referral sources, or even vendors to notify someone when they are displeased, you risk losing customers and perpetuating the problem. A threat-free environment must exist for patients or staff to feel comfortable pointing out a problem or a mistake. Although some patients are more than happy to mention their displeasure to anyone they encounter, others may withhold this information, fearing that "the bookkeeper will get in trouble if I tell someone that my supplementary insurance was billed incorrectly."

The Washington, D.C. research firm Technical Assistance Research Programs, Inc. has studied customer complaining behavior and has found that customers often don't complain because they believe the process is complex and time consuming and that the result is not worth it. Sometimes they don't complain because they believe nothing will result from it. These customers leave, taking their referral potential with them.[3]

To encourage patients to disclose problems, make it easy for them, and make it clear that effective action will follow. Offer options for identifying problems. Patient questionnaires, postvisit surveys, and suggestion boxes work well, but the best approach is a personal one. At the end of the visit, the physician, a nurse, or a technician can say to the patient, "Our practice goal is to provide good care in every way. Was everything satisfactory today? Is there anything we need to discuss?" This open-ended question can elicit a variety of responses, from the hidden agenda about a patient's health concerns to a problem with a staff member.

In larger practices, it may be wise to implement a formal system for tracking and following up on patient complaints (don't, however, use the form as an excuse for delaying immediate action whenever possible). A complaint form is used by practices such as the Cleveland Clinic in Ohio and San Luis Medical Clinic in San Luis Obispo, California to collect information about the problem, how it was resolved, by whom, and with what results along with recommendations for changes in procedures. A sample complaint form is shown in Exhibit 28-1.[4]

Exhibit 28-1 Service Recovery Action Form

Complaint Taken By: _____ Date/Time: _____

Patient Name: _____

Complainant/Relationship to Patient: _____

Telephone Numbers (Patient/Complainant): _____

Date of Incident: _____

Follow-Up Date and Action Taken with Patient/Complainant: _____

_____

_____

Describe the Problem: _____

_____

_____

Department or Individual Involved: _____

Type of Problem:
- ❏ Access to Service
- ❏ Medical Care
- ❏ Charges/Professional Fees
- ❏ Interpersonal Communications
- ❏ Billing/Insurance/Credit/Payment
- ❏ Other _____

Have you tried to resolve this problem? Please describe action(s) and results:

_____

_____

Is a change in policy or procedure needed? Please explain: _____

_____

Comments: _____

Copies to: _____

PATIENT EXIT INTERVIEWS REVEAL SOURCE OF PROBLEMS

Another way to identify service errors that might otherwise go unnoticed or deliberately hidden is by conducting an exit interview with patients who request a records transfer. Although patients may change physicians as a result of a move or a change in insurance, sometimes it is because of poor service, misunderstandings, or perceived problems with care. One physician who routinely calls departing patients found that a mass exodus of about 20 patients was caused by an new insurance clerk who, in her zeal to collect outstanding balances, was calling patients in predawn hours, calling employers, and even calling ex-spouses.[5]

The exit interview telephone call can be made by the physician or a sympathetic staff member, who should express regret that the patient wishes to leave the practice and interest in learning how the practice might improve and prevent further errors. The patient should be told that his or her honest and candid responses will be used to correct problems in action or attitude. If the patient is hesitant to respond, and if questioning does not elicit clarification, encourage the patient to put the complaint in writing and send a form and/or a stamped self-addressed envelope to make it easy to do so.

STRIVE FOR PERFECTION, BUT PLAN FOR RECOVERY

Striving for service excellence demands a service recovery process. Let's face it: Even if the minimum standard in your practice is 100% perfection, you'll seldom achieve it. Even at 99% perfection, there's a 1% chance that someone will blow it occasionally. A service recovery strategy accepts imperfection but says, "We'll fix it and keep striving." More to the point, it says, "We care about what our customers think. We aren't perfect, but we'll work continually and consistently to get there." ✐

Action Steps for Service Recovery

1. Accept that mistakes will occur, but don't accept the mistakes.
2. Institute a service recovery strategy (the Triple-A Action Plan):
   - Acknowledge the mistake.
   - Apologize, even if you are not at fault.
   - Amend. Take corrective action as a tangible indication of regret that it occurred.
3. Be sympathetic in listening to complaints and sincere in conveying regret.
4. Identify the source of the mistake to prevent recurrence. Provide methods for errors to be brought out: surveys, suggestion boxes, personal follow-up, exit interviews.
5. Create a "threat-free" environment to encourage everyone—patients, staff, vendors, and referral sources—to point out service errors.
6. Criticize and correct the process, not the person.
7. Empower employees to take appropriate action immediately.

References

1. T.J. Peters and R.H. Waterman, Jr. *In Search of Excellence: Lessons from America's Best-Run Companies* (New York, N.Y.: Harper and Row, 1982): 166.
2. R. Zemke and D. Schaaf, *The Service Edge: 101 Companies That Profit from Customer Care* (New York, N.Y.: New American Library, 1989): 319.
3. J.A. Goodman, T. Marra, and L. Brigham, Customer service: Costly nuisance or low-cost profit strategy? *Journal of Retail Banking* (Fall 1986): 7-16.
4. R. Luecke, V.R. Rosselli, and J. Moss, The economic ramifications of "client" dissatisfaction, *Group Practice Journal* (May/June 1991): 8–18.
5. G. Darrow, I learn a lot from patients who leave me, *Medical Economics* (April, 1991): 116–121.

29

What Your Patient Wants To Know

"I want to know what's wrong, not just that the doctor will fix it. When he can explain something so I can understand, I feel like he knows what he's doing."

"What I look for in a doctor is someone who takes time and is thorough. My doctor explains things verbally, but also visually, with drawings and models. This helps me understand, and I feel confident that he knows what he's talking about. When I had surgery, he took my wife aside after the operation and explained what he had done. That impressed us both."

Today's patients want information, education, and a complete understanding of their condition and treatment. The younger the patient, the more demanding he or she tends to be. No matter what the age, patients equate communication with quality. According to a 1988 National Research Corporation (NRC) survey, the key characteristics that consumers use in rating physicians they judge to be of high quality include willingness to maintain patient health through educational information and willingness to talk about the individual's illness and treatment.[1]

In another NRC survey, consumers listed willingness to explain things as the most important criterion in selecting a physician. This criterion was given a 9.6 rating on a 10-point scale;

other factors such as reasonable fees, telephone access, friendly office staff, convenient appointments, and convenient office location rated much lower.

Physicians, wrote geriatrics specialist Paul Rousseau, MD, in *Patient Care*, "toss about specialized terminology the way a cook flips hamburgers at a fast food restaurant, neglecting to translate acronyms or explain procedures. . . ."[2(p.32)] Rousseau recognizes that, especially for the elderly population, communication is often more important in ensuring quality care than the medical lingo, fancy gadgets, and high-tech tests and procedures to which physicians and the health care system are sometimes wedded. Patients need information about how the health care system works as well as the process and prognosis of their disease or condition, and it's most effective and credible if it comes from their provider.

Patient education is critical to compliance and outcome. It satisfies patient expectations as well as offering these benefits:

- Patients are more confident in their physician.
- Patient education provides tangible evidence of the visit.
- Patients look to their physician as a primary source of information.
- Informed patients make better decisions and are more compliant.
- Patient education information gives consistent quality to your message.

INFORMED PATIENTS FEEL MORE CONFIDENT IN THEIR PHYSICIAN

Patient education is critical, according to Lawrence Cohen, MD. "If you take the time to discuss your findings and your diagnostic or treatment plan with the patient, this creates an open channel of communication, it promotes good will, and it tells the patient you as the doctor respect them enough to take the time to talk with them, and you feel they are intelligent enough to understand. Patients appreciate this. It also probably helps minimize medical-legal problems."

No doubt about it, education does limit malpractice liability. It's a quantifiable and tangible component of communication that more and more patients expect and malpractice insurers are carefully scrutinizing.

A patient scheduled for a complex surgical procedure confirms Dr. Cohen's observation with the following description of a preoperative encounter with her anesthesiologist:

> *Without question, English was his second language. Medicalese was his mother tongue. No patient should meet a physician they cannot communicate with, especially when he is charged with putting you to sleep for several hours. Needless to say, my visit with him prior to surgery did not inspire my confidence. It was fortunate that my surgeon had spent considerable time carefully explaining the technical aspects of the surgery as well as the post-op course. His communication style and the depth of information he provided offset what the anesthesiologist sorely lacked.*

TANGIBLE EVIDENCE OF SERVICE AND QUALITY

Patient education provides tangible evidence of the visit and your service quality. "My doctor always gives me some sort of written information," commented one woman. "It helps me remember what he's told me. I get the feeling he's concerned about me because he wants to help me stay healthy."

Educational information—whether in the form of a computer-printed information sheet developed in the office, a custom-printed brochure, a purchased information pamphlet, an audiocassette, a video, a hand-drawn illustration, or a formal, structured class or educational session—personalizes and demystifies health care. It is tangible evidence that you are concerned and that you want your patient to be informed. And, like the hotel stationery many guests take as a memento of their stay, educational information is an after-the-visit reminder of the quality of service you provided.

PATIENTS LOOK TO THEIR DOCTOR FOR MEDICAL INFORMATION

Although newspapers, general interest magazines, and health and wellness publications such as *American Health* and *Prevention* are common sources of knowledge about new developments in the world of medicine, patients still turn to their physicians as the ultimate credible authority. Magazines, newspapers, and the evening news are impersonal and nonspecific, and they raise further questions that need personalized answers. When Frances, your patient, reads in the latest issue of *Reader's Digest* about Joe's gallbladder and the new operation called a laparoscopic cholecystectomy, she looks to you to personalize what she has read.

Giving patients a personal response needn't require a lengthy discourse. Printed information can back up a brief explanation from the physician yet still appear personalized. In computerized practices, clearly written descriptions of the most commonly treated conditions and treatment options can be stored on the computer; the physician can then note on the superbill which information form should be printed out for the patient.

Because people want information about the latest health care trends, it's a good idea to subscribe to the most popular general interest magazines and newspapers for exam rooms as well as the reception area. A staff member should be given the responsibility of reviewing these publications as they arrive and alerting the physician to articles or news reports that may generate patient comments or questions. In some cases, it may be wise to plan ahead with a written response or position paper for controversial articles. For example, when the silicone breast implant story became big news in 1991, plastic surgeon Gustavo Colon, MD, prepared a comprehensive information packet that included a "position paper." This packet was provided to every patient who expressed concern or asked questions about implant safety.

INFORMED PATIENTS MAKE BETTER DECISIONS

Patients who understand their symptoms, diagnosis, treatment, medications, and other health care details are more likely to make good decisions. They are more compliant and have a stronger commitment to wellness.

Despite everything we've said about patients as consumers, about patients who stand up to their physicians and demand complete detailed explanations, a certain number of patients will meekly accept what they are told; they will not question or press for detail, and they will leave your office without a clear understanding of what they have been told or what they have been instructed to do. These passive patients are in awe of the "physician-as-god" figure. They will benefit from additional information that they can take home to review with family members. Given this additional information, they are more likely to follow instructions because they are more likely to *understand* the instructions. They will make decisions about diet, exercise, medications, and follow-up care that are based on fact rather than whim.

Other patients are uninformed about what symptoms or conditions require professional care, what certain specialists treat, when self-care and over-the-counter medications are advisable, and so forth. For these instances, patient education yields cost-effective health care. The Sansum Clinic in Santa Barbara, California answers questions in its patient education brochures that help consumers understand the health care system. For example, its allergy brochure (Exhibit 29-1) answers questions about what an allergist does and when allergy symptoms warrant professional care as well as informing patients about the services of the allergy specialists at the clinic.

Family practice specialist Robert Bright, MD, is a warm, friendly physician with a practice that reflects his concern for patients. Yet he acknowledges, "People worry about taking too much of the doctor's time. Or they have other concerns so they don't hear what I have to say about lifestyle issues. I may have a patient who needs to be on a low-sodium diet because of hypertension. I could explain this to my patient, but he may not give me his full attention. So I'll have him sit comfortably and talk with a staff member for 10 minutes or so about diet and other patient education issues."

PATIENT EDUCATION MATERIAL GIVES YOUR MESSAGE CONSISTENCY

"Quality has to be consistent, not some of the time, but all of the time," observes Dr. Cavanaugh. "If a patient has cataract surgery in September and she is told one thing by a staff member, then in December she has the second eye done and she is told something else by another staff member, it can be disrupting. Patients need to get a unified message." Printed materials, vid-

Exhibit 29-1 Sansum Clinic Allergy Brochure

The information in this excerpt from the Sansum Clinic allergy brochure helps Sansum patients understand what an allergist does.

Adult and Pediatric Allergies, Asthma, and Immunology at Sansum

What Does An Allergist Treat?

A cardiologist takes care of your heart. A dermatologist takes care of your skin. An ophthalmologist takes care of your eyes. What do these specialties have in common? They all treat a single organ system. An allergist is different. Instead of dealing with just one organ system, an allergist diagnoses and treats disorders of a **variety** of systems ranging from sinuses to skin. To confuse you even more, many of the diseases treated by allergists aren't even **allergies!** For example, half of all cases of asthma aren't caused by allergic reactions in the first place.

The common denominator to all these diseases? **Inflammation.** If the inflamed tissues are in the bronchial tubes, it's asthma. If the skin is inflamed, it's hives or eczema. In fact, an allergist has special expertise managing a wide variety of inflammatory diseases:

❑ Hay fever
❑ Sinus problems
❑ Asthma
❑ Food allergies
❑ Drug allergies
❑ Insect sting allergies

But an allergist (actually an allergist-**immunologist**) is more than an allergy doctor. Because allergies and inflammation are all part of the immune system, the allergy specialist is also an expert in immune disorders. As a result, an allergist is often asked to evaluate and treat immunodeficiencies, defects of the immune system that result in frequent, severe, or unusual infections:

❑ Recurrent infections or pneumonias
❑ Antibody deficiencies
❑ Adults and children who are "always sick:" bronchitis, ear infections, etc.

What Does An Allergist Actually Do?

Lacking a clear-cut diagnosis, you may have had the frustrating experience of trying to hit or miss remedies for your wheezing, coughing, or sneezing. But it's rare that a patient leaves the Allergy Clinic still wondering what the problem is.

In fact, it's a little like playing Sherlock Holmes. First, an allergist gathers data based on your personal medical history and physical examination. Sometimes this is sufficient to identify the culprit. Often, however, more data are needed, such as allergy skin tests, lung function tests, X-rays, or laboratory tests. With these pieces of the puzzle in place, the diagnosis can usually be clarified so that you and the allergist can go to work on therapy.

If these steps sound complicated, they sometimes are. That's why the specialty of Allergy and Immunology requires one of the longest training programs after medical school: 3 years of training in Internal Medicine or Pediatrics, then another 2 or 3 years of specialty training.

Source: Courtesy of Sansum Medical Clinic, Santa Barbara, California.

eos, audiocassettes, and other forms of patient education provide a consistent message that can be documented. (This also points out the importance of giving a consistent message about clinical policies and procedures to staff as well as to patients.)

Susan Northrup, MD, obstetrician-gynecologist, views education as "the key to patient satisfaction. Probably 90% of my patients comment how pleased they are because 'the doctor talks to me.'" Her office is heavily stocked with educational materials ranging from pharmaceutical and specialty society booklets to videos, models, articles from journals and popular magazines, and newspapers. Patients are encouraged to browse through the information available, but Dr. Northrup's efforts go beyond encouragement. When a surgical procedure or certain other forms of treatment are recommended, patients are required to watch the appropriate video. They then sign a form acknowledging that they have seen and understood the video.

INTERACTIVE VIDEO: HIGH-TECH PATIENT EDUCATION

The newest approach to patient education is high tech. It's the patient-interactive videodisk with "shared decision programs." A landmark study by the Foundation for Informed Medical Decision Making in Hanover, New Hampshire documented the impact of interactive video. This state-of-the-art "tailored technology," first tested with men with benign prostatic hyperplasia, allows patients to learn the pros, cons, and potential outcomes of surgery according to their own conditions, lifestyles, and preferences. Use of the video at several HMOs has resulted in an annual drop in prostate surgery ranging from 44% to 60%.[3]

The interactive video concept has spread to other specialties and conditions, including low back pain, hypertension, juvenile diabetes, early-stage breast cancer, stable angina, estrogen replacement therapy, and benign uterine conditions. It's predicted to result in more satisfied patients, greater productivity for physicians and staff (the physician can see other patients while the patient is watching the videodisk), and possibly an improved bottom line as a result of reduced liability insurance costs.[4]

In 1992, videodisk equipment cost about $8,000 plus about $1,000 for each program. Videotape education doesn't have to be elaborate or costly, however. Dr. Colon created personalized videos 7 years ago to help patients understand cosmetic surgery procedures. The videos feature Dr. Colon and patients who have had surgery. Surgical candidates are given the videotape to view at home; this allows them time to think of questions for their return visit. Neil Baum, MD, develops videotapes in which he discusses common conditions; these are also available for patients to take home and view at their leisure.

SIMPLE VIDEOTAPES: EFFECTIVE FOR PATIENT PARTICIPATION

Saul Schreiber, MD, also uses videotapes for patient education. He videotapes every arthroscopic surgery he performs and has the tapes cataloged in his patient education library. Thus when a patient is scheduled for anterior cruciate ligament surgery, for example, Dr. Schreiber will explain verbally what the procedure entails. A videotape of the procedure is popped into the VCR in the patient education room. The patient watches the video and then completes an evaluation sheet that asks him or her to comment on his or her understanding of the content. This video information sheet backs up the formal preoperative consent form; it also alerts Dr. Schreiber or his staff if a patient indicates lack of understanding of the scheduled procedure.

"We don't have the patient sign the pre-op permission here in the office," Dr. Schreiber says. (That's done at the hospital.) "I don't want to introduce the lawyer into my practice." The video information form is a nonlegalese way of ascertaining the patient's understanding.

By following this procedure for patient education, Dr. Schreiber addresses the patient's "need to know" as well as legal requirements. His approach satisfies three criteria for informed consent:

- It is a visual presentation that helps patients understand what they will experience.
- It is reproducible evidence.
- It is documentable. The video information form and the legal informed consent form both are filed in the patient's medical record along with a notation of which video the patient was shown.

EDUCATION MEETS PATIENT NEEDS AND GIVES YOU AN EDGE

Education does more than meet the patient's needs. It gives your practice a marketing edge. It meets patient expectations because your patients **do** expect information and education. A 1988 Louis Harris poll found that 9 of 10 Americans consider it "very important for a doctor to be knowledgeable and competent, to answer questions honestly and completely, to explain medical problems in clear language, [and] to make sure patients understand what they've been told about their medical problems. . . ." Patient education enhances the perception of your quality, improves patient compliance, reduces malpractice risk, and increases productivity by reducing after-hours or next-day telephone calls. The more patients know about the services you offer and the conditions you treat, the more thorough their knowledge of your practice. The administrator of a large Midwestern orthopedics practice says, "I hear from patients all the time, 'I didn't know you did that' when we give them a brochure or pamphlet."

Information increases patient satisfaction even when the news is not good, according to a 1991 study reported in *Lancet,* a British medical journal. In the study, two specialists in Australia sent cancer patients a letter summarizing what had been discussed during their initial visit, including treatment choices, test results, status of the disease, and referral arrangements. Patients who got the letter rated their overall satisfaction higher than those who didn't. Satisfaction with the explanation and information they had been given was higher; letter recipients also felt that they remembered what they had been told and that they had had a chance to ask all the questions they wanted.[5]

MAKE PATIENT EDUCATION A SERVICE STRATEGY

Following are steps for making patient education a service strategy:

1. *Make a commitment to patient education.* Without a clear understanding by everyone that a practice goal is educated patients, this will become a secondary priority. (Commit-

ment, you recall, is *making* time to do something; interest is doing it when you have time.)

2. *Investigate sources for information that reflect your views and beliefs.* Most specialty societies and the American Medical Association offer a catalog of educational materials. Don't limit the material you acquire to your own specialty. People welcome information about general health topics. Purchase brochures and audiovisual materials from national organizations such as the American Heart Association, the American Lung Association, and the Arthritis Foundation. Pharmaceutical companies are a generous source of information. The National Council on Patient Information and Education (NCPIE) provides an assortment of educational assistance (NCPIE, 666 Eleventh Street N.W., Suite 810D, Washington, D.C. 20001). If what you find about a particular condition or procedure doesn't say what you want your patients to hear, write and print your own material. It doesn't have to be fancy, expensive, or elaborate. Many physicians prepare simple, typewritten instruction or information sheets to give to patients.

3. *Establish a standard and a protocol to be followed in your practice with each patient.* When you have a consistent procedure, you can be certain that every patient gets accurate, detailed information pertaining to his or her condition, treatment, surgery, or health status. The protocol should outline **what** the patient is to receive, **who** should provide it, **in what form or format** the material should be provided (print, video, audio, personal explanation, etc.), **when** it should be given (e.g., before scheduled surgery, when a condition is diagnosed, etc.), and **what documentation, confirmation, or follow-up** is required (i.e., completion of a form by the patient acknowledging receipt of the information, repetition of key information by the patient to confirm understanding, a follow-up phone call by the medical assistant to ensure understanding and compliance, etc.). Documentation of patient education should always go in the medical record, of course.

A protocol can reduce the chance of misunderstanding, such as occurred with one patient who was instructed to follow a restricted diet. The brochure he was given said to eliminate red meat from his diet. A nurse following up later found that the man was cooking his daily steak well done in the belief that "red" meat meant rare and that overcooking thus solved the problem.

4. *Remember this: to educate patients, you must first understand not only their clinical problems but their values, beliefs, and work and family situations.* Review the communication and listening techniques in Chapter 24 to be certain that you gather symptoms, lifestyle issues, underlying concerns, and other information from patients. Listen and probe for expectations. Education is a give-and-take conversation, not a lecture. It takes a special questioning approach and especially nonjudgmental "listening between the lines" to draw out details that help you make an accurate diagnosis and an appropriate treatment recommendation for your patient.

5. *Use language that your patients will understand, with words that create mental pictures, common terms, and analogies (bed sores instead of decubitus ulcers, brain wave instead of electroencephalogram, and grip strength test instead of dynamometer).* "When doctors use fancy names, it makes them feel good and builds their egos," neurologist Marvin Korengold, MD, observes. "But it just confuses patients." And if the patient nods knowingly, too embarrassed to admit he or she is baffled, you could be at risk for a malpractice suit, or at the least an unhappy, noncompliant patient.

6. *Don't let any patient leave your office without tangible evidence of your commitment to education.* Even patients who are healthy can benefit from educational information. Develop a library of health and wellness material, and pass it out freely to every patient. When you give someone a handout about the importance of dietary fiber or how to incorporate exercise into a busy schedule, the subtle message is, "I care about you." This is a powerful, virtually unbreakable thread to weave through the fabric of the physician-patient relationship.

7. *Education takes time, but it saves time in the end.* Physicians who consistently take the time to review lab tests, diagnosis, and treatment with their patients and give them information to take away report that their patients require less

follow-up time on the phone and in the office. Ray Hughes, MD, the Phoenix, Arizona family practice physician who gives patients a computerized printout of their visit, believes that this tangible proof of quality has brought him new patients.

8. *Give patients information in print and pictures, and then document your efforts to improve compliance and to reduce liability.* Use anatomical drawings filled in with details specific to your patient. Develop instruction sheets and descriptive forms. Urologist Neil Baum gives patients a fill-in-the-blank form (see Exhibit 29-2) that lists medications, dosages, symptoms and side effects to expect, symptoms that warrant a call to the doctor and other details. A completed copy goes in the medical record. One family practice physician gives patients an instruction sheet in the reception area. The patient fills in his or her name, the date, a description of the presenting problem, and any other health problems. In the exam room, the physician fills in the rest of the form while discussing instructions and diagnosis with the patient.

9. *Share your views on current hot medical topics.* Dr. Colon's position paper on breast implant safety was shared with patients, the public, and the local media. Rather than hurting his practice, the implant crisis brought people seeking factual information. Other practices prepare scrapbooks of articles from newspapers and magazines on medical and fitness subjects of interest to patients. Some physicians find that it saves time and questions to develop a one- or two-page discussion of topics that make headlines. When a patient brings up the risk of heart attack with the nicotine patch, for example, the physician can briefly review the side effects and then give the detailed discussion paper to the patient. The benefit: an informed and satisfied patient in less time than it would take to discuss the complete content of the sheet.

10. *Use staff to fill in the gaps.* Many practices have a patient coordinator or a nurse, technician, or other clinical employee who comes into the exam room when the physician leaves to answer patient questions and to provide detailed instruction. This can be more effective and more productive than relying on the physician alone.

Exhibit 29-2 Patient Instruction Form

Neil Baum, MD
Professional Medical Corporation
Urology
3225 Prytania St., Suite 614
New Orleans, Louisiana 70115
(504) 891-8454

Patient Name _____

Date_____

Your diagnosis is _____

_____

_____

Your medication is _____

to be taken (#) _____times a day at _____and
without eating/with/before/after meals (circle one).

You can expect to have (symptom) _____for (time)_____.

(symptom)_____is normal with this condition/medication.

(symptom)_____is **abnormal** with this condition/medication.
PLEASE CALL OUR OFFICE AT ONCE IF YOU HAVE THIS REACTION.

Please call our office in_____days for the results of your tests.

Notes: _____

_____

_____

_____

Source: Courtesy of Neil Baum, MD, New Orleans, Louisiana.

"I like to think I'm a pretty open and easygoing person," one physician said, "but I'll be the first to admit that my nurse gets all kinds of questions and comments that I never get. I know it's because patients feel like they just 'can't say that' to me. That's O.K. As long as they're getting the information they need, and they leave here feeling like we all care about them, that's what counts." ❧

Action Steps for Educated Patients

1. Establish a patient education program in your practice to ensure that every patient receives tangible information about his or her health or condition.
2. Purchase or prepare printed information about conditions you commonly treat, medications you prescribe, or treatment options.
3. Have a staff member review popular magazines for medical articles that may require written comment or elaboration for patients in your practice.
4. Use patient education information to help your patients understand the health care system: when to call the physician, symptoms that need attention, services provided by your specialty and your practice, limitations and requirements of Medicare or certain health plans, and so forth.
5. Remember that people learn in different ways. Don't rely on only one medium; use print, models, videotapes, audiocassettes, drawings, and computer software to help patients understand.
6. Investigate and use information available from your professional society, national health care associations, pharmaceutical companies, and other sources.
7. Incorporate documentation and follow-up whenever you or staff members provide information to patients.
8. Take time to understand your patient's values and needs to provide appropriate, personalized information.
9. Use everyday language that your patients can understand.
10. Don't forget your staff. They can fill in the blanks and often will elicit further questions and concerns that patients may hesitate to bring up to you.

References

1. National Research Corporation, Voluntary Hospitals of America, *Marketing Monitor* (1988): 6.
2. P. Rousseau, A painful lack of education, *Patient Care* (September 30, 1992): 32.
3. S. Greengard, The physician's new care companion, *American Medical News* (June 29, 1992): 7–9.
4. B. Clements, Interactive videos, *American Medical News* (November 16, 1992): 11–12.
5. J.E. Bishop, Doctors get results by sending letters after treatment, *Wall Street Journal* (October 11, 1991): B-3.

—— ࠫ ——
30

Compliance Is Good for Patients and Good for You

If physicians could be granted three wishes by a genie in a test tube, this would probably be one of them: "I wish people would follow instructions for their treatment and take better care of themselves."

"Why won't patients do what's good for them?" doctors often ask rhetorically during discussions of quality service and satisfied patients. If you weren't dignified professionals, you might be tearing your hair out and stamping your feet in frustration. We hear variations on this theme: "People spend time and money consulting a medical professional; they get tests and prescriptions and surgery and therapy, but they don't follow instructions. Then they complain because they don't get well fast enough or because they relapse."

Patients don't follow instructions because they don't think it's important to do so. Or because they don't comprehend what will happen if they don't fill the prescription, do the exercise ordered, come in for a follow-up appointment, or stick to the recommended diet. Or because they don't understand what a high-fiber diet is, or why the full 10 days of antibiotics must be taken, or the risk of not changing surgical dressings.

In other words, what we have here is a failure to communicate. Compliance depends on thorough, complete communication. There is sufficient evidence to prove a direct correlation between physician-patient communication and positive patient outcome, concluded the consensus panel of the 1991 International Doctor-

Patient Communication Conference held in Toronto, Ontario. The panel concurred with previous research that "the physician's interpersonal skills also largely determine patient satisfaction, compliance and positively influence health outcomes."[1(p.1385)]

YOUR PATIENTS HAVE GOOD INTENTIONS, BUT . . .

Patients are not programmable; they are people who stuff an assortment of personal or social problems and perspectives into their bags of good intentions. All the following can impair or prevent adherence to treatment plans: lack of medical insurance or insufficient coverage, time or transportation problems, family pressures, religious beliefs, outside opinions, work obligations, and lack of connection or relationship with the physician. Yet if the physician or a staff member listens to Mrs. Keyes and explains **why** she must give 3-year-old Liza all her antibiotic rather than save half of it "for the next time she gets a sore throat," the impact of these factors can be mitigated. Active listening and probing questions may reveal that the prescribed antibiotic is costly and that Mrs. Keyes believes she is demonstrating thrift and foresight by saving half the prescription.

"You have to know the patient's experience, cohort, and beliefs," says David Silverman, MD, a West Hartford, Connecticut physician. "You can't assume that what you ask a patient to do as part of your plan will be carried out. Patients with financial limitations may not fill a prescription for high blood pressure if you write it for a medication that costs $1.50 per pill. You have to spend time to find out if there are situations that may prevent compliance."

Dr. Silverman sees many elderly patients on fixed incomes. Rather than embarrass them by asking, "Can you afford this drug?" he asks indirect questions: "What are your typical meals like? What do you do to socialize? How do you spend any extra money? Who helps you out with shopping, housework, and caring for yourself?" This line of questioning takes time, he agrees, but "quality service is going the extra step."

Communication, compliance, and satisfaction are circular characteristics of the physician-patient relationship. According to

COMSORT, a Baltimore, Maryland academic consortium that designs continuing medical education programs, compliance and outcome are directly linked to improved patient satisfaction with the medical encounter. COMSORT's programs focus on improving clinical communication because of research indicating that when patients participate in the exchange as egalitarian members of their own health care team, satisfaction and compliance improve measurably. Additional benefits of good communication include better appointment keeping, less "doctor shopping," and lower risk of litigation.

LISTEN BETWEEN THE LINES

In communicating to gain compliance, it is especially important to listen for feedback, watch for visual cues, and to ask the patient to repeat your instructions to be certain that he or she has heard what you said and not what he or she **thinks** you said. Don't assume that patients understand the reasoning behind your treatment suggestions. The following story was related by a well-educated woman who admitted that even years later she is bitter that a lack of information from health professionals could have jeopardized her health as well as that of her unborn baby.

> When I was hospitalized during my pregnancy for pulmonary emboli, I was given oxygen therapy through uncomfortable nose prongs. Whenever I talked on the phone, which was quite frequently, I removed the tubing. After several days of this practice, my doctor came into my hospital room while I was on the phone and chided me severely for not using the oxygen.
>
> No one had explained the importance of the oxygen and certainly never mentioned the potential danger of not using it consistently. Actually, the doctor never really explained the gravity of my condition at all. I was angry at the doctor and the nurses for not letting me know why the oxygen was necessary. Since I felt no difficulty breathing, this part of my treatment did not seem particularly important. Had there been a negative outcome for either the baby or me, I

certainly would have considered legal action for withholding information.

Specific research studies have looked at patients with hypertension, diabetes, and breast cancer and found that simple adjustments in the communication interchange, such as allowing patients to talk without interruption, encouraging patients to ask questions during the visit, and using open-ended questions and motivational interjections, all lead to better compliance. For example, patients who were allowed to speak without interruptions during their doctor visit experienced significantly greater reduction in blood pressure.[2] It makes sense: If doctors and patients communicate actively and clearly with each other, listening **actively** and clarifying their understanding of what was heard, the chances improve for common agreement about the problem, cause, and appropriate course of treatment and the responsibility each has in the patient's care.

PATIENTS MUST PARTICIPATE FOR GOOD CARE

But this may be asking a lot. Remember the Boston, Massachusetts primary care clinic study in which physicians and patients were asked what problem or condition had been addressed during their most recent visit? In less than half the cases did provider and patient even agree that the problem involved the same organ system!

Patient participation is especially important in managing chronic diseases. When the disease is a daily part of their lives, patients must take long-term responsibility for sticking to the treatment plan. In essence, the chronic disease patient becomes his or her own primary caregiver. Drug therapy, diet, exercise programs, and lifestyle changes are all elements of the treatment plan requiring understanding and agreement if compliance is to occur.

Compliance is more likely to occur if the patient is given options rather than rigid rules. Dr. Silverman says, "I try to give people choices and consequences without risking their lives. I'm not their mother; I treat them like adults. If a patient needs to reduce salt intake, I'll suggest a low-salt diet plan and let him know the consequences of following it. I'll also explain the consequences of following his regular diet, and let him know it's his decision, but I'm there to help."

Most physicians agree that if patients have participated in decisions relating to a specific regimen, they will be more likely to carry it out. You and your staff play an important role as educators, negotiators, motivators, and coaches. Physicians and practice staff (especially nurses, therapists, technicians, and assistants) can influence a patient's willingness to stick to a care plan. You also can change your patients' perceptions and self-confidence regarding their ability to influence their health status through their own actions.[3]

Your staff have a pivotal role. If they are well acquainted with your typical treatment plans, they can reinforce and provide greater detail for your instructions. After you have left the exam room, your nurse, technician, or assistant should ask the patient if he or she understood everything you reviewed. Often, a patient is less hesitant to admit uncertainty to a nurse than to the physician. Thus your staff members offer a safety valve by double-checking whether the patient accurately heard your instructions—or by determining whether **you** heard your patient's perceptions and fears accurately—if at all.

YES, SOMETIMES YOUR PATIENTS FRUSTRATE YOU

Compliance is a topic that frustrates many physicians, including most of those we interviewed. Lifestyle changes such as diet and exercise are critical in controlling many conditions, yet they are the most difficult to initiate successfully and even harder to maintain. Sustaining patient commitment and motivation in these areas requires more than effective education. It's critical that you encourage positive action and compliment even small improvements. Asking patients to demonstrate what they've learned or accomplished shows interest on your part; it also is a clue to how well patients are following instructions.

"I try to explain not only what is the proper therapy but why it is important," remarks one surgeon. "Many patients just want to take a pill rather than participate in a treatment plan. But in most cases, pills just aren't the answer. When I prescribe postsurgical exercises for joint mobility, I ask for a demonstration at the follow-up visit. In this way, I can see if they have been performing the exercise properly and I reinforce the importance of doing it."

This same surgeon recalls a diabetic patient with foot ulcers who was not following the prescribed regime for the ulcers or overall management of the systemic disease: "I'm not the first doctor to explain to this patient the need to control his diabetes. I'm sure he has heard it from his family doctor and his endocrinologist. It's frustrating for me because the patient must take some responsibility if he is to have a reasonable outcome." In cases like this, try drawing up a contract with the patient, specifying through mutual agreement what the patient's obligations are and what you and your staff will do to help motivate him or her. Look for systems that will help patients comply, such as community support groups, other patients in your practice with the same condition who are willing to offer encouragement by phone or visit, or a weekly phone call from your nurse or you to check on progress.

UNDERSTANDING IS KEY TO COMPLIANCE

Noncompliance with prescription medications is widespread and well documented across all specialties. Patients often ignore or misuse drug therapy regimes. Patients rarely volunteer to their physician that this may be the case, and physicians don't often ask.[4] Studies document that a significant portion of patients use prescriptions in ways that threaten their health. Much of the problem can be attributed to poor instruction.

"Again and again, the most important contribution to patient compliance with drug prescriptions appears to be the patient's understanding of the illness, the rationale and importance of the drug therapy, and instructions for use," according to Debra Roter, DrPH, of the Johns Hopkins School of Hygiene and Public Health. Yet physicians don't always explain clearly or completely why they've prescribed a particular medication or how to take or use it. In their book *Doctors Talking with Patients/Patients Talking with Doctors,* Debra Roter and J. Hall suggest things to discuss with patients and/or family members when medications are prescribed. The checklist can be found in Exhibit 30-1.

Exhibit 30-1 Prescription Pointers for Patients

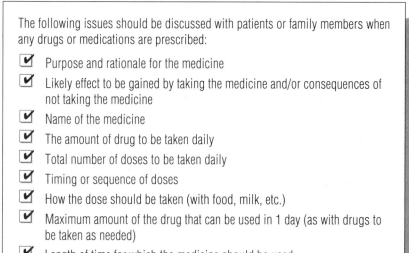

The following issues should be discussed with patients or family members when any drugs or medications are prescribed:

☑ Purpose and rationale for the medicine

☑ Likely effect to be gained by taking the medicine and/or consequences of not taking the medicine

☑ Name of the medicine

☑ The amount of drug to be taken daily

☑ Total number of doses to be taken daily

☑ Timing or sequence of doses

☑ How the dose should be taken (with food, milk, etc.)

☑ Maximum amount of the drug that can be used in 1 day (as with drugs to be taken as needed)

☑ Length of time for which the medicine should be used

☑ Other drugs, specific foods, or activities that should be avoided

☑ Proper storage techniques

☑ Possible or likely side effects

Several physicians find that preprinted information sheets about the most commonly prescribed drugs are time saving and effective patient education. "I leave blank spaces for dosage and strength so that the information forms can be customized for each patient as I review it with him," one physician said (see Exhibit 29-2 for Dr. Neil Baum's personalized information sheet). These forms are also available through some pharmaceutical firms and medical vendors.

Personalized information sheets reinforce instructions given by the physician; they also help reduce calls from patients who may have forgotten what they heard in the office. And they are tangible evidence that you care about your patient's well-being.

Edward Buchbinder, DPM, an Arizona podiatrist, said that when he sees patients for a follow-up exam after giving them a new prescription, he asks them to bring the prescription container so that he knows how many pills are left. If too many pills remain (or if the patient hasn't filled the prescription), he reviews the proper dosage and necessity for completing the medication. Another physician lamented, "If the problem clears up before the medication is gone, many patients become lax about taking the rest of the prescription or using a topical cream. They don't realize that the treatment may fail when it is not properly completed." Of course, this points to the significance of good communication about the purpose of the medication and the importance of completing it.

Knowing that patients are apt to forget to take medications, some physicians suggest that patients store their medications next to their toothbrush or near the coffee maker. "Little suggestions like this let the patient know that I think it's important for them to take the medication," a physician explained.

NO GENIE, NO MAGIC, JUST COMMUNICATION AND EDUCATION

Because the arrival of a health care genie magnanimously granting your wishes is unlikely, the task of encouraging patients to comply is in your hands, with the assistance of your staff. Use education, communication, choices, and, when needed, a little concerned nagging to help your patients understand **why** taking their medicine and following instructions are good for them. Call on their partnership responsibilities: "I'm doing my part; now here's your assignment." Taking the time to gain compliance saves time and frustration for you and your patients, and needless to say, will take you and your practice a long way on the road to patient satisfaction. ✒

Action Steps To Gain Compliance

1. Compliance is more likely to occur if your recommendations reflect your patient's experience, income, and beliefs. Ask questions that give you this information.
2. Have patients repeat your instructions to be sure that they understand them. Back up verbal instructions with printed or taped information.
3. Try to give patients options and consequences and to gain their agreement regarding the best choices for them individually.
4. Use your staff to reinforce your instructions and to validate (or correct) patient perceptions.
5. Have patients demonstrate or explain what they've learned or accomplished during a follow-up visit.
6. A contract that spells out the patient's obligations and what you and your staff will do to assist may help compliance, especially with patients with chronic conditions.
7. Emphasize to your patients that the doctor-patient relationship is a partnership in which the patient has an equal responsibility with the physician to gain the best outcome.

References

1. M. Simpson, R. Buckman, M. Stewart, P. Maguire, M. Lipkin, D. Navack, J. Till, Doctor-patient communication: The Toronto Consensus statement, *British Journal of Medicine* 303 (1991): 1385.
2. J.E. Orth, W.B. Stiles, L. Scherwitz, D. Hennritus, and C. Vallbona, Patient exposition and provider explanation in routine interview and hypertensive patients' blood pressure control. *Health Psychology* 6 (1987): 29–42.
3. S.H. Kaplan, S. Greenfield, and J.E. Ware, Jr., Assessing the effects of physician-patient interactions on the outcomes of chronic disease, *Medical Care* 27 (3) (March 1989 supplement): S110–127.
4. D.J. Steel, T.C. Jackson, and M.C. Gutmann, Have you been taking your pills? The adherence-monitoring sequence in the medical interview, *The Journal of Family Practice* 30, (3) (1990): 294–299.

31

Special Attention to Special Populations

In 1990, 80% of Americans were white, down from 83% in 1980, according to the U.S. Census. The remainder were racial and ethnic minorities, ranging from . . . Puerto Ricans, African-Americans, and Asian-Americans to . . . refugees from Latin America, Southeast Asia, and other regions.[1(p.28)]

Some 43 million Americans—17% of the population—are considered disabled (defined as limited in one or more of life's major activities).[2]

The whole world is fast becoming a melting pot as international borders crumble and once-intact countries and communities assimilate new ways, new attitudes, and new looks. Add to this cultural and ethnic diffusion an older population that may have physical impairments; and a federal law designed to allow access for the disabled, people with acquired immunodeficiency syndrome (AIDS) and individuals with other impairments or special needs; and it's apparent that groups once easily segmented and categorized are throwing researchers into a tizzy.

This "diffused homogeneity" brings a mixture of special needs. Pocket communities with unique cultures and values have sprung up across North America and around the world. The people who make up these international neighborhoods may be your patients. How do you address the language and cultural differences, as well as the medical needs and expectations, of a Lebanese woman with high blood pressure, a Vietnamese man with dietary deficiencies, or a Haitian patient with diabetes?

Elderly individuals are often viewed and dealt with in the same way as 40-year-olds. If they are given any special attention, it's only because of their increased number of medical problems and the greater complexities of their medical care, which are due to multisystem conditions and multiple medications. Yet the elderly person has unique physical and psychosocial characteristics that surround and may affect his or her medical condition, attitudes, compliance, and behavior. These characteristics often require special attention.

Individuals with disabilities want and need access to your office. There may be special circumstances related to their disability. How does your office welcome the 25-year-old athlete who happens to use a wheelchair to get around? The Americans with Disabilities Act (ADA) specifies certain modifications that businesses must make. Are you familiar with these modifications required for disability access? More important, do you and your office staff have an enlightened attitude about disabilities of any kind?

People with AIDS represent an increasing portion of the health care population. Are you and your staff sensitive to their concerns and special needs, beyond what the Occupational Safety and Health Administration says you must do to make your office a safe environment? Do you seek educational and dialog opportunities to ensure compassion and knowledge on the part of everyone in the practice?

Practices that don't specialize in children often are at a loss when a youngster becomes a patient in the practice. Do you make an effort to treat children with dignity while understanding and accommodating their age-appropriate emotional reactions to the sometimes frightening health care setting? Do you address questions and comments to the child as well as to the accompanying adult? Do you pay attention to truthfulness and trust building, for example saying, "You'll feel a little stick; it'll hurt a tiny bit, but then it goes away" rather than, "This won't hurt" when indeed it will?

PERSONAL SERVICE MEANS ADDRESSING INDIVIDUAL NEEDS

When all members of the practice staff acknowledge and take pains to address the characteristics and needs of every individual in the practice, true personal service takes place. And, as we have seen, attentive individualized service also can result in more appropriate medical care. In Chapters 13 and 14 we pointed out the importance of knowing the specific needs and expectations of each patient in the practice if you are to meet and surpass those expectations. We said that you must know on a personal level what each individual wants and expects. Nowhere does this requirement become clearer than where patients with ethnic, cultural, religious, social, physical, or age diversity are concerned.

MEET NEEDS WITH KNOWLEDGE

To meet and exceed the needs and expectations of these individual patients, however, you must understand certain characteristics of the cultural, demographic, or ethnic group to which a patient may belong. For example, a 72-year-old Native American woman who has severe arthritis may bring with her these special needs when she comes to your practice:

- impaired vision and inability to distinguish certain colors due to age
- hearing loss due to age
- reduced agility and mobility due to arthritis and age
- hesitation about taking medication or undergoing surgery due to cultural beliefs
- inclination to adhere to the traditional ways of her people, but pressure from younger family members to use "modern" medicine
- high-fat diet due to low income
- difficulty communicating due to language barrier

To adequately serve this patient, you and your staff must be familiar with more than the bone and joint deterioration of her arthritic condition. You must find some means of learning about the cultural beliefs of her people, perhaps adapting some of the Native American medicine practices where appropriate and adjusting your recommendations and treatment plan to encompass the diet and home environment to which she will return. You must also be familiar with the physical limitations that come with age as well as specific diseases or conditions that may be more common in certain ethnic groups.

Obviously, it is not possible to turn a practice into a miniature United Nations of translators and ethnic/cultural anthropologists on the off chance that a Navajo or Vietnamese may become a patient. What quality service means in this context, however, is that practices must have methods for providing appropriate, knowledgeable care *that will be understood, agreed to, and complied with* by the patient. This is the ultimate goal for all medical care: understanding, agreement, and compliance by the patient. Accomplishing this with a patient from a socioeconomic or ethnic group unfamiliar to the practice may simply mean requesting that the patient bring along a family member or friend who can translate language, explain cultural beliefs, and interpret patient concerns.

INVESTMENT IN CULTURAL AND ETHNIC AWARENESS

If you consistently treat patients of an ethnic or cultural group unfamiliar to you and your staff, however, it's not only wise but necessary to invest in continuing education to familiarize everyone with the history, values, traditions, and beliefs as well as the nutritional and medical needs of this group. For example, some Hispanic patients may not ask questions, no matter how confused or concerned they may be about their diagnosis or treatment, because they believe it challenges your authority. If you see a significant number of Hispanics in your practice, you need to be aware of cultural behaviors like these if you are to find acceptable ways to meet their needs.

Without acknowledgment and understanding of the cultural diversity of your patients, the essential element of patient satisfaction—effective communication—can't take place. Communication, we know, entails more than words. For example, a certain amount of eye contact is considered a sign of mutual trust in the mainstream American culture. But in other countries direct eye contact is inappropriate, and in some Arab and African cultures eye contact is prolonged to show interest. For many Americans, lengthy eye contact would be uncomfortable.

Here are some techniques for learning about the ethnic and cultural beliefs of your patients:

- Hire bilingual employees and/or employees who represent the ethnic or cultural group(s) that you serve in your practice.
- Contact the language or other appropriate department of a local community college or university for someone who is familiar with the cultural differences and influences of a particular ethnic group in your practice service area. Invite this expert to present an educational seminar for your practice physicians and staff.
- Contact a local hospital for the names of volunteer interpreters you can call on who may be knowledgeable in the language and culture of ethnic or racial groups in your community.
- Contact the Chamber of Commerce for a particular group, (e.g., the Chinese-American Chamber, the Hispanic Chamber, or similar organizations).
- Some larger cities have consulting firms that specialize in workplace or cultural diversity. Consider this if yours is a large practice with a fair number of patients of nonwhite North American heritage.
- Ask a patient or the family member of a patient to speak to the practice staff in an educational setting about his or her ethnic and cultural beliefs, particularly those that directly or indirectly may affect attitudes and beliefs as well as overall health or medical treatment.

Meeting the special needs of the ethnic, cultural, or age groups commonly seen in your practice is an effective service strategy. The Neurology Center in Chevy Chase, Maryland brings together employees to role play patient situations, events, and interactions and to talk about appropriate responses. Standard practice policies and procedures are adjusted to accommodate older patients. The same is true of Arthritis and Rheumatism Associates, whose patients are not only often older but frequently physically debilitated, with limbs painfully contracted and deformed. "Our employees have been taught to love the physically unlovable," says office manager Margaret Dieckhoner.

Here's Help

Additional resources for understanding and meeting the psychographic and multicultural needs of your patients:

The American Academy of Family Physicians
8880 Ward Parkway
Kansas City, MO 64114
(800) 274-2237
Videotape on racial and cultural biases in medicine

The National Coalition of Hispanic Health and Human Services Organizations
1501 16th Street, NW
Washington, DC 20036
(202) 387-5000
Provider's guide as well as workshops for providing health care to Hispanics

The Boston Area Health Education Center
c/o Boston City Hospital
818 Harrison Avenue
Boston, MA 02118
(617) 534-5258
Tapes on conducting general and geriatric bilingual medical interviews

The Western Journal of Medicine
Order from:
Circulation
P.O. Box 7602
San Francisco, CA 94120-7602
(415) 882-5177
Special issue devoted to cross-cultural medicine.

The Merck Manual
P.O. Box 2000
Mail Code WBS-435
Rahway, NJ 07065
The Merck Manual, long a reference on Western medicine, introduced a section on cross-cultural medicine in 1993.

WALK IN THEIR SHOES, SEE THROUGH THEIR EYES

The office staffs in many practices with a significant number of elderly patients learn the special needs of this demographic group by personally experiencing them. An eye-opening role play exercise that's easy to duplicate by practice staff involves simulating the physical impairments of advanced age. By experiencing the effects of cataracts, hearing loss, and arthritis, staff members begin to understand why Mr. Leebov clings to his spouse as he walks slowly down the hall or why he looks on blankly as soft-spoken Robert, the physician's assistant, explains pre-op procedures. "It made me see our older patients in a whole new light," admitted the receptionist in an internist's office who participated in this role play. "We became much more understanding once we saw and felt what our patients do." This elderly sensitivity exercise is described in Appendix 31-A at the end of this chapter.

DISABILITY AWARENESS AND ETIQUETTE

People with disabilities don't want pity, they want access and awareness. ADA protects the civil rights of all individuals with disabilities and provides for access to the public as well as to employees of an organization. The public accommodation section of the ADA became effective in 1992. Public access refers to the right of your patients and visitors who have physical or mental conditions or disabilities to be served in an equal and integrated manner.

This right to public access means that a medical practice, regardless of size, must:

- Do those things that are "readily achievable" to eliminate architectural barriers
- Meet the communication needs of persons with vision, hearing, or other impairments
- Train staff to provide service to patients with disabilities in a sensitive, respectful, and appropriate manner
- Provide necessary aids and modify policies, practices, and procedures as appropriate

Effective in 1992, a practice with 25 employees or more is required to make reasonable accommodations for disabled employees as well. Complying with the ADA calls for changes in hiring practices, including questions that may be asked during the interview.

Complying with the ADA is important not only because it's a legal requirement but because doing so (and perhaps doing more than the law requires) is physical evidence of the commitment of a practice to its patients—all of them. While you are investigating the environmental adaptations that may be required in your practice to ensure access, take time to educate physicians and staff to dispel misconceptions and inaccuracies. At the same time, clarify physical and attitude expectations of patients with disabilities, cancer, and other conditions. Some resources are listed below.

For materials on disability etiquette, misconceptions and facts, and building access, write for a catalog of publications:
National Easter Seal Society
2023 West Ogden Avenue
Chicago, IL 60612

For general information about the ADA and architectural accessibility information, write or call:
U.S. Department of Justice
Office of Americans with Disabilities Act
P.O. Box 66118
Washington, DC 20035-6118
(202) 514-0301, (202) 514-0381, or *(202) 514-0383 (TDD)*

Architectural and Transportation Barriers Compliance Board
1331 F Street N.W., Suite 1000
Washington, DC 20004
(202) 272-5434 (Voice/TDD), (202) 272-5447 (FAX),
or 1-800-USA ABLE

For a copy of the Federal Register ADA provisions, call: U.S. Equal Employment Opportunities Commission *1-800-669-4000.*

The American Medical Association offers information about practice compliance with the ADA in their booklet Physician's Guide to ADA. *For information, call 1-800-621-8335.*

DON'T BE IGNORANT OF AIDS UNDERSTANDING

It's almost impossible to pick up a journal or newspaper without reading about AIDS research, treatment, and epidemiology. Nevertheless, societal ignorance and lack of understanding about the disease are all too common. Medical practices, even those that do not routinely treat AIDS patients, should be especially sensitive to the need for compassion, understanding, and knowledge not only for the benefit of patients but also to help educate others who have misinformation or inaccurate perceptions. Patient satisfaction increases when patients and family or friends see active, ongoing evidence of concern and compassion toward all groups and individuals, no matter what their background, beliefs, condition, or limitations. Contact a local AIDS support organization or hospice for more information about ways to enhance AIDS awareness and sensitivity in your practice.

HIDDEN DISABILITIES CAN AFFECT YOUR CARE

Some patients may have hidden disabilities that can affect their physical and emotional well-being and how you care for them. For example, posttraumatic stress disorder (PTSD) affects war veterans as well as victims of car accidents, natural disasters, and other traumatic events. Survivors and current victims of physical and sexual abuse have special needs that may go unrecognized if physicians and staff are not knowledgeable of and alert for symptoms and clues. Stress reactions and depression can be expressed in physical, emotional, behavioral, and cognitive ways, and people with these hidden disabilities have special communication as well as medical needs. You can provide both reassurance and appropriate treatment, but only if you search for, recognize, and understand the true problem. To meet the needs of these patients, you may need to probe deeper, in a sensitive, nonjudgmental manner, to uncover the medical and emotional issues hidden beneath the surface. Many local and national organizations offer information and training in identifying symptoms of PTSD, physical or sexual abuse, depression, and other hidden disabilities.

UNDERSTANDING ETHNIC, CULTURAL, AND PHYSICAL DIVERSITY

As nations exchange ideas, goods, and knowledge across borders, as medical science improves the life span through education about diet, fitness, and disease, and as diseases are eliminated and new ones are discovered, the diversity of people and problems encountered in society and in medicine will expand. Certainly some assimilation will take place, but it is human nature for people to cling to traditional behaviors and values, and in the case of age or physical impairment, some of the changes or differences cannot be changed. Society, including medical practices, physicians, staff, and others, must accommodate to these individuals with special needs to provide high-quality medical care and service.

The further a practice goes in understanding, adapting to, and meeting or exceeding the needs of these groups and individuals, the greater the level of satisfaction that is likely to be encountered by **all** the patients in the practice. When physicians and staff become attuned to the unique needs of certain groups or cultures and seek to address these needs, patients, family members, referral sources, vendors, and others spread the word that your practice is keenly customer sensitive and responsive to patients. What better image can a practice have and what more satisfying role could you and your staff play?

Action Steps for Meeting Special Needs

1. If you have a patient group with special requirements due to culture, ethnicity, age, or medical condition, make a sincere effort to learn about this group's values, beliefs, ideals, and heritage as well as these patients' specific medical conditions.
2. If you have a large number of patients of a particular ethnic origin, consider hiring one or more staffers of the same ethnic or cultural background.
3. Sensitize everyone in the practice to the diversity of your patient population through role playing, staff meeting discussions, and sensitivity exercises.
4. The hospital with which you are affiliated may offer programs on cultural diversity; if not, suggest them.
5. Contact national organizations for information about making your practice physically accessible and physicians and staff socially aware and compassionate to the needs of every patient group.

References

1. C.M. Solomon, A world of difference, *American Medical News* (November 9, 1992): 27–29.
2. L. Sharn, Accessibility means a whole new life, *USA Today* (January 24–26, 1992): 6A.

Appendix 31-A

Elderly Sensitivity Exercise

Supplies

- Spectacles
- Petroleum jelly
- Cane
- Walker
- Thick cotton gardening gloves
- Several elastic bandages
- Wooden rulers
- Cotton
- Childproof pill containers
- Multicolored candies to serve as "pills"

Procedure

1. Staff members should take turns playing the role of the elderly person. To simulate the physical limitations of age, the individual should wear the glasses, which have been smeared with petroleum jelly. Place cotton in both ears. Wrap bandages around hands, elbows, and knees, placing a ruler behind one knee to immobilize the joint. Wear the gloves, and walk with either the cane or the walker. Discuss the sensations and impairments noticed.
2. Ask the "elderly" staff member to go outside the office building and follow the routine a patient would, from the parking lot

into the practice. A staff member should accompany the patient from the reception area to the exam room, X-ray suite, lab, or other locations if that is normal procedure. By using the questions below as a checklist, evaluate how well the practice meets the needs of elderly, disabled, and other patients:

- Are there handrails on all staircases?
- Is the building easily accessible for cane, walker, and wheelchair users?
- Is the practice signage (exterior and door) visible, legible, and readable?
- Is the door to your office easy to open?
- Is there a clear path from the doorway to the reception desk?
- (Sit in a chair in the reception area.) Are there straight arms to help you get out of the chair? Is the chair firm and not overly plush?
- (Read a magazine.) Is the lighting adequate for easy reading? Does the lighting cause glare? Can the magazine print be easily read?
- (Fill out the patient information form.) Is the type large and easy to read?
- (Find the bathroom.) Is it well marked? Is it easy to get to? Does the door open without difficulty? Is there room for a walker or wheelchair? Are there grab bars? Is the sink low enough?
- (Get a drink from the fountain or coffee or tea from the refreshment cart, if available.) Are refreshments accessible but safely located? Is there a place to set cups while you wait in the reception area? Does the drinking fountain have a cup dispenser as an option?
- (Open the pill container.) Can you find the yellow (or red, or brown) "pill?"
- (Ask the receptionist a question.) Is there a seat nearby if you are weary or physically debilitated?
- As you walk back to the treatment area with a staff member, do you feel rushed, or does the staff member slow his or her pace to yours?
- Does the staff member shout at you to be heard, or does he or she use a slightly raised voice, looking directly at you to ensure understanding?

3. Note the following:
   - Does the reception desk or check-out counter have a place for patients to place personal belongings while scheduling a follow-up visit?
   - Are discussions about account balances or medical conditions conducted in a private location, rather than at the check-out or reception desk, where others may overhear?
   - Can all signs be easily read?
   - Are presurgery, postsurgery, and other educational materials readable by patients with poor vision?
   - Is there seating for patient companions in all exam and treatment areas?
   - Is the companion made to feel welcome?
4. When staff members have completed the simulation portion of this exercise, get together as a group and discuss changes that would enhance the experience and service that patients encounter in the practice. Develop an implementation plan with action steps and dates to complete the quality improvement process. It might be wise to hold a focus group of elderly patients in the practice to learn their perceptions and experiences and what changes they would recommend.
5. Communicate with your patients after making physical and service adjustments and improvements so that they are aware that you are interested in their needs and expectations. ❧

---------- ào ----------

32

Benchmarking: What You Can Learn from Others

"These people have been places I'll never go and done things I'll never do; they also have solutions to problems I haven't yet solved."

—Charles Attwood, MD

Benchmarking once was a technical term that meant a surveyor's reference point. In the quality-focused corporate world, it refers to adopting or adapting the best practices and strategies for a particular activity from other businesses and industries. Or, as quality guru Juran defines it, "setting goals based on knowing what has been achieved by others.[1(p.35)] He points out that benchmarking implies that the goal is attainable because it has already been achieved by others.

In the late 1970s and 1980s, a series of changes took place that dragged hospitals into the world of competition and commerce. With payments limited under DRGs and consumers exercising choices about where they would have surgery, babies, and other inpatient services, hospitals became more customer-focused. In the process, they discovered the practice of benchmarking. One of the first industries they looked to for customer-pleasing ideas was hospitality. From Marriott and other successful hotel chains they adapted the lobby concierge. In hospitals, the concierge became a knowledgeable staff member who could answer questions and guide visitors. Many hospitals also implemented valet parking, VIP suites, colorful decor in patient rooms, and special restaurant style dinners for new parents in the maternity units. Although these superficial touches generated favorable reactions, hospitals found that they needed to go further. Like hotels and restaurants, they implemented customer satisfaction surveys. They instituted "guest relations" programs for employees, a somewhat limited but significant step toward quality management.

COMPETITION CREATES CHALLENGES

This surge of hospital interest in the patient as customer occurred during a time when health care was at risk of becoming a commodity. Physicians faced growing and unfamiliar pressure from competition and declining reimbursement; in response, they frantically focused on administrative and cost issues, sometimes at the expense of patient satisfaction. Gradually, physicians and office managers in solo and group practices realized that patients were comparing them, sometimes unfavorably, with the restaurants, retail stores, auto dealers, and even other doctors and dentists they patronized.

Thus, following the example of hospitals, surgicenters, and other health care providers, medical practices began to try out some radical ideas—radical because heretofore it was rare for physicians to be very concerned about service or quality unless the terms preceded or followed the words *patient care*. *Quality* referred to medical care; *service* referred to the promptness with which recall cards were mailed or, occasionally, how the practice phone was answered.

But then came the widespread success of *In Search of Excellence* by Peters and Waterman in 1982, of *Service America!* by Karl Albrecht in 1985, and of *Marketing Strategies for Physicians* by Brown and Morley in 1986, which discussed the role of non–health care customer satisfaction strategies in medical practice. These books heralded, or accompanied, heightened consumerism and a more educated and demanding public. Many physicians and office managers took a page from these books and listened more carefully to their sometimes impatient patients. They heard their customers say things such as this:

- "We *hate* waiting."
- "Why does your office have to look like a government waiting room, complete with dog-eared magazines from 6 months ago?"
- "We want to know more about our conditions and treatment plans."
- "We're customers, even if we don't pay the bill ourselves."
- "Why can't you run your office like a business but still treat us like human beings instead of 'cases?'"
- "Why don't you and your staff get together and agree on things? We hear one thing from you and something entirely different from your nurse or receptionist or office manager."

PERSONAL SERVICE IS CUSTOMER SATISFYING

Your patients have become more vocal about their needs and concerns because **other** businesses have begun listening when customers complain. And customers like it. They like the personal attention they get from the salesclerk at Nordstrom, from the service advisor at the Saturn dealership, from the Wal-Mart "greeter," and from the friendly waitress at the coffee shop around the corner, who knew long before the advent of total quality management that paying attention to her customers paid off in bigger tips as well as a more enjoyable work day.

Customers—your patients—have learned that they don't have to take poor service. Their expectations have escalated as service standards have risen (unfortunately not uniformly—there's still plenty of poor service available in the retail world), and they bring these rising expectations into your office.

Mindful of what's taking place in the service world, what can you learn from other medical practices, from the businesses you and your patients deal with every day, and even from the corporations you read about in *Fortune, Forbes,* and the *Wall Street Journal*? Plenty. For starters, here are a few things done by non–health care businesses that you might adapt in your practice.

PRACTICE "MANAGEMENT BY WALKING AROUND"

We've mentioned it in previous chapters, citing "management by walking around" as a leadership trait, but it bears repeating. Internist Richard Abrams, MD, knows the value of strolling through the group practice in which he's a partner, talking to his staff, and especially noticing the good things they're doing: "People want to know that what they do has value." "Management by walking around" is a concept practiced by many big businesses and retailers, from Wal-Mart to American Express, where executives may spend a day at the computer keying in applications to learn what clerical workers confront. Get around in your practice. Listen. Watch. Learn. It's the best way to pay attention to the little things that affect patient satisfaction, things you might not notice or hear of otherwise. When you notice poor quality or poor service, don't walk on; do something about it. When you see good service or extra effort by an employee, say so. Recognizing it reinforces and perpetuates quality service.

HIRE SMART, SHARP, FRIENDLY PEOPLE

Hire people who are just a little smarter, friendlier, and more professional. Expect the best from the top employees you've hired and trained, and reward them with praise and recognition and better pay than they can get elsewhere. It works for Marriott; it works for Dr. Stephen Hales, the pediatrician; it can work for you. When you go to medical conferences, talk to your colleagues from other locations and learn their "success secrets." Consider bringing your office manager or practice administrator to these major meetings. Most have sessions for administrative staff, and they will learn a lot that can benefit your practice by meeting with their peers. Look at what other businesses do. Many have profit-sharing plans; why not offer a bonus plan so that your staff share in the financial rewards when your practice thrives as a result of their good work?

STAY IN TOUCH WITH YOUR CUSTOMERS

Many practices have already learned the value of surveying patients and referral sources. Don't forget your first-line customers as well: your employees. Ask for their opinions and ideas. They know your patients as well as (or better than, in many cases) you do. Listen to all your customers. The idea for Wal-Mart's "people-greeter," who welcomes every customer, was suggested by a $5-an-hour sales associate. If staff members know their ideas and concerns will get a hearing, they're more likely to look for solutions.

BECOME FANATIC ABOUT SERVICE

Nordstrom, the Seattle, Washington–based department store, will go to any length to accommodate a customer's needs. Nordstrom knows that customer loyalty stems from its service orientation. When you experience service fanaticism in your daily life, whether at the dry cleaners, the supermarket, or your bank, pay attention to what happens, how, why, and who provides it. Tell the story of your experience to your staff. It emphasizes to them that you take service seriously, and it shows what a strong impact service extras can have. Your patient loyalty will flourish if patients sense a strong, sincere, and **personalized** service attitude on the part of everyone in the practice.

EDUCATE AND ORIENT YOUR STAFF

Orient your employees to new services, new equipment, and new concepts. Every major corporation has an employee orientation program as well as ongoing in-services. Companies such as IBM and Ritz-Carlton® understand that knowledgeable employees perform better. Make sure your staff know your practice, your services, and your expertise. When you return from a national conference or CME program or when you start performing a new test or procedure, review what you've learned with your staff and point out the significance of this information to patients. When you purchase new equipment, in-service those who will be using it, but also make certain that **everyone** in the office understands how the equipment benefits the practice **and** patients.

FOLLOW OTHER INDUSTRIES AND BUSINESSES

Familiarize yourself with what other industries are doing to improve customer service and to increase satisfaction by reading about them. Publications such as *Fortune, Forbes, Business Week, Inc.,* and *USA Today* and business best-sellers are full of the latest service trends as well as time-tested techniques for satisfying customers and improving business productivity and efficiency. Read, share, and use information in books and articles that may be applicable to your practice.

A SYSTEMATIC APPROACH TO BENCHMARKING

These are just a few concepts that health care can (and has) adopted from non–health care industries. There are plenty of others. Just ask pediatrician Charles Attwood, MD, of Crowley, Louisiana. Not only does he understand benchmarking, he has systematized it. He keeps a computer file of "advisors"—several hundred medical and nonmedical experts from a cross-section of industries. "These people have been places I'll never go and done things I'll never do; they also have solutions to problems I haven't yet solved," he says.[2(p.35)]

"Doctors need to understand how to use benchmarking concepts," Dr. Attwood insists. "Unfortunately, too many of them don't even know what the term means. We need to find the best of every industry and use it." He has benefitted from his "advisors" in a number of ways, most of them in patient relations. For example, he met a restaurant owner who cooked specially requested dishes for good customers no matter how busy he and the staff were. The restaurateur's reason? "These customers may spend over $50,000 in a lifetime here." Dr. Attwood heeded the lesson: He makes a special effort to retain pediatric patients from birth to college-age and beyond by learning what they or their parents want and expect in sickness and in health.

A hotel manager taught him that special requests should never be declined, that problems should be quickly fixed, and that service extras are always a good idea. So lower-income patients in Attwood's practice who have transportation problems have their taxi fare paid. Patients who ask to use the phone in the office are handed a cordless phone, an idea he picked up from the restaurant owner.

Attwood's practice FAX, once reserved for receiving lab reports and hospital records, is now used to send drug and office supply orders to the supplier, thus saving staff time, mistakes, and inventory. That idea came from a cafeteria manager. An attorney came up with the time-saving suggestion that Attwood make hospital rounds only once a day at noon instead of morning and evening, as he had been doing.

THIS PHYSICIAN'S NETWORK WORKS!

Dr. Attwood's network includes automobile dealers, college professors, retailers, computer programmers, and even an IRS agent who audited his tax return one year. He says, "My advisers may not know clinical medicine, but they are experts in meeting and exceeding customer expectations. I pick their brains, usually on the phone, sometimes at conferences and seminars. Occasionally I'll take one out to lunch. Hiring them is out of the question, but when they need medical advice, I'm their man."[3(p.35)]

Benchmarking is an effective tool for service quality improvement because the "reference points" are everywhere. Walk into any Gap store and you'll be assaulted with ideas any practice could adapt. For example, the first thing that happens when you walk in the door is a friendly greeting from a good-natured salesperson, who may ask, "What do you think of our new colors?" instead of the more typical and impersonal "May I help you?" This prompts a real response from the customer instead of "No thanks, I'm just looking."

What service strategies can you take away from a business like the Gap? For starters, just the greeting itself. Despite the emphasis on customer orientation, there are still too many medical practices with the Plexiglass window insulating the receptionist from patients. And if any greeting occurs, it's a quick sliding of the window just long enough for the receptionist to glance at the confidentiality-violating clipboard on which the patient has just signed in followed by, "Have you changed address, employers, insurance? Have a seat." And the window slides back. The Sansum Clinic in Santa Barbara, California, like many of the practices we visited, understands the value of a personal greeting. Their "hospitality hostess" is the first person you see, and talk to, when you enter the lobby (they *don't* call it a waiting room).

At the Gap, Nordstrom, and other service-focused businesses, employees know their product and show it with service. Ask a question about stone-washed jeans, cotton polo shirts, or support pantyhose in taupe, and the service personnel at these stores can answer your questions. On the rare occasions that they can't, they'll find an answer for you. Quickly. Are **your** staff members familiar with all the services you provide and your patient care philosophy? Can they answer patient questions about what laboratory you use, how often you recommend mammograms for women over 35, at which hospitals you have privileges, when you make return phone calls, or your stance on the excimer laser?

THERE ARE IDEAS EVERYWHERE

Plastic surgeons were among the first physicians to look beyond health care for service ideas. Their patients may have imposed this attitude on the specialty: plastic surgery patients tend to look upon themselves as customers rather than patients because most pay the bill themselves. Some of the retail ideas that started in plastic surgery practices have caught hold and spread to ophthalmology, obstetrics and gynecology, and even urology. Refreshment corners stocked with everything from coffee and cookies to frozen yogurt and juice have been successfully adopted (and enjoyed by appreciative patients). In-office surgery patients are offered headphones and their choice of music, from jazz to classical, to divert their attention from the procedure. Offices and exam rooms are more homelike in appearance, with soothing colors and non-clinical artwork and reading material. Vans and limos provide convenient transportation for same-day surgery patients.

Some surgeons and physicians, however, may have gotten carried away by the surplus of marble and expensive furnishings they encounter in exclusive resort lobbies. The result is benchmarking excess. One patient recalled the contrast between the practice ambience of his internist, whose X-ray room doubled as a storage area, and another physician to whom he was referred whose office was in a posh, high-rent location with ornate and overdone furnishings. Although the first physician was very competent, "Having an X-ray amid boxes of copy paper and bathroom products was not a confidence builder," the patient admitted.

NORDSTROM: A MODEL FOR THIS PHYSICIAN'S PRACTICE

Sometimes health care can learn from the overall attitude found in other businesses. Susan Northrup, MD, recalls that when she and her partner were setting up their practice, A Woman's Place for Health Care, in Scottsdale, Arizona, "We went to Nordstrom in California. We both were impressed with the quality of service we encountered, and agreed that this was the model for our practice."

Similarly, the Heart Center uses concepts from organizations such as Disney, from whom the practice picked up the "74 and 1 rule." (The rule says that each Disney customer averages 74 interactions or "moments of truth." Employees are trained and counseled to make sure that each of these interactions or customer contacts with the organization is positive.) "We emphasize with our staff all of the opportunities our patients have during their visit, and how one bad interaction can mess up their perception of the practice," says Alan Kaplan, MD, Heart Center cardiologist.

For radiologist Lawrence Cohen, MD, benchmarking comes naturally. His family background is in retailing, which gives him a "basic instinct for sales and marketing." He says that in the family business, his father treated clientele "like family," so that many have been customers for 30 years. Cohen grew up believing that "the customer is always right, no matter what," a doctrine he carries out at the Washington Imaging Center, the 14-physician practice to which he belongs.

It may be his familiarity with the retail field that drives Cohen's insistence on personalizing the traditionally high-tech, no-touch specialty of radiology. He pointed out that many radiologists often have little or no direct contact with patients; thus patients tend to view their encounter as "faceless and cold." To counteract this perception, Cohen attempts to greet his patients when they arrive; if this isn't possible, he consults with them after the procedure. He believes that this personal approach builds repeat business, and he's right. Terri Goren, marketing director in the practice says, "When his patients return for even a very brief procedure, they always ask for Dr. Cohen and they're very disappointed if they don't get to say hello to him." You can bet these satisfied patients communicate their pleasure to referring physicians.

PAY ATTENTION TO SERVICE EXPERIENCES WHEREVER YOU ARE

Benchmarking can enhance **your** pleasure in medicine. Try it. Pay attention to service experiences when you travel, dine, or shop. Read magazines you ordinarily don't read. Encourage staff members to bring up ideas and encounters from outside health care. Subscribe to the CASE principle (Copy And Steal Everything). Benchmarking is a quality strategy for improving service and patient satisfaction while widening the horizons of everyone in the practice. ✿

Action Steps for Benchmarking Success

1. Pay attention to other industries, and learn from the customer-sensitive and service-oriented things they do.
2. Talk to physicians in your own and other specialties to learn their service and success secrets; adopt or adapt the best ideas to your practice.
3. Solicit your employees for ideas. They hear patient comments and complaints and can be a storehouse of suggestions for improving service.
4. Develop a network of experts in other industries with whom you can trade information and ideas.
5. Read the *Wall Street Journal, Fortune, Business Week,* and other business publications and best-sellers as well as the *Journal of the American Medical Association, Medical Tribune,* and the *New England Journal of Medicine.*
6. Remember that your patients compare the service experiences they have in other physicians' offices and other businesses. Don't permit their experience in your office to fall short on service.

References

1. J.M. Juran, *Juran on Quality by Design: The New Steps for Planning Quality into Goods and Services* (New York, N.Y.: The Free Press, 1992): 35.
2. C. Attwood, For practice tips, solicit an informal network of advisers, *American Medical News* (August 10, 1992): 35.
3. C. Attwood, For practice tips, 35.

Part 5

Final Thoughts and Comments

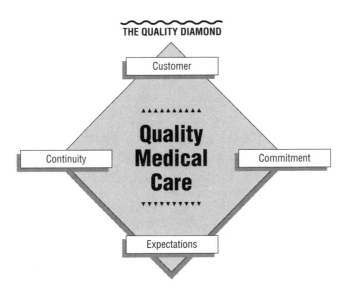

You're on the home stretch. We have just a final few thoughts and ideas on patient satisfaction and quality service. But think of this as the beginning rather than the end, because meeting the needs of your patients, as you know now, is a day-to-day, moment-to-moment process. You provide quality care with your medical expertise and technique, but it's borne on attentive, personal interaction. Ensuring satisfied patients is the role and responsibility of everyone in the practice, and the rewards of practice success belong to everyone who participates: patients, staff, and physicians.

33

A Round-Up of Thoughts and Suggestions for Quality Service

---

*"What are we gonna do with all this **stuff?** We have too much information. Too many good ideas! What are we going to leave out?"*

This was the dilemma we faced as we sorted through the interviews and research we compiled for *Patient Satisfaction Pays.* We had done our homework too well. We had far too much to be able to use it all. What to eliminate?

In the end, we eliminated a great deal: strategies and suggestions that were routine or not applicable to a broad number of physicians and practices, and techniques that were more sales than patient satisfaction. But we still had a great many good ideas and powerful points left. And we didn't want to leave them out. Instead, we decided to wrap up what was left in a "round-up" chapter. So that's what you have here: a treasure chest of tips that may work for your practice, nuggets that may nurture change, and tales to get you and your staff thinking—and acting.

But we want to start out by once again emphasizing a point we and other physicians have made throughout this book: Quality service and patient satisfaction are worth the effort. You'll see the payoff in the practice bottom line and professional satisfaction. But they begin and end with your belief and your commitment. A continuing, visible commitment is the only way to achieve service that consistently satisfies and frequently surpasses expectations. What we're saying is that you must know what you believe. Sound simple? Perhaps, but in far too many practices the employees (and sometimes the physicians) can give no specific, consensus response to the question, "What are you here for?"

If a practice team is to provide quality service, strive to exceed expectations, and give quality medical care, they must agree and sincerely believe that the patient comes first. And this belief must be shared by everyone in the practice: the bookkeeper, billing clerk, medical assistant, physician's assistant, nurse, technician, part-time janitor, patient education coordinator, receptionist, and of course the physicians.

WAL-MART SUCCESS WORTH A SECOND LOOK

Some time ago, one of us wrote a column for *American Medical News* about lessons physicians can learn from companies such as Wal-Mart. The point of the article was that the principles that Sam Walton used to create "the darling of Wall Street" apply to medical practices as well. These principles are scattered throughout this book. They include management by walking around; hiring the best and then training, listening to, and rewarding them; listening to your customers; being obsessed with service; and practicing top-down management (e.g, leadership by example).

In his book *Made in America*, Sam Walton offered 10 rules for success. We think that, once again, Sam makes sense for physicians. Walton's rules are given on the next page.

Sam Walton's Rules for Success

1. Commit to your business (see Chapter 6 for details).
2. Share your profits with your "associates"—your staff. Treat them as partners, and they will reflect your values (see Chapter 8).
3. Motivate your employees—your practice partners. Keep them challenged not just with money but with new responsibilities and new ways to achieve objectives (see Chapters 11 and 28).
4. Communicate everything you possibly can to your team.
5. Appreciate everything your team does for the business. Say "thank you" often.
6. Celebrate your successes. Take time for fun.
7. Listen to everyone in your company. Get people talking about what's going on out there and how to do it better. This is what total quality is all about.
8. Exceed your customers' expectations (see Chapters 13 and 14 if you've forgotten how or why).
9. Control your expenses better than your competition, or at least as well as they do. With RBRVS for Medicare reimbursement, managed care, and increased government, third party, and employer regulation and intervention, you can't afford not to.
10. Swim upstream. Ignore the conventional wisdom. Do things your way.

Source: From *Sam Walton: Made in America* by Sam Walton. Copyright © 1992 by Estate of Samuel Moore Walton. Used by permission of Doubleday, a division of Bantam Doubleday Dell Publishing Group, Inc.

We encountered plenty of physicians and practices with a unique style in everything from scheduling and billing to their interaction with patients. There's no one perfect way to practice medicine, except to concentrate on providing the best quality of medical care and service. What works for you and exceeds patient expectations is the best way.[1]

One Physician's Quality Prescription

Timothy Cavanaugh, MD, of the Hunkeler Eye Clinic, says he believes that quality service has four elements. We like the way he packaged it neatly. These are Dr. Cavanaugh's "Big Four for Service":

1. **Staff interaction:** How staff respond to and interact with patients has a strong impact on how patients perceive the physician and practice. For example, when a patient is told, "I don't know" by an employee in response to a question, there's a very strong message. In contrast, consider the message that accompanies this response, "I don't know, but I'll find out for you."

2. **Waiting time:** "It **is** a big deal," Cavanaugh recognizes. "Patients are consumers; they expect the same quality of service they encounter in non–health care encounters."

3. **Communication:** It's a must between physician and patient. And when communication includes education about a condition or procedure, you get better results: more compliant patients and better surgical candidates.

4. **Quality of medicine:** Surgical, diagnostic, and treatment ability have to enter the picture, even though patients can't fully evaluate technical and clinical components. The burden is on the physician to hone his or her skills and continually upgrade his or her knowledge.

ATTENTION TO DETAIL COUNTS

What impressed us about the practices we visited? Attention to detail. Communication and smiles. Lots of them. Wherever we went in these extremely busy practices, people were courteous, friendly, and helpful. We had the sense that employees in these customer-sensitive practices enjoyed their work. Moreover, we felt that they truly wanted to ensure a positive experience for all their customers: patients, visitors, family members, and each other. We were also struck by the strong sense of professional satisfaction and fulfillment among the physicians in practices with a patient-satisfaction focus. For example, Carol Gilmore, MD, of Denver, Colorado ticked off an assortment of frustrations she has encountered in building her practice: reimbursement, managed care limitations, clinically superb referral physicians with lousy bedside manners, and a desire to do more but not enough time or money with which to do it. She concluded by saying, "I'm not where I want to be at this point in my life. But on a scale of 1 to 10, I rate my satisfaction a 10."

Other details we noticed: Orthopedic surgeon Saul Schreiber's reception area is furnished with upholstered straight-back chairs with ottomans. He specializes in knees. Obviously he's thought about his patients' comfort. His reception area also has a large, circular sculpture. It revolves to depict a colorful underwater scene that changes constantly, soothing and captivating waiting patients (who don't wait long, as we pointed out in Chapter 21. He monitors waiting time carefully). The rest of his office has the same attention to detail. The X-ray room has a huge map of the world covering one wall, so that patients have something interesting to look at during a procedure. Exam rooms were designed with built-in corner seating to allow family members accompanying patients to observe but not interfere with the exam. There are no sticky notes, memos, or scrawled messages taped to walls anywhere in the practice. Bulletin boards are neat and current. Information is sorted, filed, or posted for quick but not messy access. We asked a staff member how they maintain such a neat appearance. She seemed bewildered by the question: "We just do. It's the way we do things."

DISTINCTIVE STYLES WORK, TOO

Dr. Hales does everything in his practice: Work-ups. Complete exams. Return phone calls to patients. He estimates that he talks to 60 to 80 patients a day on the phone. "Telephone contact forms part of the relationship I have with patients," he says. He doesn't do "protect the doc," believing that people are turned off when they have to jump over the hurdles of receptionist, nurse, and others. It's his unique style of practice, and it works for him. He says that the traditional pediatric practice style is not his way: "You come in and the child is screaming because they don't like being stripped and they don't like being on the exam table. You either write a prescription or scribble in their chart, then leave the chart outside the door, the nurse comes in and gives the shot to the screaming child. It's efficient. I hate it." Instead, he comes in with the loaded syringe in his pocket, puts the child on his lap, and quickly does the injection. No screaming. "I slip a Band-Aid™ on and give them their sticker."

IN-DEPTH STAFF AWARENESS

A four-physician ophthalmology practice in Philadelphia requires all staff—front and back office—to watch a cataract surgery video to help them understand the technical expertise required of the surgeons. According to the office manager, without this knowledge there's a tendency for staff to regard the ophthalmologists as "quality control inspectors of the eyes." We think that this is a good idea but would recommend that surgical practices allow or encourage practice staff members to observe an actual surgery rather than a video. The real-life experience is far more dramatic and impressive than watching a video (which usually leaves out the preparation and teamwork required to accomplish the surgery).

STAFF EDUCATION RITZ-STYLE

Practices that are patient centered understand that an educated, informed staff give better care and better service. This commitment to education and training is also prevalent in America's most respected service companies. Employees of the Ritz-Carlton Hotel Company, for example, go through an average of 126 hours of training each year. The practices we visited make a significant commitment to staff development with monthly educational programs on clinical as well as personal growth topics. The Heart Center encourages (and pays for) appropriate seminars, courses, and educational programs for staff. Each employee has an individualized plan for growth and development that is based on his or her goals as well as opportunities and plans by the practice management and leadership that affect him or her. They hold noon in-services for clinical staff, taught by a physician in the practice, and invite clinical staff from other practices to attend.

Ray Hughes, MD, a family practitioner in Phoenix, Arizona, has a unique continuing education program for his staff. Each Friday afternoon the staff (all of whom are cross-trained in administrative as well as basic clinical tasks) are tested on clinical terms, symptoms, and diagnostic tests. Employees are told in advance the topics and page numbers in the reference manual from which the test is taken. Each correct answer earns at least $1; a recent test had a potential $47 bonus per employee. According to Dr. Hughes' office manager, the weekly test is a very effective incentive to encourage staff members to study and be well informed. A set of typical test questions for Dr. Hughes' staff is seen in Exhibit 33-1.

Dr. Hughes is described by a staff member as "a great boss." His patients might give similar glowing reviews. Dr. Hughes sponsors a free musical recital during the holidays for his patients and guests. Featured performer: Dr. Hughes himself, who has a degree in voice and piano. He's offered classical and ragtime performances to audiences of more than 600 for the past 7 years. "It's a token of appreciation for my patients' support," Dr. Hughes says.

THE VALUE OF COMMUNICATION

Quality-oriented practices understand the value of communication. They communicate up, down, and across all lines and segments of the practice. They hold regular staff meetings, department meetings, and unit meetings. Physicians and staff meet together and separately. They talk formally and informally. Casual hallway meetings and formal weekend retreats are typical. They emphasize quality by reviewing and praising incidents that were handled well and by discussing those that were not (then they figure out what they should do next time). They bring in speakers from other industries and businesses to import the quality message. They compliment each other when things go right and help each other out when times are tough. As one practice administrator said, "We try to recognize the Disney concept of interdependence—that everyone's day depends on everyone else."

These practices not only communicate but have fun and celebrate together. High-quality practices often are places where stress sometimes reaches outrageous levels; these practices de-stress with laughter. They understand that humor distracts and provides a new perspective. Tom Peters (co-author of *In Search of Excellence)* advocates frequent celebrations, plenty of little events as well as big blow-outs,

Exhibit 33-1 Dr. Ray Hughes' Clinical Test for Staff

Dr. Ray Hughes gives a simple clinical test to his staff each week similar to the one below. Each correct response is worth $1 per point.

Sample Test

Define "renal tubular acidosis"—Page 1626	1 Point
Define "renal glycosuria"—Page 1627	1 Point
Define "nephrogenic diabetes insipidus—Page 1628	1 Point
Define "polycystic renal diseases"—Page 1630	1 Point
Define "hydronephrosis"—Page 1633	1 Point
Define "BPH"—Page 1635	1 Point
Define "neurogenic bladder"—Page 1637	1 Point
Define "urinary incontinence"—Page 1639	1 Point
Describe the probable signs and symptoms of urinary calculi. pt—Page 1641	1 Point
What is the usual treatment for kidney stone?—Page 1642	2 Points
What are the usual symptoms and signs of carcinoma of the kidney?—Page 1648	2 Points
What are the usual symptoms and signs of bladder CA?—Page 1649	2 Points
What are the usual symptoms and signs of prostatic cancer?—Page 1650	2 Points
What are the primary diagnostic tests and procedures needed for diagnosing prostatic CA?—Page 1650	2 Points
What are the usual symptoms and signs of testicular cancer?—Page 1651	2 Points
What are the signs and symptoms of advanced hydronephrosis?—Page 1634	2 Points
What are the usual signs and symptoms of BPH?—Page 1636	2 Points
5 Point Bonus Question: What is "paradoxical incontinence?"—Page 1640	5 Points

Source: Courtesy of Ray Hughes, MD, Phoenix, Arizona.

semispontaneous events (planned into the calendar but fresh and new), and lots of variety. Celebrate small attempts as well as big successes, Peters says; it's important to acknowledge when someone tries, even if he or she doesn't succeed at first. Celebrating keeps the service and quality momentum going, he believes. Most of all, he counsels (and we concur), that the "top dogs" must participate with the rest of the team.[2]

COMPACT MEETING FORMAT ENHANCES COMMUNICATION

We came across a communication forum that has merit for any organization. We call it the Speak-Up/Follow-Up meeting. It lasts 10 to 20 minutes maximum and is held every 2 to 4 weeks in every department for a large practice or practicewide for a small practice. The purpose of the meeting is to resolve problems, build morale, establish trust, quell rumors, provide quick in-service, and generate ideas. In other words, to communicate. Led by a strong facilitator, the meeting includes brief statements of needs, information, problem situations, or questions. Each statement or question is followed by a desired action, agreement about the person(s) responsible for the action, and an assigned completion or follow-up date. Minutes are kept and reviewed quickly at the end of the meeting so that there's group consensus on the statements, actions, and responsibilities. A copy of the minutes goes to each department as well as individuals responsible for action. It's an effective approach for a practice that claims, "We don't have time for meetings."

THERE'S NO COOKIE CUTTER FOR QUALITY

Do you get the impression that you don't create patient satisfaction and quality service by using a cookie cutter? You're right. Every practice and every physician has a unique style, and you can maintain that style **if** you've first determined that it does not undermine your ability to provide excellent medical care and superior service and to exceed patient expectations. ✄

References

1. S. Walton with J. Huey, *Made in America* (New York, N.Y.: Doubleday, 1992): 245–249.
2. P. Cohen, ed. Hard work/hard play makes Chiat/Day/Mojo a dull place—not! *On Achieving Excellence* 7, no. 9 (1992): 2–4.

34

Take the First Step to Practice Success

We originally planned to call this chapter **"This Won't Hurt a Bit."** It was going to focus on the future.

But we changed our plan. The future of medicine is too unpredictable for us to say it won't hurt. No matter what happens to health care in the next decade, it's likely to be somewhat painful for everyone: patients, payers, employers, and physicians.

It will be painful in the sense that change is *always* painful. And although no one can predict with certainty what the future will bring, it's fairly safe to assume that the transformations witnessed in the past decade are only the beginning of change. Despite these uncertainties, we feel confident about this prediction: Satisfying patients will be the hallmark of successful medical practices and professionally fulfilled physicians through the next century. It's the one stable characteristic of medicine: Good physicians care for their patients by caring for their patients (yes, we know that Sir William Osler said it first). A continuing drive to achieve patient satisfaction will be the constant in the turbulence of the medical delivery system.

In successful practices, however, patient satisfaction won't be constant; it will be continually escalating because the quality of service that these practices offer will continually improve. It's how successful practices get that way. They aren't satisfied with how good they are today; they're always looking for ways to get better. Successful physicians listen to their patients. They talk to their colleagues. They pay attention to what's going on in the world around them. They anticipate trends rather than try to catch up with them.

WATCH FOR THESE TRENDS

What are the trends you should be anticipating? What are the trends that will influence your practice in the coming years? What are the **realities** that may be affecting your practice now? Here's what you can expect:

- The continued growth and influence of managed care
- Increased influence by employers and patients on managed care
- Group practice as the predominant form of practice
- The continued explosion of technology—medical technology as well as information technology—available to physicians and consumers
- Government regulations that increasingly limit payment for medical coverage and potentially restrict types and levels of care
- Continued adaptation by state and private payers of governmental approaches to reimbursement
- Changing demographics and psychographics of society with the aging of the Baby Boom generation, the burgeoning number of elderly people, and increased multicultural diversity.

Each of these trends will affect how medical services are developed, delivered, and assessed. They will influence how you practice medicine and how patients find providers and pay for their services. Through all these changes, consumers will continue to expect quality service and treatment. In fact, as you've seen, those consumers—your patients—will expect better quality service and treatment than any previous generation (that's a trend that's already reality in most practices).

How you respond to these changes will determine not only how successful you will be financially but how satisfied you will be in your chosen profession. There were times during our interviews when physicians expressed disillusionment with the "business of medicine." Time after time, they told us that treating patients is still rewarding but that the regulations, restrictions, documentation, and paperwork are draining some of the pleasure out of medicine.

It is our sincere belief that, by centering your practice around your patients, you will renew the satisfaction and fulfillment that compelled you to choose medicine as a profession. By viewing your patients as customers and caring about them as people, you center your own life professionally and personally.

When we were discussing this patient-centered philosophy—used by all the successful physicians and practices in this book—a physician still groping with what patient satisfaction is and how to measure it said, "But every patient is different! You can never be sure of what someone wants." Essentially what he was looking for was a "one-size-fits-all" formula for satisfying patients.

CUSTOMIZED PATIENT SATISFACTION SCORES BEST

Is there a one-size-fits-all approach to patient satisfaction? By now, you know the answer. You satisfy your patients one by one, moment by moment. As you know by now, you must step into your patient's shoes and walk through your practice, seeing through your patient's eyes and hearing with your patient's ears.

You must adopt your patient's perspective because what you may consider a satisfactory or successful outcome may not be how your patient perceives it (it's that perceptual gap you learned about in Chapter 3). You know what a serious impact it can have when you and your patient don't see eye to eye. You know by now that patient satisfaction affects not only how he or she evaluates you and the care you've given them, but also his or her compliance and even outcome. You know that your staff are important in this picture because patients judge you by your staff, and sometimes they'll even stick with a physician **because** of the staff.

TIME FOR A TEST!

Now that you know all this, you qualify as an expert—a Certified Patient-Satisfying Physician (that's a CPSP if you're into lots of letters after your name). So perhaps you're ready to take your

"Patient Satisfaction Certification" Examination. We've made it easy: no essay questions. You might even call it an open-book test. For this test, you need to evaluate your practice just as your patients would. The answers are in your practice.

Take a few minutes to answer the following questions. Be truthful. You're the only one who has to see your answers, and there are no grades given (other than your patients' evaluations). How you answer this quick quiz may help you focus on where you want to go with your practice when you have turned the final page of this book.

1. **Do you want your practice to be focused on customer satisfaction and driven by quality service?**
   ❏ Yes, definitely.
   ❏ Things are fine the way they are.
   ❏ I **am** quality.
   ❏ It sounds like a good idea. Someday, when I have the time . . .
2. **Do you know your patients' expectations?**
   ❏ Yes   ❏ No
   ❏ I know what quality medical care is. That's what counts.
3. **Is your staff a source of information about patient expectations?**
   ❏ Yes   ❏ No
   ❏ Their job is to keep things running, not to chit-chat with the patients.
4. **Is there a concise, written statement of your practice mission or service quality strategy that's shared by everyone in the practice?**
   ❏ Yes   ❏ No
   ❏ I'm working on it.
5. **Does every staff member understand your practice service strategy and his or her role in carrying it out?**
   ❏ Yes   ❏ No
   ❏ Their job descriptions spell out their tasks.
6. **Do you have a system for measuring how well you are meeting the needs of your patients?**
   ❏ Yes   ❏ No
7. **Do you have a system for determining how well you meet the needs of other physicians and health professionals who refer patients to you?**

❑ Yes ❑ No
❑ Why do I need one?

8. **Are your employees recruited for their people skills as well as their technical skills?**
   ❑ Yes ❑ No

9. **Does your staff have the *authority* as well as the responsibility to meet the needs of your patients?**
   ❑ Yes ❑ No

10. **Overall, how patient centered and quality service oriented would you say your practice is today?**
    ❑ We have a perfect system, a model of excellence in action.
    ❑ We're getting there, moment by moment.
    ❑ Someday, when we have time, we'll work on it.

If you answered "yes" to the first question, then your answers to the next nine questions will help you understand your weaknesses and opportunities. For every answer that wasn't affirmative in questions two through nine, you need to work at developing systems and processes to attain these fundamental elements of a patient-focused, service-oriented practice. In the preceding chapters we've given you the basics for accomplishing these tasks. In truth, your colleagues across North America gave you the techniques for achieving patient satisfaction. We simply organized their ideas.

The last question is really a trick question. Even if you answered "yes" to each of the previous nine questions, the right answer is, "We're getting there." Practices that are far above the norm in delivering quality care and patient-centered service are never satisfied. Quality and service excellence represent a moving target. Think back to Chapter 28, where we said that the better you are, the better you must be because as the level of quality in your practice soars so, too, do the expectations of your patients. No system is perfect, at least not in this universe.

To maintain quality, you must keep moving, continually improving. So don't let your reading stop here. There are numerous journals, newsletters, books, videotapes, and seminars on service, quality, and other topics that will help you reach your destination of practice success. Although few publications currently available are focused on health care, the principles of quality and service are easily transferred from one industry to the next, as you learned in Chapter 32 (and if predicted trends prevail, you can expect an explosion of publications and books specific to service quality in health care in the coming years).

You've taken the first step of the quality journey by completing this book. In doing so, you've earned your CPSP designation (or CPSMD if you like **lots** of letters after your name). Our goal was to give you an overview of customer satisfaction and quality service concepts as well as to introduce you to the techniques and tactics other physicians are using and succeeding with. We sincerely hope that you will consider investing in a one-way ticket—because once you begin the journey to quality service and practice success, you will never want to turn back. ❧

Index

—— ?♠ ——

About the Authors

Stephen W. Brown, PhD, is an internationally recognized authority on services marketing and a past president of the 50,000-member American Marketing Association. A prolific author, he has written more than a hundred articles in professional journals and 11 books. He is co-author of *Marketing Strategies for Physicians: A Guide to Practice Growth,* a reference text which was among the first on the topic of physician marketing, and the book *Promoting Your Medical Practice: Marketing Communications for Physicians.* He is a lead editor of the first multinational book on service quality, *Service Quality: Multidisciplinary and Multinational Perspectives* and co-edits the annual series, *Advances in Services Marketing and Management.*

He is professor of marketing and executive director of the First Interstate Center for Services Marketing at Arizona State University, as well as senior advisor to The HSM Group, Ltd., a Scottsdale, Arizona health care consulting firm. In 1988, he was awarded the Academy for Health Services Marketing's coveted Philip Kotler Award. Dr. Brown obtained his doctoral degree in marketing from Arizona State University.

* * *

Anne-Marie Nelson is vice president of The HSM Group. During more than 20 years in the fields of public relations, marketing, and internal communications, she has held positions as hospital public relations director, marketing director for the Arizona operations of a national long-term care chain, and communications director for a dental group. A frequently published writer and a columnist for the *American Medical News,* she was editor of the HSM text, *Promoting Your Medical Practice: Marketing Communications for Physicians.*

An accredited business communicator, she has a bachelor of arts degree in journalism from Northern Arizona University in Flagstaff.

* * *

Steven D. Wood, PhD, has been an active researcher, educator, and consultant in services marketing industries for more than 20 years. He has published in excess of 70 papers in professional journals and texts and given over 150 presentations to various organizations. He is co-author of the text, *Promoting Your Medical Practice: Marketing Communications for Physicians.*

Dr. Wood obtained his master's degree in business, with mathematics minors, from San Diego State University, and a doctoral degree from the University of Wisconsin-Madison in quantitative business analysis, with minors in strategy and computer science. In addition to being vice chairman of The HSM Group, he is professor of Decision Information Systems and former dean of graduate programs in the College of Business at Arizona State University.

* * *

Sheryl J. Bronkesh, MBA, is president of The HSM Group. Ms. Bronkesh has headed public relations and marketing departments for a 700-bed teaching hospital, a community hospital, and a major multihospital system. In addition to her management and consulting activities, Ms. Bronkesh shares authorship of the resource text, *Promoting Your Medical Practice: Marketing Communications for Physicians.* She has authored numerous professional articles and is a frequent speaker at national conferences and seminars. She has won several national and regional awards for her work, and is active in a number of health care marketing associations on national and local levels.

Ms. Bronkesh was graduated *magna cum laude* with a bachelor of arts degree in communications from American University and earned a master of business administration degree from Arizona State University.

* * *

The authors are associated with **The HSM Group, Ltd.,** a Scottsdale, Arizona consulting firm specializing in health care marketing and management issues. For information, call or write: The HSM Group, Ltd., 6908 East Thomas Road, Suite 201, Scottsdale, Arizona 85251, 602/947-8078. ❧